For _____,

with my best wishes,

Krishna Dronamraju

HALDANE

AND

MODERN BIOLOGY

K. R. Dronamraju, Editor

HALDANE
AND
MODERN BIOLOGY

The Johns Hopkins Press, Baltimore

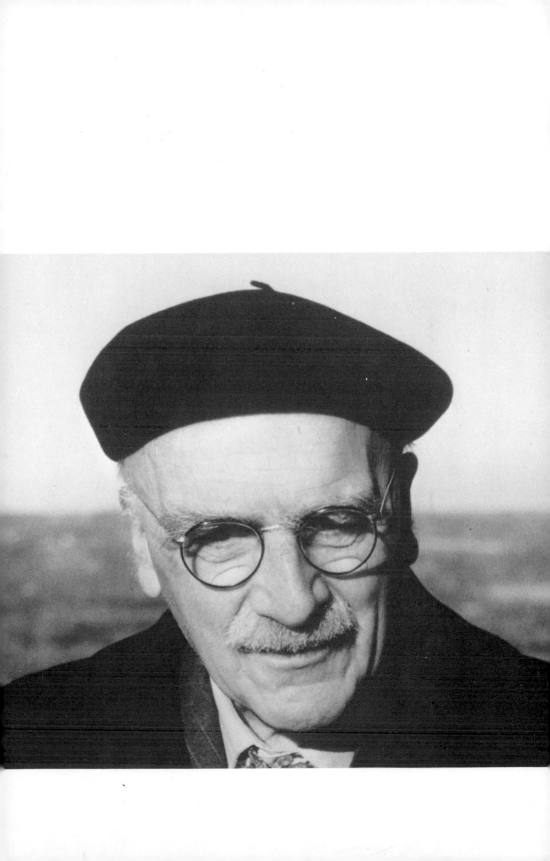

Title page photograph of Haldane courtesy of Dr. K. Patau, Univ. of
Wisconsin, Madison, Wis.

To
Raj Gopal

PREFACE

This book is a memorial to the late Professor J. B. S. Haldane. Contributions by distinguished scientists on certain aspects of Haldane's work reflect the versatile talent for which he was well known. Accounts are given of Haldane's early fundamental work as well as later extensions by himself and others. Biographical aspects of Haldane's life are discussed by his sister, Naomi Mitchison; Mrs. Mitchison's son, N. A. Mitchison, is the author of Chapter VII ("Antigens") in this volume.

Haldane made fundamental contributions to genetics, evolutionary theory, biochemistry, physiology, and biometry, and influenced the growth of biology as a whole during the past fifty years. He was prominent among the founders of population genetics and biochemical genetics. Distinguished as a classical biologist, he put forward so many novel ideas and predictions that his influence on the development of biology will continue for many years in the future. His concepts of the origin of life and his experiments in human physiology will continue to play a prominent role in future research on space travel and planetary explorations. He is truly a central figure in modern biology and will go down in history as a great synthesizer of the twentieth century.

John Burdon Sanderson Haldane was born in Oxford, England, on November 5, 1892. He was educated at Eton and Oxford where he studied mathematics, classics, and philosophy. His formal university education thus involved no branch of science. While still at school, however, he assisted his father, Professor J. S. Haldane, in research on respiratory physiology, in particular with those aspects concerning deep-sea diving and safety in mines. His first scientific paper in 1912, in collaboration with his father and C. G. Douglas, was entitled "The Laws of Combination of Haemoglobin with CO and Oxygen." His first paper on genetics was published in the *Journal of Genetics* in 1915, in collaboration with his sister N. M. Haldane (now Naomi Mitchison) and A. D. Sprunt. The authors discovered one of the first cases of partial linkage in mammals. During World War I Haldane served in the Black Watch, and, after being wounded in Mesopotamia, he was sent to Simla to recuperate; later he spent a year in Central India directing a bombing school at Mhow. His research in genetics and physiology was continued on his return to Oxford. In 1923 he was appointed to the newly created Sir William Dunn Readership in Biochemistry at Cambridge which he held until 1933 when he resigned to accept the chairs, first of genetics, and later of biometry, at University College, London. During the later part of his Cambridge period Haldane held part-time appointments as officer-in-charge of genetic investigations at the John Innes Horticultural Institution and Fullerian Professor of Physiology at the Royal Institution. In 1957 Haldane resigned from the Weldon Chair of Biometry at University College, London (not retired, as stated in the obituary in *Nature*, April 17, 1965), to migrate to India where he accepted a research professorship at the Indian Statistical Institute, Calcutta, and became an Indian citizen in 1961. He resigned in 1961 and headed for some time a research unit of the Council of Scientific and Industrial Research, Government of India, before making his final move in 1962 to become the director of the Genetics and Biometry Laboratory, Government of Orissa, Bhubaneswar, where he died on December 1, 1964.

Haldane believed that the years he spent in India were among the best of his life. He felt freer in many ways than he had in England, and he found the cultural and political life compatible with his interests. The richness of Indian fauna and flora excited his interest, stimulating him to suggest numerous problems for research. He took great interest in human genetic research and encouraged, among other projects, studies of consanguineous marriages in Andhra Pradesh. He advised numerous individuals, departments, and governments on problems ranging from coconut breeding and animal behavior to statistics and national planning. He continued, until death, his earlier work on the mathematical theory of natural selection. His popular articles in the English dailies and magazines and their translations into local languages made him known to millions of people.

It is a matter of particular pleasure to me that this book is being published by The Johns Hopkins Press. Haldane, in intellectual lineage, was a "grandson" of the late W. K. Brooks, of The Johns Hopkins University. Bateson (whose protégé Haldane was) spent the summers of 1883 and 1884 at Hampton, Virginia, and Beaufort, North Carolina, studying the embryology of *Balanoglossus* under Brooks. Bateson has recorded that it was Brooks who gave him the idea that heredity is a subject worth studying for itself. (A. H. Sturtevant, *A History of Genetics*, Harper & Row, 1965, p. 29.)

Acknowledgements

For much encouragement and useful advice, I am greatly indebted to Naomi Mitchison, Cedric Smith, A. G. Searle, and Ernst Caspari. Part of the work was supported by the Institute for Advanced Learning, City of Hope Medical Center, Duarte, California. In the preparation of the book, Dr. James Silvan of The Johns Hopkins Press has given me much valuable advice.

K. R. Dronamraju

Department of Genetics, University of Alberta,
Edmonton, Alberta, Canada

CONTENTS

CONTENTS

CONTRIBUTORS

Dr. A. C. Allison, National Institute for Medical Research, Mill Hill, London, N.W.7, England.

Professor M. S. Bartlett, F.R.S., Professor of Biomathematics, University of Oxford, Oxford, England.

Dr. Albert R. Behnke, 2865 Jackson Street, San Francisco 15, California.

Dr. Ralph W. Brauer, Director, Wrightsville Marine Bio-Medical Laboratory, Wilmington, North Carolina 28401.

Dr. T. C. Carter, Director, Agricultural Research Council, Poultry Research Centre, King's Buildings, West Mains Road, Edinburgh 9, Scotland.

Professor Ernst W. Caspari, Chairman, Department of Biology, University of Rochester, Rochester, New York 14627.

Mr. Arthur C. Clarke, 47–5, Gregory's Road, Colombo–7, Ceylon.

Professor F. A. E. Crew, F.R.S., Upton's Mill, Framfield, Sussex, England.

Professor James F. Crow, Department of Medical Genetics, University of Wisconsin, Madison, Wisconsin 53706.

Professor T. A. Davis, Indian Statistical Institute, Calcutta-35, India.

Dr. Motoo Kimura, Head, Department of Population Genetics, National Institute of Genetics, Yata 1.111 Mishima, Sizuoka-ken, Japan.

Professor A. Lacassagne, Fondation Curie, 26 Rue d'Ulm, Paris-V^e, France.

Professor Joshua Lederberg, Department of Genetics, Stanford University Medical School, Palo Alto, California.

Professor I. Michael Lerner, Department of Genetics, University of California, Berkeley, California 94720.

Mrs. Naomi Mitchison, Carradale House, Campbelltown, Argyll, Scotland.

Dr. N. A. Mitchison, F.R.S., Head, Department of Experimental Biology, National Institute for Medical Research, Mill Hill, London, N.W.7, England.

Dr. A. E. Mourant, F.R.S., Director, Serological Population Genetics Laboratory, St. Bartholomew's Hospital, West Smithfield, London, E.C.1, England.

Dr. Joseph Needham, F.R.S., Gonville & Cauis College, Cambridge, England.

Dr. A. I. Oparin, Director, A. N. Bach Institute of Biochemistry, Academy of Sciences of the U.S.S.R., Moscow, U.S.S.R.

Dr. N. W. Pirie, F.R.S., Head, Biochemistry Department, Rothamsted Experimental Station, Harpenden, Herts., England.

CONTRIBUTORS

Professor Sheldon C. Reed, Director, Dight Institute for Human Genetics, University of Minnesota, Minneapolis, Minnesota.

Professor William J. Schull, Department of Human Genetics, University of Michigan School of Medicine, Ann Arbor, Michigan.

Dr. A. G. Searle, Medical Research Council, Radiobiological Research Unit, Harwell, Didcot, Berks., England.

Professor Cedric A. B. Smith, Weldon Professor of Biometry, Galton Laboratory, University College, London, W.C.1, England.

Dr. J. Sutter, Institut National d'Etudes Démographiques, Ave. Franklin D. Roosevelt, 23-25, Paris-V^e, France.

Dr. Yu. M. Svirezhev, Department of General Radiobiology and Genetics, Institute of Medical Radiology, Obninsk, Kaluga Region, U.S.S.R.

Professor Sewall Wright, Department of Genetics, University of Wisconsin, Madison, Wisconsin 53706.

Professor René Wurmser, Institut de Biologie Physico-Chimique, 13 Rue Pierre Curie, Paris-V^e, France.

Dr. N. W. Timoféeff-Ressovsky, Department of General Radiobiology and Genetics, Institute of Medical Radiology, Obninsk, Kaluga Region, U.S.S.R.

Frontispiece supplied by Dr. K. Patau, Department of Medical Genetics, University of Wisconsin, Madison, Wisconsin.

Co-authors Inouye, MacCluer, and Svirezhev have the same addresses as their senior authors, Lerner, Schull, and Timoféeff-Ressovsky, respectively.

xvi

GENETICS

The permeation of biology by mathematics is only beginning, but unless the history of science is an inadequate guide, it will continue. . . .

J. B. S. Haldane, *The Causes of Evolution*
(Longmans, Green & Co., 1932, p. 215).

As a disciple of Hopkins I believe that biochemists should attempt to trace the fate of individual molecules and atoms. If they do so they will be brought to recognize that the chemical structure of the chromosomes is as detailed as that of a book or a picture, and that the key to a knowledge of that structure is the science of genetics.

J. B. S. Haldane, *The Biochemistry of Genetics*
(Allen & Unwin, 1954, p. 126).

SEWALL WRIGHT
Department of Genetics,
University of Wisconsin,
Madison, Wisconsin

I. CONTRIBUTIONS TO GENETICS*

Haldane's contribution to genetics was of a unique sort. He conducted no systematic breeding experiments, yet few geneticists have had more influence on the steady course of development of the subject than he during his long career. He contributed by numerous critical analyses of data, often involving novel statistical methods, and by numerous syntheses of the findings in all branches of genetics and of biology in general which frequently suggested fruitful lines of research. His analytical studies added to our knowledge of the genetics of many kinds of plants and animals, especially to that of man, where methods to extract the maximum amount of information from unusual family histories must take the place of experiment. His outstanding scientific contribution, however, was to the quantitative theory of natural and artificial selection.

Haldane's first genetic paper (1915; co-authors, A. D. Sprunt and N. M. Haldane) was on what was then called reduplication, now linkage, in mice. The authors noticed that certain data presented by Darbishire in 1904, before recognition of the phenomenon, indicated linkage between two loci of which the recessive alleles determined, respectively, albinism and a pink-eyed pale variety. They confirmed this by new experiments. This case and one that had been reported very shortly before on experiments with rats (probably involving a homologous chromosome) were the first recognized cases of partial linkage in mammals.

After World War I, he again took up the subject of linkage in a paper (1919a) on the most accurate method of determining its amount and the probable error, and in one (1919b) in which he gave a formula for the relation of map distance to amount of recombination. He called attention (1920) to the occurrence of linkage in data of Nabours on the genetics of the grouse locust, *Paratettix texanus*. He reported the first case of partial

*Brief excerpts of this article have appeared in the *Biographical Memoirs of Fellows of the Royal Society*, Vol. 12 (1966), pp. 219-49.

SEWALL WRIGHT

linkage in the fowl (1921) and collaborated with Crew (1925b) in demonstrating an important effect of age on the amount of recombination, in this case in male gametes. He worked with Gairdner (1929, 1933c) to demonstrate balanced lethals in *Antirrhinum majus*.

Haldane's most important contribution to linkage theory was the development of the complicated theory for polyploids (1930c) and its application, in collaboration with DeWinton (1931c, 1933b, 1935a) to experiments involving three linked loci of tetraploid *Primula sinensis*. In comparison with the results from diploids, the crossover percentages were similar.

In another notable paper (1931d), he gave a cytologic demonstration of the hitherto purely genetic phenomenon of interference by analyzing the frequency distributions of the number of chiasmata in chromosomes of *Vicia faba*, reported by Maeda. The variances of these distributions were found to be much smaller than the means in contrast with the equality expected if chiasmata occurred along the chromosomes at random as in the Poisson type of distribution.

Some years later (1944, 1946a) Haldane worked with Whitehouse in interpreting the pattern of spores in the asci resulting from meiosis in certain ascomycetes, and with Lea (1947a) on a mathematical theory of chromosome rearrangement. His last contribution to the subject of linkage in an organism other than man had to do with the mosquito, *Culex molestus*, in collaboration with Gilchrist (1946b, 1947d). The authors demonstrated partial sex linkage (6.3 ± 0.6 per cent) between a white-eyed mutation and the male determining gene, heterozygous in males. There was no visible differentiation of X and Y chromosomes in this case.

Because his synthetic papers depended on the reliability of data reported by many authors, Haldane was acutely aware of the danger that genetics might become bogged down in uncertainties unless the proportion of authors whose published data are warped by wishful thinking, or selection, or are downright fraudulent, remains very small. He applied tests of credibility. In one notable case, he and Philip (1939b) tested data of Moewus, which had been widely acclaimed as of major importance for several aspects of genetic theory, and found that the agreement with expectation was so extraordinary that the probability of a better fit by accidents of sampling was only 1 in 3.5×10^{22}. Their warning that the results should be confirmed by an independent observer was fully justified by subsequent events.

Haldane's capacity for coming up with an interesting generalization from scattered data was demonstrated in an early paper (1922) based on all available reports on first generation hybrids between animal species.

2

He found that in all cases in which one sex was absent or rare or sterile, that sex was the one that is heterozygous with respect to the X chromosome (female in birds and lepidoptera, male in mammals and diptera). He gave a possible evolutionary interpretation in terms of greater disturbance of balance in hybrids of the heterozygous sex than in those of homozygous sex with respect to genes that have come to differentiate the two species. Exceptions to this rule have since been found, but it still remains the prevailing situation.

Haldane's knowledge of physiology and biochemistry enabled him to discuss the relations of genes to characters in a fruitful way in many papers. His assemblage of the scattered information on genes with demonstrable biochemical effects and the discussion of the implications for physiological genetics in his book *The Biochemistry of Genetics* (1954) were very useful at a time when biochemistry was becoming the center of interest in genetics.

At this point it will be well to go back to his most widely quoted series of papers, those on "The Mathematical Theory of Natural and Artificial Selection," of ten papers published between 1924 and 1934. The purpose was indicated in the opening sentences of Part I: "A satisfactory theory of natural selection must be quantitative. In order to establish the view that natural selection is capable of accounting for the known facts of evolution, we must show not only that it can cause a species to change, but that it can cause it to change at a rate which will account for present and past transmutation."

At the time this was written, the precise effect of selection on the composition of a Mendelian population had been presented in only the simplest cases. Haldane proceeded to make a comprehensive investigation of the subject. Part I was concerned with 13 relatively simple situations for which he gave formulas for the number of generations required to produce any given change in the frequency of the favored type, and gave concrete examples. Thus, for a dominant gene with a selective advantage of .001, he showed that it required 6,920 generations to pass from a frequency of .001 to 1 per cent, 4,819 generations to pass from 1 to 50 per cent, 11,664 generations to pass from 50 to 99 per cent, and 309,780 generations to pass from 99 to 99.999 per cent. In later parts, he investigated the effects of self-fertilization and less intense inbreeding, assortative mating, and selective fertilization in relation to those of selection; the effects of selection on systems of multiple interacting factors, on metastable systems, and on polyploids; the consequences of overlapping instead of discrete generations; the balancing of adverse selection by recurrent mutation; and the effects of partial isolation and rapid selection, among others.

3

One important result was the finding (1927*b*) that the probability that a single mutation with selective advantage k will not be lost by accidents of sampling but will ultimately become established is only about 2k, if more or less dominant, and only of the order $\sqrt{k/N}$ if completely recessive, where N is the population size.

Haldane's book *The Causes of Evolution* (1932*d*) has become a classic for its lucid examination of the status of Darwin's theory from the standpoint of twentieth century knowledge of heredity and variation and of his own and other mathematical analyses of the quantitative aspects.

Two other mathematical theories of evolution were being developed at about the same time as Haldane's. The mathematics of all three agreed essentially in spite of superficial differences in the formulas. Haldane expressed his results in terms of the ratio, u, of the frequency of the mutant gene (A′) to that of its type allele (A), (distribution 1A:uA′). R. A. Fisher (1922) preferred a function of the gene frequency distribution $(1 - p)A:pA'$, viz., $\theta = \cos^{-1}(1 - 2p)$, which has the property that its sampling variance is constant, $1/(2N)$, but he shifted later (1930) to the gene frequency itself which was used systematically by Wright (1929, 1931).

There were, however, great differences in the application to evolution. Haldane assigned selective values, usually constant, sometimes variable, to each gene or, in some cases each genotype involving two or more interacting loci, and deduced deterministically the number of generations required to bring about a specified change in the gene frequency ratio under many alternative assumptions relating to the genetics of the character. Fisher aimed at general theorems with respect to the course of evolution, applicable regardless of the number of loci or their inter-actions. The most important was his fundamental theorem of natural selection (1930): "The rate of increase in fitness of any organism at any time is equal to its genetic variance in fitness at that time." Genetic variance was here defined as the additive component of the total genotypic variance. It was tacitly assumed that the species is essentially homo-geneous. This theorem implies that selection is always according to the net effect of each gene and thus that there can be no selection among inter-action systems. In such a species, interactional effects among unfixed loci are significant only in reducing the rate of progress by reducing the amount of additive variance, although, of course, a particular interactional system, more or less favorable, tends to be built up step by step, because any mutant gene is advantageous only if it fits in with the genome already established.

4

Fisher's theory was essentially similar to Haldane's in its deterministic character under given external conditions for genes with more than a few representatives in the population. Both authors, however, recognized that the fate of a single mutation is decided by a stochastic process. Fisher (1922) attempted to derive the stochastic distribution for his function θ, but obtained incorrect results (Wright, 1929), which he corrected in 1930. For the case of a semidominant favorable mutation, he gave the exact probability of ultimate fixation which Haldane's 2k, referred to above, closely approximated in large populations.

My theory was directed toward ascertaining whether some way, after all, might exist in which selection could take advantage of the enormous number of interaction systems provided by a limited number of unfixed loci. It was maintained that this is possible in a large population subdivided into many small, local populations, sufficiently isolated to permit considerable random differentiation of gene frequencies, but not so isolated as to prevent gradual diffusion of the more successful interaction systems from their centers of origin. The process involves three phases.

The first phase is stochastic variability of all gene frequencies in each local population about its set of equilibrium frequencies. The sort of selection involved in determining these equilibrium values was assumed to be, in most cases, that directed toward an optimum not far from the current mean of each quantitatively varying character instead of toward fixation of particular genes. Since many genotypes determine nearly the same intermediate grade under multifactorial heredity, selection toward such a grade implies the existence of many selective peaks in the "surface" of selective values, separated by saddles, and at various heights because of secondary effects on other characters (pleiotropy). The occasional crossing of a saddle between a lower and a higher peak as a result of extreme stochastic variation leads to the second phase, in which selection is directed toward the set of equilibrium frequencies of the higher peak, a process to which Haldane's formulas (and also Fisher's fundamental theorem) apply. The final phase is the spreading of this superior system by excess population growth and emigration to neighboring populations and ultimately, perhaps, throughout the species as a whole. It was recognized that local selection in a different direction from that prevailing may sometimes lead to superior general adaptation and replace the first two phases. This theory applies in pure form only if there is a favorable state of subdivision of the species and external conditions are relatively stable over a period of many generations.

When external conditions change drastically, many genes that have been less favorable than their type alleles become more favorable, and the more deterministic process of Haldane (and Fisher) dominates the situation until there is approximate adjustment to the new conditions. The concrete cases to which Haldane applied his theory were ones that involved such change. One of these cases (1942*a*) was based on data assembled by Elton on the steady decline in the proportion of silver fox pelts among fox pelts marketed in various parts of Canada in the century preceding 1933. Silver is due to a simple recessive gene; Haldane calculated that this gene must have been at an average selective disadvantage of about 3 per cent per year (6 per cent per generation if generation length is taken as two years) compared with its allele in red and cross foxes, presumably because of excess shooting of the much more valuable silvers. Another case (1924, 1956*b*) involved the nearly complete replacement of light colored moths, *Biston betularia*, by a semidominant dark mutant form (which in the end became completely dominant, presumably by direct selection of modifiers) in industrial districts of England in the course of half a century. He found that the selective value of the original light form must have averaged only two-thirds that of the dark, and much less at times and places in which selection was most severe, an estimate that seemed to some to be excessive when first made in 1924. It was quite in accord with the later observations of Kettlewell (1956) on the relative amounts of destruction by birds of the two color varieties on soot-covered, compared with clean, tree trunks.

If change of environment keeps pace with major changes in gene frequencies, evolution essentially according to Haldane's theory may continue indefinitely, and a case can be made for this as a major evolutionary process. It is somewhat of the nature of a treadmill, however, as each new rough adaptation accompanies the undoing of an old one. The process is deterministic only during each period of adjustment, since the changes in conditions on which continuance of the evolution depends introduce an indeterminate aspect.

The situation is unfavorable for either type of theory if external conditions are stable over very long periods of time and population structure is unfavorable for the stochastic process. Such evolution as there is would be of Haldane's type, limited by the exceedingly rare occurrence of novel (nonrecurrent) favorable mutations.

If population structure is favorable and external conditions are changing at a tempo compatible with evolutionary adjustment, a compound process should occur that probably leads to more rapid evolution than either by itself. In his later papers (e.g., 1949*b*) Haldane recognized the importance of fine-grained subdivision of the species.

Haldane continued throughout his career to make mathematical contributions in the field of population genetics. Among these were studies (1934a, 1935c) in collaboration with M. S. Bartlett in which the changes in the frequencies of types of matings were determined for diverse systems of inbreeding from the characteristic equation of a matrix representing the recurrence formulas for each type. This procedure gives a more complete account of the consequences of a system of inbreeding than the path analysis method I had used (Wright, 1921) for systems in general, but it is more cumbersome than mine in arriving at the most significant parameter, the rate of decrease of heterozygosis. For example, analysis of a relatively simple system, continued mating of double first cousins, requires a 12 × 12 matrix by Bartlett and Haldane's method and solution of an equation of the 12th degree (Fisher, 1949), whereas path analysis had led to a cubic equation, a factor of the above 12th degree equation (Wright, 1921, 1933). The most important novel results Bartlett and Haldane obtained by their method concerned the effects of self-fertilization and sibmating in tetraploids (1934a) and of various systems under forced heterozygosis at a linked locus (1935c). Haldane (1937a, 1955a) also gave a complete analysis of the consequences of brother-sister mating in terms of types of mating and any number of alleles.

Of special importance for evolutionary theory were Haldane's comprehensive discussions, largely verbal, but mathematical where necessary, of such matters as the evolution of dominance (1930a, 1939a), a subject introduced by Fisher in 1928, selection in relation to the time of action of the gene in the life cycle or reproductive cycle (1932b), the evolutionary consequences of recurrent mutation (1933a), residual heterozygosis in pure lines (1936a), and the reduction in fitness when equilibrium is attained between recurrent mutation and selection compared with fitness in the complete absence of the mutant gene (1937b). In this last case he arrived at a simple principle (sometimes known as Haldane's principle) that at first sight seemed rather surprising, viz., that the fitness at equilibrium, $1 - v$, for a completely recessive mutation or $1 - 2v$ for a more or less dominant one, depends merely on the rate, v, of recurrence of the mutation and not at all on the severity of the selection (although, of course, the latter has a great deal to do with the number of generations required to approach equilibrium after a change in mutation rate).

This principle has been interpreted as implying that practically all mutations from barely deleterious to lethal are essentially equivalent in the load they impose on the population, an interpretation which has played a major role in recent attempts to evaluate the genetic damage to populations from mutations induced by high energy radiations from

7

nuclear explosions or other sources. Haldane himself, however, stressed mostly lethal or nearly lethal mutations because of the rapidity with which the genetic damage is manifested. He proposed methods to determine the rate of induction of such mutations in mice from linked marker genes (1956a, 1956c, 1957b, 1960). He suggested (1955c) that the effects probably would be much more serious than had been estimated on the basis of experiments with *Drosophila* because of the likelihood that nearly all spontaneous mutations in long-lived forms, such as man, are due wholly to high energy radiation (instead of a small fraction of 1 per cent in *Drosophila*), as a result of evolutionary protection from low energy agents that otherwise would prevent all reproduction. He indicated that the amount of radiation required to double the spontaneous rate in man might well be as low as 3 röntgens instead of 50 to 80 röntgens, as deduced from *Drosophila* experiments.

Among other evolutionary topics that he analyzed with his usual lucidity were: the theory of clines (1948a); the various mechanisms that may be responsible for the presence of two or more alleles in a population (1942b; 1954b; 1955b; 1962; and, in collaboration with S. D. Jayakar, 1963a); the quantitative measurement of the rate of evolution (1949a); and the measurement of the severity of natural selection (1954a). In discussion of what he called the cost of natural selection (1957a, 1961), he started from the principle, painfully familiar to livestock breeders, that the number of things which can be strongly selected for at the same time are limited severely by reproductive capacity. It should be noted that the "cost" here is not to the species (which always profits from a favorable mutation) but to the effectiveness of selection at other loci.

In his final years in India, he returned, in collaboration with Jayakar, to some especially difficult problems of the sort that he had treated in developing his mathematical theory in the 1920's (1963a, b, c, d; 1964a; 1965).

As noted earlier, Haldane became more and more concerned with the implications of genetics for mankind. His first paper on human genetics (1932a) was a mathematical study of the corrections necessary, in investigating possible recessive characters, to overcome the bias in data resulting from omission of sibships from heterozygous parents that happened to produce no recessive offspring (taken up again in 1938a).

One of his most notable factual contributions to human genetics was the first determination of a mutation rate, that for the sex-linked trait hemophilia, which he based on the assumption of equilibrium between recurrent mutation and strong adverse selection (1935b). His first estimate 2×10^{-5} was raised by additional data to 3.2×10^{-5} (1947b).

8

He and Bell (1936c) made the first estimate of partial linkage in man—between the two sex-linked conditions, hemophilia and color blindness. Their 5 per cent estimate was raised by Haldane and Smith (1947c) to 10 ± 4 per cent.

Following evidence by Koller and Darlington for pairing and formation of chiasmata between segments of the X and Y chromosomes of the rat, Haldane made an intensive search for possible partial sex linkage in man. In 1936b he listed six abnormal traits that appeared to exhibit this phenomenon, at least in some of the family histories, and he added another possible case in 1941. He recognized, however, that none of the cases could be considered to be firmly established. His tentative interpretation has not been substantiated by more recent data, and the existence of partial sex linkage in man is now considered doubtful.

He summarized his views on the formal genetics of man in his Croonian Lecture (1948b).

Haldane wrote frequently on eugenics (e.g., 1938b, 1949b, 1964b). He accepted the value of negative eugenics as a means of reducing the frequencies of dominant and sex-linked recessive abnormalities and of autosomal recessives where means can be found for identifying heterozygotes. He emphasized, however, the impossibility of ever doing more than shifting the equilibrium between recurrent mutation and adverse selection by strengthening the latter.

He was skeptical of the possibility for successful positive eugenics, partly because he doubted whether anyone has enough wisdom for decisions on goals but also because of his strong belief in the positive value of a high degree of diversity both within populations and among them.

REFERENCES

A. Publications by J. B. S. Haldane

Haldane wrote 23 books, more than 400 scientific papers, and many popular scientific articles. Among the scientific papers, more than 100 were on population genetics, and some 85 were on other aspects of genetics (especially linkage), excluding book reviews. He also made many contributions to the theory of mathematical statistics, physiology, and other fields of biology. The following list includes only papers referred to here.

1915. (with A. D. Sprunt and N. M. Haldane) Reduplication in mice. *J. Genet.*, 5:133–35.

1919a. The probable errors of calculated linkage values and the most accurate method of determining gametic from certain zygotic series. *J. Genet.*, 8:291–97.

1919b. The combination of linkage values and the calculation of distances between the loci of linked factors. *J. Genet.*, 8:299–309.

1920. Note on a case of linkage in Paratettix. *J. Genet.*, 10:47–51.
1921. Linkage in poultry. *Science*, 54:663.
1922. Sex ratio and unisexual sterility in hybrid animals. *J. Genet.*, 12:101–9.
1924a. A mathematical theory of natural and artificial selection. Part I. *Trans. Camb. Phil. Soc.*, 23:19–41.
1924b. A mathematical theory of natural and artificial selection. Part II. *Proc. Camb. Phil. Soc.* (Biol. Sci.), 1:158–63.
1925. (with F. A. E. Crew) Change of linkage in poultry with age. *Nature*, 115:641.
1926. A mathematical theory of natural and artificial selection. Part III. *Proc. Camb. Phil. Soc.*, 23:363–72.
1927a. A mathematical theory of natural and artificial selection. Part IV. *Proc. Camb. Phil. Soc.*, 23:607–15.
1927b. A mathematical theory of natural and artificial selection. Part V. Selection and Mutation. *Proc. Camb. Phil. Soc.*, 23:838–44.
1929. (with A. E. Gairdner) A case of balanced lethal factors in Antirrhinum majus. *J. Genet.*, 21:315–25.
1930a. A note on Fisher's theory of the origin of dominance and on a correlation between dominance and linkage. *Amer. Natur.*, 64:87–90.
1930b. A mathematical theory of natural and artificial selection. Part VI. Isolation. *Proc. Camb. Phil. Soc.*, 26:220–30.
1930c. Theoretical genetics of autopolyploids. *J. Genet.*, 22:359–72.
1931a. A mathematical theory of natural and artificial selection. Part VII. Selection intensity as a function of mortality rate. *Proc. Camb. Phil. Soc.*, 27:131–36.
1931b. A mathematical theory of natural and artificial selection. Part VIII. Metastable populations. *Proc. Camb. Phil. Soc.*, 27:137–42.
1931c. (with D. De Winton) Linkage in the tetraploid Primula sinensis. *J. Genet.*, 24:121–44.
1931d. The cytological basis of genetical interference. *Cytologia*, 3:54–65.
1932a. A method for investigating recessive characters in man. *J. Genet.*, 25:251–55.
1932b. The time of action of genes and its bearing on some evolutionary problems. *Amer. Natur.*, 64:5–24.
1932c. A mathematical theory of natural and artificial selection. Part IX. Rapid selection. *Proc. Camb. Phil. Soc.*, 28:244–48.
1932d. *The Causes of Evolution.* Harper, New York and London. 235 pp.
1933a. The part played by recurrent mutation in evolution. *Amer. Natur.*, 67:5–19.
1933b. (with D. DeWinton) The genetics of Primula sinensis. II. Segregation and interaction of factors in the diploid. *J. Genet.*, 27:1–44.
1933c. (with A. E. Gairdner) A case of balanced lethal factors in Antirrhinum majus. *J. Genet.*, 27:287–91.
1934a. (with M. S. Bartlett) The theory of inbreeding in autotetraploids. *J. Genet.*, 29:175–80.
1934b. A mathematical theory of natural and artificial selection. Part X. Some theorems on artificial selection. *Genetics*, 19:412–29.
1935a. (with D. DeWinton) The genetics of Primula sinensis. III. Linkage in the diploid. *J. Genet.*, 31:67–100.
1935b. The rate of spontaneous mutation of a human gene. *J. Genet.*, 31:317–26.
1935c. (with M. S. Bartlett) The theory of inbreeding with forced heterozygosis. *J. Genet.*, 37:327–40.

1936a. The amount of heterozygosis to be expected in an approximately pure line. *J. Genet.*, 32:375–91.

1936b. A search for incomplete sex-linkage in man. *Ann. Eugen.*, 7:28–57.

1936c. (with J. Bell) Linkage in man. *Nature*, 138:759.

1937a. Some theoretical results of continued brother-sister mating. *J. Genet.*, 34:265–74.

1937b. The effect of variation on fitness. *Amer. Natur.*, 71:337–49.

1937c. (with J. Bell) The linkage between the genes for colour-blindness and haemophilia in man. *Proc. Roy. Soc. Lond., B.*, 123:119–50.

1938a. The estimation of the frequencies of recessive conditions in man. *Ann. Eugen.*, 81:255–62.

1938b. *Heredity and Politics*, W. W. Norton and Co., New York. 202 pp.

1939a. The theory of the evolution of dominance. *J. Genet.*, 37:365–74.

1939b. (with U. Philip) Relative sexuality in unicellular algae. *Nature*, 143:334.

1941. The partial sex-linkage of recessive spastic paraplegia. *J. Genet.*, 41:141–47.

1942a. The selective elimination of silver foxes in Eastern Canada. *J. Genet.*, 44:296–304.

1942b. Selection against heterozygosis in man. *Ann. Eugen.*, 11:333–43.

1944. (with H. L. K. Whitehouse) Symmetrical and asymmetrical postreduction in Ascomycetes. *Nature*, 154:704.

1946a. (with H. L. K. Whitehouse) Symmetrical and asymmetrical reduction in Ascomycetes. *J. Genet.*, 47:208–12.

1946b. (with B. M. Gilchrist) Sex-linkage in *Culex molestus. Experientia*, 11(9):372.

1947a. (with D. E. Lea) A mathematical theory of chromosomal rearrangements. *J. Genet.*, 48:1–10.

1947b. The mutation rate of the gene for haemophilia and its segregation ratios in males and females. *Ann. Eugen.*, 13:262–71.

1947c. (with C. A. B. Smith) A new estimate of the linkage between the genes for colour-blindness and haemophilia in man. *Ann. Eugen.*, 14:10–31.

1947d. (with B. M. Gilchrist) Sex-linkage and sex-determination in a mosquito Culex molestus. *Hereditas*, 33:175–90.

1948a. The theory of a cline. *J. Genet.*, 48:277–84.

1948b. The formal genetics of man. *Proc. Roy. Soc. Lond., B.*, 135:147–70.

1949a. Suggestions as to quantitative measurement of rates of evolution. *Evolution*, 3:51–6.

1949b. Human evolution: past and future. *In* G. L. Jepsen, E. Mayr, and G. G. Simpson (eds.), *Genetics, Paleontology and Evolution*. Princeton Univ. Press, Princeton.

1954a. *The Biochemistry of Genetics*. G. Allen and Unwin, London. 144 pp.

1954b. The measurement of natural selection. *Caryologia* 6 (Suppl.):480–87.

1954c. The statics of evolution, pp. 109–21. In J. S. Huxley, A. C. Hardy, and E. B. Ford, *Evolution as a Process*. Allen & Unwin, London.

1955a. The complete matrices for brother-sister and alternate parent-offspring mating involving one locus. *J. Genet.*, 53:315–24.

1955b. On the biochemistry of heterosis, and the stabilization of polymorphism. *Proc. Roy. Soc. Lond., B.*, 144:143–221.

1955c. Genetical effects of radiation from products of nuclear explosions. *Nature*, 176:115.

1956a. The estimation of mutation rates produced by high energy events in mammals. *Current Sci.*, 25:75–6.

1956b. The theory of selection for melanism in lepidoptera. *Proc. Roy. Soc. Lond., B.*, 145:303–8.

1956c. The detection of autosomal lethals in mice induced by mutagenic agents. *J. Genet.*, 54:327–42.

1957a. The cost of natural selection. *J. Genet.*, 55:511–24.

1957b. Methods for the detection and enumeration of mutations produced by irradiation in mice. *Proc. Int. Genet. Symp.*, *1956, Cytologia (Suppl.)*, Vol. 22.

1960. The interpretation of Carter's results on the induction of recessive lethals in mice. *J. Genet.*, 57:131–36.

1961. More precise expressions for the cost of natural selection. *J. Genet.*, 57:351–60.

1962. Conditions for stable polymorphism at an autosomal locus. *Nature*, 193:1108.

1963a. (with S. D. Jayakar) Polymorphism due to selection of varying direction. *J. Genet.*, 58:237–42.

1963b. (with S. D. Jayakar) The elimination of double dominants in large random mating populations. *J. Genet.*, 58:243–51.

1963c. (with S. D. Jayakar) The solution of some equations occurring in population genetics. *J. Genet.*, 58:291–317.

1963d. (with S. D. Jayakar) Polymorphism due to selection depending on the composition of a population. *J. Genet.*, 58:318–23.

1964a. (with S. D. Jayakar) Equilibria under natural selection at a sex-linked locus. *J. Genet.*, 59:29–36.

1964b. The implications of genetics for human society. *Proc. XI Int. Congr. Genet.*, pp. xci–cii.

1965. (with S. D. Jayakar) The nature of human genetic loads. *J. Genet.*, 59:53–9.

B. *Other Publications*

ELTON, C., 1942. *Voles, Mice and Lemmings; Problems in Population Dynamics*. Oxford Univ. Press, Oxford.

FISHER, R. A. 1922. On the dominance ratio. *Proc. Roy. Soc. Edinburgh*, 42:321–41.

———. 1928. The possible modification of the response of the wild type to recurrent mutations. *Amer. Natur.*, 62:115–26.

———. 1930. *The Genetical Theory of Natural Selection*. Clarendon Press, Oxford. 272 pp.

———. 1949. *The Theory of Inbreeding*. Oliver and Boyd, Edinburgh. 120 pp.

Kettlewell, H. B. D. 1956. Further selection experiments on industrial melanism in the Lepidoptera. *Heredity*, 10:287–301.

Wright, S., 1921. Systems of mating. *Genetics*, 6:111–28.

———. 1929. Evolution in a Mendelian population. *Anat. Rec.*, 44:287.

———. 1931. Evolution in Mendelian populations. *Genetics*, 16:97–159.

———. 1933. Inbreeding and homozygosis. *Proc. Nat. Acad. Sci.*, 19:411–20.

F. A. E. CREW
(formerly of) University of Edinburgh,
Edinburgh, Scotland

II. HALDANE AS A GENETICIST

During the lifetime of J. B. S. Haldane, no science pursued a more rapid development or exerted a more profound influence upon other spheres of human thought and action than did genetics. The years that followed the rediscovery of Mendelism in 1900 were remarkable for the abundance of elegant experimentation and exciting theorizing in this field; no sooner had one surprising discovery been announced than it was followed by another one even more surprising. As the major interest in genetics moved from the biological toward the molecular level; as the hunt for ratios gave place to the search for the actual vehicles that carried the elements of Mendel, the factors of Bateson, the genes of Johannsen; as this emphasis in its turn gave way to efforts to disclose the actual nature of the gene and of the mode of genic action; as the mouse, the guinea pig, the rabbit, the garden plant and the like came to be replaced as the experimental material of choice by *Drosophila* and maize and as these made room for the bacterium, the virus, the mold, and the fungus; as genetics branched out into the specialties of animal, biochemical, bio-metrical, epi-, human, medical, immuno-, microbial, pharmaco-, physio-logical, plant, population, and radiation genetics, and as it came to be recognized that genetics had much of great value to offer to the anthro-pologist, the educator, the evolutionist and the social scientist, among others, new investigational methods and tools were constantly in demand. The geneticist who was active in the second decade of the present century and who hoped to keep abreast of these developments as they occurred was required continually to add to his intellectual equipment; he had to be, or to become, competent not only in the biological sciences but in the physical as well. Of the very few who were sufficiently equipped to play a leading part in the development of genetics during the whole of the last fifty years, J. B. S. Haldane was an outstanding example.

He was one of the most erudite scientists of his generation; he was exceptionally well-endowed genetically, highly intelligent, and possessed of a prodigious memory. The atmosphere of his home was such as to encourage the full expression of his many talents as was the formal education he received at school and university. He graduated in 1915, having taken a first in mathematics and done equally well in classics and philosophy. While he was a student, exciting developments were taking place; the Morganian school in Columbia University was fashioning the chromosome theory of heredity; the Batesonian school of genetics was very active at the John Innes Horticultural Institute, and the first chair of genetics in Great Britain was created at Cambridge, its occupant being Punnett. That Haldane was well aware of these events and was affected by them is revealed in his first genetic paper (with Sprunt and his sister Naomi) which appeared in 1915 on linkage, which is discussed in Chapter I. Haldane was already interested in and knowledgeable concerning genetic phenomena, was already reading the literature and examining data obtained by others, and was already employing his considerable mathematical skill to disclose their meaning. During the years he spent in World War I service, he must have given much thought to genetic problems, for, on his return to Oxford with a fellowship at New College, he at once began to publish further papers on linkage, as described in Chapter I.

In 1922, in his paper on the sex ratio and unisexual sterility in hybrid animals, he displayed his remarkable ability to formulate a generalization from data widely scattered in the literature. He examined all the available records of interspecific crosses with particular reference to the fertility of the F_1 individuals. His "law" stated that if in such cases one sex was absent, rare, or sterile, that sex was the heterogametic (XY or XO). He thought that a greater degree of genic imbalance existed in the heterogametic than in the homogametic sex with its two X's. A few exceptions to this rule have since been encountered but, in general, it still holds.

He contributed much to the development of biochemistry in Great Britain and can rightly be regarded as one of the founders of biochemical genetics. During the period 1927–36 when he held a part-time appointment at the John Innes Horticultural Institute as officer-in-charge of genetic investigations, he came into contact with the work on plant pigments being carried out by Scott-Moncrieff, Robinson, Lawrence, and Price. This appointment also brought him in close touch with Darlington who was exceedingly active and productive at that time in cytology. This attachment to the John Innes was a very interesting and an important one; Bateson had died in 1926 and had been succeeded as director of the institute by Sir Daniel Hall, who was not a geneticist. Haldane thus became Bateson's real successor and was soon to become an acknowledged leader in the genetic field.

He was to be the author of nearly 200 papers dealing with genetics and to write half a dozen books that presented his considered views concerning genetic phenomena or the application of genetic knowledge to human and social affairs. His interests ranged very widely, and he contributed to almost every genetic specialty, particularly to human genetics. From among these papers and books, individuals with different interests will choose differently when selecting those that seem to possess the greatest and most enduring value. All that can now be attempted is to refer to a number of his papers that illustrate the breadth of his interests and the variety of his talents.

In 1924 the first of his papers on a mathematical theory of natural and artificial selection appeared; the tenth in the series was published ten years later. In them he proceeded to make a comprehensive examination of the precise effects of selection on the composition of a Mendelian population. The subject is expanded in his book *The Causes of Evolution* (1932), which is remarkable for its lucid examination of Darwin's theory from the standpoint of twentieth century ideas on heredity and variation, together with an evaluation of the mathematical analyses by Fisher, Sewall Wright, and himself of the quantitative aspects of the subject. Possibly Haldane's contribution to the quantitative theory of natural and artificial selection will come to rank as the most important of his many contributions to biological science. It was a fortunate happening that these three gifted men should be coevals and should focus their interest upon the same problem, for each served as a whetstone on which the others sharpened their developing hypotheses.

His other contributions to evolutionary theory in these early years included papers on the evolution of dominance (1930, 1939), a subject introduced by Fisher in 1928; on selection in relation to the time of action of the gene in the life or reproductive cycle (1932), on the evolutionary consequences of recurrent mutation (1933), on residual heterozygosis in pure lines (1936); and on the loss of fitness when equilibrium between recurrent mutation and selection is attained in the complete absence of the mutant gene (1937).

At the John Innes Horticultural Institute, he collaborated with Gairdner (1929, 1933) in demonstrating the existence of balanced lethal genes in *Antirrhinum majus* and with de Winton in applying his ideas concerning linkage to polyploids (1931, 1933, 1935), which is discussed in Chapter I. In a paper in 1931 making use of Maeda's data on *Vicia faba*, he showed that the discrepancy between the observed and the calculated (Poisson) frequencies of bivalents with different numbers of chiasmata could be used as a measure of interference. Another of his papers on incomplete sex linkage in man (1936) was based upon the cytological work of Koller and Darlington on the XY bivalent of the rat. In his paper on the genetic evidence for a cytological abnormality in man (1932), he developed the hypothesis that chromosomal aberration played a significant role in the causation of phenotypic abnormality, long before the cytological evidence of this following the development of new cytological techniques in 1952.

In 1933, when Haldane resigned his Cambridge post to take, firstly, the chair of genetics and later the Weldon Chair of Biometry at University College, London, his academic title came to be in harmony with his major scientific interest. In 1933 he wrote on the genetics of cancer, the disease that was to destroy him thirty-one years later. In 1934, in collaboration with Penrose, he considered the mutation rates in man. In his *Causes of Evolution* he had shown that as a consequence of the low degree of fitness of hemophiliacs, the loss of the hemophilia gene in each generation must be balanced by recurrent fresh mutation, since, if this were not so, the disease would eliminate itself. He argued that about one-third of all the known cases of the disease must have arisen by mutation of the gene in each generation. If the incidence of the disease among the male population was one in 30,000, the mutation rate must be around 10^{-5} per gene per generation. In this 1935 paper a formula for sex-linked genes generally is given, $2\mu + v = (1 - f)x$, where μ and v are the mutation rates in females and males, respectively, x the frequency of the disease among males at birth and f the fitness of the affected males as a fraction of the normal. Twenty-one years later he was to bring the sex-linked recessive form of muscular dystrophy into the scheme (1956).

Save for 1945, 1950, and 1962, every year up to 1957, when he resigned from University College and went to India, produced its crop of genetic papers, all bearing the stamp of his remarkable personality and many of them contributions of very considerable merit. He continued to be interested in rates of change in evolution and in changes in gene frequency. In 1949 in his contribution to the book *Genetics, Paleontology and Evolution*, he proposed the term "darwin" for a unit of evolutionary change, one darwin standing for the rate of change of 10^{-6} per year. He showed that the average rate for the teeth of the horse was around 40 millidarwins and that, whereas the rate of one darwin was exceptional in the wild, the rate of change under conditions of artificial selection could reach kilodarwins or more. In his address to the Ninth International Congress of Genetics in 1953, he dealt with the measurement of natural selection (published in

Caryologia in the following year). He proposed to measure the intensity of selection by $I = \ln s_0 - \ln S$, where s_0 is the fitness of the optimum phenotype and S is that of the whole population. Applying this relation to the data obtained by Karn and Penrose on birth weight and mortality, by Rendel on duck eggs, and by Weldon and Di Cesnola on snails, he found that the selection intensity involved was around 2.4 per cent and pointed out that natural selection tends to reduce variance by eliminating extreme forms. As early as 1924 (in his first paper on a mathematical theory of natural and artificial selection) he had realized that the intensity of selection must be very great in the case of industrial melanism in moths. His findings when he returned to this subject in 1956 are described in Chapter I.

In 1942, making use of the data assembled by Elton on the steady decline in the proportion of silver fox pelts among the pelts marketed in Canada during the century preceding 1933, he calculated that the recessive silver gene must have been at an average selective disadvantage of around 3 per cent per year as compared with its dominant allele in the homozygous and heterozygous red foxes, the selective agent in this case being the gun of the hunter. In his 1937 paper on the effect of variation on fitness, Haldane derived a principle that the loss of population fitness due to recurrent deleterious mutations depends entirely upon the mutation rate and not upon the degree of harmfulness of the mutant genes, provided that this effect is large enough to keep the gene rare. He estimated that the loss of fitness due to such mutations amounts to about 3 or 4 per cent in *Drosophila* and about 10 per cent in man. The same principle was discovered later independently by Muller who expressed it in terms of "genetic death." In the same 1937 paper Haldane considered a case in which the heterozygote was fitter than either homozygote and showed that such a gene pair plays a far greater role in lowering the fitness of a species than recurrent harmful mutations. In this way he created the basis from which the concept of genetic load was later developed. He returned to this topic in several later papers. In 1957 he published a paper of exceptional note on the conditions necessary for co-adaptation in polymorphism for inversions, and in the same year another important paper on the cost of evolution, a mathematical treatment of genetic loads in phylogeny appeared.

In 1957 he became a member of a biometry research unit in the Indian Statistical Institute, Calcutta, but soon resigned and with several of his colleagues established in his own house a research unit financed by the Indian Council of Scientific and Industrial Research. When, in 1961, he made his final move to become the head of a laboratory of genetics and biometry established for him by the Government of Orissa in the Agricultural College, Bhubaneswar, around him and Helen Spurway, his wife, gathered a number of graduate students who were deeply influenced by him. He was at his best when surrounded by a group of young researchers, ready to communicate his ideas without reservation, to listen, and to exercise his powerful and fertile intellect on any subject. He took to India with him the *Journal of Genetics*, which he had edited since 1945, and continued as its editor until the time of his death.

The number, the quality, the originality of Haldane's contributions to genetics are very impressive, and it is surprising to find that his is not included in the list of the names of those whose work in the field of genetics is regarded as being of special significance. No major discovery of a new genetic phenomenon is associated with his name, which is remarkable when the quality of his intellectual equipment is considered. Possibly the very breadth of his interests and activities precluded his complete and continued concentration upon one particular subject or field of inquiry. He seemed to be content to cultivate novel genetic ideas and to devise neat and clever mathematical tools for their investigation; he enjoyed applying his own analytical methods to material collected by others. He himself was not an experimentalist in genetics.

Certainly he foresaw developments in genetics long before they occurred. For example, in his *Causes of Evolution* (1932), he stressed the significance of the roles of disease and disease resistance in selection and evolution, but the first clear evidence of the role of infectious disease in shaping the human genetic constitution was not forthcoming until it was provided by Allison in 1954 in his study of the relation of malaria and the gene for sickle hemoglobin. Quite rightly, therefore, it is Allison's name and not that of Haldane that is associated with this important discovery. His experience as a biochemist in Cambridge had had him to accept the one-gene-one-enzyme hypothesis, originally formulated by Garrod, long before Beadle and Tatum, in their work on *Neurospora* in 1941, raised it to the level of a principle in experimental genetics. At one time it seemed that Haldane's ideas concerning partial sex linkage were to lead to a discovery of first rank. In 1936 he gave a formal analysis of the consequences of partial sex linkage in man. However, he himself remained skeptical, and later investigations have tended to show that most of his conclusions about special conditions were not valid. He was using data amassed by other people, in this case by medical men, which proved to be unreliable.

Nevertheless, no one exerted a greater influence on the development of the science of genetics or served it more faithfully than did Haldane. His books, his scientific papers, his lectures and addresses, and his broadcasts made him one of the best-known scientists in the world. He wrote popular articles about genetics to persuade people to treat social and political questions in an objective and rational manner, and his ability to make complicated matters seem relatively simple was truly astonishing.

Haldane never built up a "school" of genetics in England; he was too much given to abstraction and preoccupation to make an efficient administrative head of a department. In England he was never really in harmony with his environment. He migrated to India at the age of sixty-five in search of this harmony. Possibly he might have found that which he sought in Bhubaneswar, but death came too soon.

His place in the history of genetics is secure.

Note: For Bibliography, see *References* following Chapter I.

T. C. CARTER
Agricultural Research Council's Poultry Research Centre,
Edinburgh, Scotland

III. HALDANE'S CONTRIBUTIONS TO MAMMALIAN RADIATION GENETICS

The 1915–16 volume of *Journal of Genetics* contains a short paper entitled "Reduplication in Mice." The authors are listed as J. B. S. Haldane, B.A., Lieutenant, 3rd Black Watch; A. D. Sprunt, B.A., late 2nd Lieutenant, 4th Bedfordshire Regiment; and N. M. Haldane,[1] Home Student, Oxford. The paper describes breeding experiments with mice carrying the recessive mutants for albinism (*c*) and what is now called pink-eyed dilution (*p*). They were undertaken to test the hypothesis, based on data of A. D. Darbishire (1904), that these two mutants show non-Mendelian segregation in double heterozygotes. The experiments were not simple, because *c* is epistatic to *p*: albinos cannot be classified visually for pink-eyed dilution, and test-crosses, therefore, had to be used to classify some of the progeny of segregated matings. Despite this difficulty and others, the experiments established beyond doubt that the segregation of *c* from *p* is non-Mendelian and thereby demonstrated, for the first time, the occurrence of autosomal linkage in a mammal. Haldane's interest in linkage in the mouse, shown in this paper written at the outset of his scientific career, remained with him to the end of it. Haldane, Sprunt, and Haldane interpreted their data on the basis of the hypothesis of primary and secondary germinal reduplication (Trow, 1913), but Morgan put forward the chromosomal recombination hypothesis of linkage at about the same time (Morgan and Bridges, 1916).

Haldane returned to the problem of linkage in 1919, with a paper entitled "The Combination of Linkage Values, and the Calculation of Distances between the Loci of Linked Factors" on tests of the germinal reduplication and chromosomal recombination hypotheses. Characteristically, his approach was mathematical: he constructed a mathematical model of chromosome recombination, derived inferences from it, and tested them with biological data. He recognized that if there were two crossover points (or any greater even number) in the chromosome strand between a pair of loci, the occurrence of the second would vitiate

---

[1] Now Naomi Mitchison

the effect of the first, and no recombination would be apparent in the zygote; recombination would be seen only if there was one crossover point, or any greater odd number. This implied that recombination in a very long chromosome, with a large average number of crossover points, would be limited to 50 per cent. He introduced the concept of map distance, as opposed to recombination frequency, and showed that, provided the existence of one crossover point did not affect the probability of another occurring in its neighborhood, recombination frequency (y) would be related to map distance (x) by the equation

$$y = \tfrac{1}{2}(1 - e^{-2x}).$$

He showed that the published data on recombination in *Drosophila* were incompatible with the germinal reduplication hypothesis but were compatible with the hypothesis of chromosomal recombination, provided one assumes that the existence of a crossover point reduces the probability of another occurring in its neighborhood; in other words, that there is some degree of chiasma interference. In honor of Morgan, he named the unit of map distance the centimorgan. The concepts of recombination frequency, map distance, and chiasma interference formed the basis of all later theoretical work on linkage, the only subsequent substantial change being the addition of the concept of chromatid interference following recognition that the formation of a chiasma involves two strands in a four-strand bivalent.

After the atomic bombs were exploded over Hiroshima and Nagasaki in 1945, Haldane took an intense interest in the implications for mankind of exposure of human populations to ionizing radiations. He examined the genetic problems in several theoretical papers (Haldane, 1947, 1955, 1956a), but his attempts at quantitation were limited—as were all attempts at that time—by lack of knowledge of the radiation doses accumulated by human germ cells and of the relation between accumulated dose and mutation rate. In 1955 when the effects of bomb-test fallout became a subject of world-wide public concern, Haldane was sounded informally about his willingness to become a member of the Committee on the Hazards to Man of Nuclear and Allied Radiations set up by the British Medical Research Council. He refused the invitation, as he felt that he could serve the community more effectively as an external critic and spur than as an internal advocate.

Critic and spur Haldane was, but always constructive. In the role of constructive critic, he suggested experiments to determine the relation between accumulated radiation dose and mutation rate in an organism which, though not human, was at least a mammal: the laboratory mouse.

These suggestions arose out of his earlier work on linkage theory and linkage in the mouse, and they were taken up by the official British group working on radiation genetics of mammals. This group had been formed in 1947 at the Institute of Animal Genetics, in Edinburgh, and was transferred in 1954 to the Medical Research Council's Radiobiological Research Establishment, at Harwell. It faced many difficulties. No mutation-detection stocks of mice (or, indeed, of any laboratory mammal) comparable to the ClB and Muller-5 stocks of *Drosophila melanogaster* were available. Attempts to induce chromosome inversions in the mouse, with the object of constructing such stocks, proved unsuccessful. No sex-linked marker gene then was known in the mouse. Many gene-tagged chromosome translocations were induced with X-rays, but they proved to have little, if any, crossover-suppressing effect. Litter size could be, and was, used to study the average induction rate of recessive lethals, but it was an unsatisfactory measure, partly because of the risk in a polytocous mammal that the death of one embryo may enhance the probability of survival of another, and also because the individual lethal genes could not be retrieved and their presence confirmed by further tests. The one reliable technique was to search for mutation to a recessive allele at a specific locus. The progeny of irradiated and un-irradiated wild-type parents were crossed with recessive homozygotes and their progeny examined for the recessive phenotype. The technique was reliable and objective, but it suffered from the drawback that only about seven loci could be scanned, since this was the greatest number of recessive visible mutants for which a mouse stock could be made homozygous while remaining viable and reasonably fecund. As the information required from the experiments was the *relative* increase in mutation rate after irradiation, the spontaneous mutation rate had to be measured accurately; to do this when only seven loci were scanned, enormous numbers of mice had to be bred. Furthermore, as the radiation dose accumulated by the average man and woman of reproductive age is low, interest lay mainly in low experimental radiation doses, at which the rate of induced mutation was expected to be low; this meant that huge numbers of mice had to be bred from irradiated ancestors. The efficiency of the technique for detecting mutation, therefore, was of great practical importance. A further disadvantage of the specific-locus method was that it was capable of detecting only two classes of mutation: recessive visibles at the specific loci and dominant visibles at any locus. It could not detect recessive lethals or sublethals (other than those at the specific loci), but, as Haldane (1947) had pointed out, these classes were likely to constitute an important component of the genetic hazard to man of radiations.

It was in suggesting methods that might be more efficient than the specific-locus one and would enable recessive lethals and sublethals to be detected, that Haldane made his main contributions to experimental mammalian radiation genetics. His approach was mathematical and stemmed from the thinking in his 1919 paper, coupled with the concept of the "swept radius" in a linkage test that had been introduced by Carter and Falconer (1951). If mutation in a chromosome segment tagged by two genes with visible effects could not be detected with certainty by suppressing crossing-over throughout it, he argued, it would be necessary to adopt a probability approach to the detection of mutation. One method was to follow through the generations a chromosome segment of unknown length tagged by a single marker gene; the presence of a new lethal gene linked to the marker would be inferred if the marker gene appeared in the progeny at a lower-than-Mendelian frequency. But before this method could be used, two difficult mathematical problems had to be solved. First, criteria had to be devised to distinguish the progenies in which the frequency of the marker gene was lower than Mendelian because of a linked lethal from those in which it was lower by chance. Second, the average radius of the genetic map swept in such a test had to be estimated. Haldane gave the solutions to these problems in a paper (1956*b*) entitled "The Detection of Autosomal Lethals in Mice Induced by Mutagenic Agents."

When Haldane had solved the mathematical problems, the next step was to try the technique in a pilot experiment designed solely to compare its efficiency with that of the specific-locus method. For this purpose a high accumulated radiation dose was desirable to minimize the size and duration of the test. The experiment was done at Harwell (Carter, 1959). The main object was achieved in that it was established beyond doubt that there is a difference in efficiency between the specific-locus method and Haldane's method, but it was Haldane's method that proved to be the less efficient. The experiment, however, was of great value because of another, quite unexpected result: though two lethals were detected in the control series and a very high accumulated radiation dose had been used (the equivalent of 1200 R of X-rays to spermatogonia of adult males), only one lethal was found in the experimental series. Haldane (1960) subsequently contested the interpretation of some of the data and put forward reasons for believing that two lethals or even three, were present in this series. I am not convinced by his argument, which failed to take account of the supplementary evidence from litter size. Whichever interpretation is right, it is highly improbable, in the face of the data, that the mutation rate in the irradiated series was higher than that in the control series by a factor of 40, the rate expected on the a priori assumption that the dose to double the mutation rate might be of the order of 30 R. Thus, what had been intended solely as a pilot experiment gave a result which, while quite unexpected, was very reassuring and rendered the planned main experiment unnecessary.

Following Haldane's lead, Auerbach, Falconer, and Isaacson (1962) developed a method for detecting sex-linked mutations in the mouse, using sex-linked marker genes (which were available by then), and Carter (1957) suggested a method for detecting autosomal recessive lethals, using linked autosomal markers. Haldane subsequently extended Carter's method, pointing out (Haldane, 1957) that it could be used for the detection not only of recessive lethals but also of recessive sublethals, a class of mutation not detectable by the methods described previously.

So far as I am aware, Haldane never carried out an experiment in mammalian radiation genetics. His importance in this field lay in the influence of his thinking on those who were doing the experimental work. It was a great loss to British workers when, after his move to India, Haldane ceased to be available for discussion and penetrating criticism.

REFERENCES

AUERBACH, C., D. S. FALCONER AND J. H. ISAACSON. 1962. Test for sex-linked lethals in irradiated mice. *Genet. Res.* (Camb.), 3:444–47.

CARTER, T. C. 1957. The use of linked marker genes for detecting recessive autosomal lethals in the mouse. *J. Genet.*, 55:585–97.

———. 1959. A pilot experiment with mice, using Haldane's method for detecting induced autosomal recessive lethal genes. *J. Genet.*, 56:353–62.

CARTER, T. C., AND D. S. FALCONER. 1951. Stocks for detecting linkage in the mouse, and the theory of their design. *J. Genet.*, 50:307–23.

DARBISHIRE, A. D. 1904. On the result of crossing Japanese waltzing mice with albino mice. *Biometrika*, 3:1–51.

HALDANE, J. B. S. 1919. The combination of linkage values, and the calculation of distances between the loci of linked factors. *J. Genet.*, 8:299–309.

———. 1947. The dysgenic effect of induced recessive mutations. *Ann. Eugen.*, 14:35–43.

———. 1955. Genetical effects of radiation from products of nuclear explosions. *Nature*, 176:155.

———. 1956a. The estimation of mutation rates produced by high energy events in mammals. *Current Sci.*, 25(3):75–6.

———. 1956b. The detection of autosomal lethals in mice induced by mutagenic agents. *J. Genet.*, 54:327–42.

———. 1957. The detection of sublethal recessives by the use of linked marker genes in the mouse. *J. Genet.*, 55:596–97.

———. 1960. The interpretation of Carter's results on induction of recessive lethals in mice. *J. Genet.*, 57:131–36.

HALDANE, J. B. S., A. D. SPRUNT, AND N. M. HALDANE. 1915. Reduplication in mice. *J. Genet.*, 5:133–35.

MORGAN, T. H., AND C. B. BRIDGES. 1916. Sex-linked inheritance in *Drosophila*. Carnegie Inst. Wash., Pub., No. 237. 87 pp.

TROW, A. H. 1913. Forms of reduplication: primary and secondary. *J. Genet.*, 2:313–24.

A. G. SEARLE
M. R. C. Radiobiological Research Unit,
Harwell, Berkshire, England

IV. COAT COLOR GENETICS AND PROBLEMS OF HOMOLOGY

Forty years ago, Haldane (1927) wrote a classic paper which helped to lay the foundations of comparative genetics. In it he discussed the principles of genetic homology and showed how these could be applied to the coat color genetics of rodents and carnivores. He drew certain conclusions on the types of mutations found, on the basic genotype within the mammalian orders studied, and on the evolutionary implications of his findings. My purpose is to discuss this important paper in the light of present knowledge of rodent and carnivore coat color genetics to show its relevance today.

It can hardly be doubted that the subject of comparative genetics is still relevant, even though the rate of growth of knowledge in this field is slow, perhaps understandably; for genetic comparison implies knowledge of at least two related species, yet genetic studies are usually concentrated on one species in a taxonomic group. For example, very much more is known about the genetics of the house mouse than of any other rodent. Yet, if we really want to understand what happened and is happening in evolution, what types of genetic change persist over very many generations, to what extent loci are lost, duplicated, transmuted, and so on, we must search for and study homologous genes. As a rule, these can only be identified with confidence by study of their mutant alleles, although comparative biochemical methods are becoming increasingly useful.

Haldane's reason for applying the principles of homology to genes is still valid today: "Structures in two species are said to be homologous when they correspond to the same structure in a common ancestor." Genes appear to be "definite structures in or on the chromosomes"; therefore genes may show homology. Now that we know so much about the chemical basis and mechanism of heredity, we can define what we mean somewhat more precisely by stating, for instance, that the sequence of nucleotides comprising a cistron in one form is homologous with the sequence in another when both are descended by replication from a

27

sequence in a common ancestor. Zuckerkandl and Pauling (1965) distinguish between duplication-dependent and duplication-independent homology, the former resulting from duplication as well as replication, while the latter depends on replication alone. The duplication-dependent type of homology seems to exist between the genes controlling the α and β chains of hemoglobin, for instance, but as far as coat color genetics is concerned it can only be surmised as one probable cause of genocopies. It seems legitimate (and is certainly common practice) to regard as homologous the mutant alleles of homologous genes in different species which have a very similar effect (for example, Siamese dilution in the cat and Himalayan dilution in the rabbit and the mouse), even though no common ancestor may have carried the same allele.

Haldane pointed out that there was no absolute criterion of homology, no way of being certain that genes in different forms were descended from a common ancestral gene. A gene might conceivably be independently evolved on several occasions. Validity of the criteria for homology depends on the uniqueness of genes and on the unlikelihood of the same gene becoming part of the genome of two different species except as a result of descent from a common ancestral gene. We now believe that a gene may consist of a sequence of hundreds or thousands of di-nucleotides of four different types with respect to base-pairing. Thus the chances of elaboration of even approximately similar genes except by duplication seems very low indeed. However, there will be further discussion of the homology concept later.

With his usual foresight, Haldane raised the question of whether a relation may exist between genes more fundamental than homology, namely chemical "identity." He pointed out that linkage studies suggested that genes were the same size as protein molecules. If this could be established, "comparative genetics and ultimately comparative morphology could be placed on a new basis."

A new molecular basis for comparative genetics is indeed emerging, especially as the result of the complete unravelling of the structure of certain proteins, such as hemoglobin and cytochrome-c, which are direct products of gene action. Ingram and co-workers have shown that substitution of a single amino acid for another is the basis of the difference between hemoglobins A and S, as well as between A and C; results with many other abnormal hemoglobins parallel these findings. The altered hemoglobin structure is the result of a change from one allele to another at the hemoglobin locus; in fact, it seems that the amino-acid change occurs because of the substitution of one base pair for another in the triplet coding for the amino acid. The biochemical nature of the original mutation thus can be deduced from the resultant change in structure of a polypeptide chain, while the detailed course of evolution of homologous genes from an ancestral gene can be unravelled by analysis of the amino-acid changes in the polypeptide chains concerned. Such an analysis cannot yet be attempted on the proteins involved in melanin synthesis, but this achievement is only a matter of time.

MAIN CRITERIA OF HOMOLOGY

Haldane suggested two main criteria of homology, but unfortunately neither has proved of much practical use in mammals. The first criterion is that the genes concerned should "produce the same effects when brought in from either side in a species cross." Accordingly, if similar genes A and B are present in two species, they can be regarded as homologous if AA in the one species, BB in the other, and AB in the hybrid all have the same phenotypic effect. It is, of course, possible that A and B might be geno-copies with one epistatic over the other, but this possibility is perhaps rather remote. The evidence is most convincing when A and B are similar recessive mutants, like the white-eyed mutants of *Drosophila melanogaster* and *D. simulans*, which Sturtevant (1929) showed were homologous by this criterion. In mammals, however, hydridization between different species is seldom possible (even with the help of artificial insemination, as suggested by Haldane), whereas hybridization between two genetically well-studied species seems practically nonexistent. The best-known example of mammalian hybrid formation is the horse-donkey cross, but very little is known of donkey genetics. Studies of F_1 mules and hinnies, however, have shown that both parental species possess a sex-linked gene for glucose-6-phosphate dehydrogenase (G6PD) as does man (Trujillo *et al.*, 1965; Mathai *et al.*, 1966). Ohno *et al.* (1965) have found a sex-linked G6PD locus in hares, again by analysis of a species cross.

Haldane considered that a second fruitful but less direct line of attack might stem from the work of Onslow (1915) on the biochemical effects of skin extracts. Onslow had shown that an extract could be prepared from the skin of black, blue, agouti, or chocolate rabbits which behaved as a tyrosinase does to tyrosine in the presence of hydrogen peroxide, forming a black pigment on incubation. The addition of skin extracts from rabbits with a dominant white coat color, however, prevented pigment formation, as if dominant whiteness was caused by a tyrosinase inhibitor. It seemed possible that skin extracts from different species might interact in essentially the same way as do extracts from different genotypes of the same species, with the product of interaction giving information on the genetic relation of the color genes concerned. In fact, Onslow himself showed that skin extracts from albino mice behaved just like those from albino rabbits when added to extracts of black rabbit skin. The nearest approach to this subsequently has been the extensive use of the "dopa reaction" to determine the melanogenic activity of skin and, in particular, the presence or absence of tyrosinase, which is essential for both eumelanin and phaeomelanin production. Dopa (3,4-dihydroxyphenyl-alanine) activates tyrosinase and also acts as substrate, being formed from tyrosine by oxidation and in turn forming dopa quinone by further oxidation; both processes are catalyzed by tyrosinase. There are many links in the chain of reaction between dopa quinone and melanin, but no further enzyme catalyzing the oxidation, rearrangements, or polymerization has been discovered (cf. Foster, 1965). Tyrosinase production, however, is known to be under the control of the albino locus, so the inability of albino skin from various species to form pigment when incubated with dopa is additional evidence for homology.

Some other ingenious methods for overcoming the species barrier are proving valuable in confirming homologies. For instance, Silvers (1965) has grafted mouse skin onto partially tolerant infant rat hosts carrying a different allele at the agouti locus. The rat melanocytes responded to the agouti locus genotype of the mouse follicles, for hair of the mouse agouti allele phenotype was produced. This result was completely in line with those from intraspecific transplants, which had shown that the follicular environment controls the expression of agouti alleles in both species. Silvers' experiments showed that the behavior of a cell in one mammalian species can be completely determined *in vivo* by the genotype of an entirely different host species. They also furnished compelling evidence for homology of the agouti locus in the two species.

SECONDARY CRITERIA OF HOMOLOGY

Haldane outlined four secondary criteria which, if satisfied, allowed one to suspect homology of the genes being compared. All four are still relevant today and will be dealt with in turn.

Similar, but Not Necessarily Identical, Somatic Effects

The rapid growth in our knowledge of the genetics of coat color in the mouse has shown that great caution must be exercised in the use of this criterion. Over forty different loci are now known to affect coat color in the mouse. These include a number of pairs or trios of independent genes with similar phenotypic effects, for example (1) color-diluting genes such as dilute, leaden, and misty, (2) at least three recessive genes which darken the agouti coat, (3) dominant spotting genes such as W, patch, steel, and splotch, and (4) recessive spotting genes such as piebald and lethal spotting. Some of these may be examples of duplication-dependent homology, so that a similar gene in another species may be homologous with more than one member of a set of genocopies. Most, however, almost certainly have evolved independently, although they may affect different stages of the same developmental pathway.

A detailed study of similar mutants often reveals fundamental differences or resemblances which may make homology less or more probable. For instance, there are two independent, dominant spotting loci in mice called W and Sl; alleles at these have almost identical pleiotropic affects, including macrocytic anemia, sterility, coat dilution, and white spotting. McCulloch et al. (1964, 1965) have shown, however, that anemic WW^v and $SlSl^d$ mice differ very greatly in their ability to form hemopoietic colonies in the spleens of heavily irradiated host mice. WW^v hemopoietic cells had less than $1/200$ the normal ability to form such colonies, whereas $SlSl^d$ cells behaved normally in this respect. On the other hand, WW^v spleens had the normal capacity to support growth of colony-forming units derived from bone marrow of other mice, while $SlSl^d$ spleens had a reduced ability in this respect. This test of colony-forming ability successfully discriminates, therefore, between the functions of these two loci and thus may make it easier to establish the homologies of similar genes in other species, such as white face (W) in the fox (Johansson, 1947).

Another example of successful phenotypic discrimination between two mimic genes concerns dilute and leaden in the mouse, which both dilute coat color to the same extent. This dilution is caused by a clumping of pigment granules in the hair resulting from abnormalities in the melanocyte, which is "nucleopetal" (Markert and Silvers, 1956) with fewer and finer processes than the normal nucleofugal type and with pigment granules concentrated around the nucleus instead of being dispersed through the cell and its processes. Furthermore, it has now been discovered that *retinal* melanin granules are clumped in dilute but not in leaden mice (Moyer, 1966). This finding also may well be useful in differentiating between possible homologies in other species.

The techniques of skin transplantation and of electron micrography are proving particularly valuable in determining whether particular coat color genes in the mouse are acting via the tissue environment or directly on the pigment cell itself, as well as the extent to which the detailed structure of the developing melanin granule is affected. The extension of these techniques to other mammals, such as rat, rabbit, and guinea pig, should provide information of great value for comparative genetics.

A. G. SEARLE

Only One Gene per Species with a Certain Effect

Haldane pointed out that only one gene was known per mammalian species which was able to convert chocolate pigmentation into black. Thus, grounds for suspecting homology were greater than if several genes could produce a certain effect, such as the conversion of piebald into self-colored. The examples given by Haldane are still valid, for in the mouse, brown rat, deer mouse, guinea pig, rabbit, cat, and dog only the dominant wild type of allele at the *B* locus is able to convert brown into black eumelanin. Although in the Syrian hamster and the mink, more than one mutant gene has been reported to give a brownish coat color, yet close study of pigment granules probably will show that in only one is the color of individual granules changed to a brown eumelanin.

Parallel Mutations to Multiple Allelomorphs

Multiple allelomorphic series provide perhaps the most convincing evidence for homology of genes in different species. The best-known series in mammals are still those described by Haldane, namely, the A (agouti), C (albino), and E (extension). I shall discuss each of these in turn, so as to give some idea of what is known about them now in the rodent and carnivore species which have been studied genetically.

Table IV-1 shows the present position with respect to the main alleles of the A series. Species in which no mutant alleles are definitely known have been omitted, even though the existence of the locus can often be inferred from the presence of banded agouti hairs in the wild type. The mouse has by far the largest number of agouti alleles known in a mammal, now totalling 13. It is, therefore, surprising that in the much-studied deer mouse *Peromyscus maniculatus* and the Syrian hamster *Mesocricetus auratus* only the wild type of agouti allele is known. In the mink *Mustela*

TABLE IV-1

DISTRIBUTION OF SOME AGOUTI ALLELES IN RODENTS AND CARNIVORES[a]

MAMMAL	ALLELE				
	Viable Yellow	Light-bellied Agouti	Gray-bellied Agouti	Light-bellied Non-Agouti	Non-Agouti
House mouse	A^{vy}	$+^b$	$+^b$	a^t	a
Brown rat	—	+	—	—	a
Black rat	—	$+^b$	$+^b$		a
Guinea pig	—	$+^b$	$+^b$	—	a
Rabbit	—	+	—	a^t	a
Cat	—	—	+	—	a
Dog	a^y	+	—	a^t	A^s

[a] + = wild type of allele; gene symbols given for mutant alleles.
[b] Different wild populations of house mice and black rats may be gray-bellied or light-bellied agouti; the same seems true of the wild cavy species.

32

vison the agouti locus itself, with the ability to make yellow pigment in the form of phaeomelanin, seems to have been lost entirely.

Only in the mouse do any of the agouti alleles have pleiotropic effects, for yellow A^y causes adiposity when heterozygous and early embryonic lethality when homozygous, while the recessive allele a^x is also lethal when homozygous (Russell *et al.*, 1963). Russell *et al.* also have shown that this agouti locus is a complex one, with about 0.5 per cent crossing-over between a^x and A^y. Phillips (1966) has confirmed this finding and has demonstrated that a pseudoallele A^s gives different phenotypes when in the *cis* and the *trans* position relative to other alleles. Silvers and co-workers (cf. Billingham and Silvers, 1960) have shown clearly that agouti alleles act on the melanocyte mainly via the follicular environment, as the pleiotropic effects of some alleles would lead one to suspect. In formation of the banded agouti hair the same melanocytes apparently are able to secrete both eumelanin and phaeomelanin pigment granules; the change in product is associated with a change in mitotic activity of hair bulb cells (Cleffmann, 1963).

In different populations of mice, black rats, and wild cavies, the wild type of allele at the agouti locus may be gray-bellied agouti A^+ or light-bellied agouti A^w. A similar phenomenon occurs with respect to the albino locus (Table IV-2), for the wild type of allele of the South American chinchillas does, indeed, seem to be homologous with the chinchilla

TABLE IV-2

DISTRIBUTION OF SOME ALBINO ALLELES IN RODENTS AND CARNIVORES[a]

MAMMAL	ALLELE					
	Full Color	Dark Chinchilla	Chinchilla	Light Chinchilla	Acro-melanic (Himalayan)	Albino
House mouse	+	—	c^{ch}	—	c^h	c
Brown rat	+	—	—	c^r	—	c
Black rat	+	—	—	—	—	c
Deer mouse	+	—	—	—	—	c
Syrian hamster	+	—	—	—	c^d	—
Vole (*Microtus arvalis*)	+	c^i	c^{ch}	—	—	c
Coypu	+	—	—	—	—	c
Chinchilla	—	+	—	—	c^h	—
Guinea pig	+	c^k	c^d	c^r	c^a	—
Rabbit	+	c^{chd}	c^{chm}	c^{chl}	c^h	c
Cat	+	—	c^{ch}	—	c^s	$c?$
Mink	+	—	—	—	c^h	—
Dog	+	—	c^{ch}	—		$c^a?$

[a] + = wild type of allele; gene symbols given for mutant alleles.

mutant allele in other forms. It is interesting to note that mutations to acromelanism have occurred in nearly as many members of this group as have mutations to albinism when the gene is completely inactivated. Yet no acromelanistic mutations have been reported outside the rodents and carnivores. The lack of mutations to albinism in fairly well studied species, such as the guinea pig and hamster, probably is not a chance effect. It may mean that complete inactivation of the gene concerned has a lethal effect in some species. On the other hand, it seems possible that the extreme type of acromelanism found in the guinea pig and hamster is really homologous with albinism in other species. Thus, slight pigment formation might occur in these species even in the absence of c locus tyrosinase.

In the extension series (Table IV-3), dominant alleles for extension of black are known or believed to be present in a number of forms, that of the black rat being responsible for the black coat of the *rattus* subspecies. It is still by no means certain that the extension locus exists in the mouse, but a dominant black mutant called sombre (So) may well turn out to be homologous with E^d (Bateman, 1961).

The most interesting allele at this e locus is undoubtedly that for partial extension of yellow, which results in a mosaic phenotype of black and yellow found in the guinea pig (tortoiseshell), rabbit (Japanese), dog (brindled), cattle, and swine. An almost identical phenotype also occurs in female cats and Syrian hamsters heterozygous for a sex-linked gene for yellow coat color. The mosaicism found with these sex-linked mutants is readily explicable by the Lyon (1961, 1962) hypothesis of sex-chromosomal inactivation, otherwise known as the single-active-X hypothesis.

TABLE IV-3

DISTRIBUTION OF SOME EXTENSION ALLELES IN RODENTS AND CARNIVORES[a]

MAMMAL	Dominant Extension of Eumelanin	Normal Extension	Mosaic	Extension of Phaeomelanin
Black rat	$+$[b]	$+$[b]	—	e
Deer mouse	—	$+$	—	y
Syrian hamster	—	$+$	—	e
Guinea pig	—	$+$	e^p	e
Rabbit	E^d	$+$	e^j	e
Dog	E^m	$+$	e^{br}	e

[a] $+$ = wild type of allele; gene symbols given for mutant alleles.

[b] The subspecies *rattus* carries dominant black E^d; others have the allele for normal extension, E.

This postulates that in female mammals one or the other X chromosome is normally inactivated early in embryonic development, this process being random with respect to paternal and maternal X. When a female is heterozygous for a sex-linked mutation, therefore, clones of mutant and of normal cells are formed, leading to a mosaic pattern if gene action is autonomous.

The problem arises as to how homozygosity for an autosomal e locus allele can produce the same mosaic phenotype as heterozygosity for a sex-linked allele. Various lines of evidence suggest that in the autosomal as well as the sex-linked mosaicism the different colored patches represent clones of cells in which different alleles are active. For instance, white-spotting genes tend to make the dark and light patches more distinct, similar to the situation in sex-linked mosaicism. This agrees with the idea that the white-spotting gene reduces the number of "stem-cells" from which clones of pigment cells are derived, so that the clones tend to intermingle less and completely fail to colonize some parts of the skin. It is also interesting to note that the dark patches are always solid black in the rabbit, in which a dominant black allele, E^d, is known at this locus, but they may be either black or agouti in the guinea pig, which does not possess such a dominant allele (Table IV-3). Thus, the Japanese rabbit looks as if it is a mosaic of phenotypically E^d and e pigment cells, and the tortoiseshell guinea pig, a mosaic of E and e.

On this basis, it would appear as if the "alleles" for partial extension of yellow had arisen as a result of unequal crossing-over in heterozygotes for e, so that the E (or E^d) and e alleles came to lie on the same chromosome, as postulated by Komai (1951). If a method of dosage compensation operates similar to that proposed by Lyon for the two X chromosomes, so that one or other of the contiguous alleles had been inactivated at random, then the expected phenotype would resemble closely that actually observed. For example, a homozygous tortoiseshell ($e^j e^j$) guinea pig would be genotypically Ee/Ee. As a result of random inactivation, one would expect clones of cells of the genotypes EE, Ee, and ee in the ratio of $1:2:1$, or phenotypically $\frac{3}{4}$ black or agouti to $\frac{1}{4}$ yellow hair. This expectation agrees well with observations, as do all the other predictions which can be made on the basis of this idea. It seems probable, therefore, that a random inactivation process can occur with some autosomal as well as with X-linked genes.

Similar Linkages in Different Species

Although nearly all the expected twenty linkage groups have been fully established in the mouse, the position in other rodents is far from

35

satisfactory, while no linkages are known in carnivores apart from those involving the sex chromosomes. So there have been few opportunities for using this criterion. As when Haldane wrote, the best example of the phenomenon is the linkage between the albino and pink-eyed dilute loci in the house mouse, Norway rat, and deer mouse, estimates of map distance being 14, 19, and 16 units, respectively. Thus, we can be confident that a segment of linkage group I in these species has remained unchanged for much of the period during which myomorph rodents were evolving. There is also, however, evidence for the occurrence of translocations, especially with regard to the brown locus. This is closely linked to the diluting gene misty in the mouse, but to silver in the Norway rat and to albino in the rabbit. Since the loci for silver, misty, and albino are known to be on different chromosomes in the mouse, it follows that interchanges involving these chromosomes must have occurred during rodent evolution, if the genes concerned are really homologous.

Information with respect to sex linkage has increased markedly since Haldane's paper, when yellow in the cat was the only example among coat color genes. A very similar sex-linked gene for yellow has now turned up in the Syrian hamster (Robinson, 1966). This species has another sex-linked mutant known as mottled-white (Magalhaes, 1954) which closely resembles members of the mottled series of alleles in the house mouse. Several other sex-linked genes affecting the coat are now known in the mouse, but so far they have no homologues elsewhere.

CONCEPT OF HOMOLOGY

By the use of these four criteria, we can clearly discern a fairly small group of coat color genes (including *A, B, C, E,* and *P*) which are definitely present in many mammalian species, as well as a much larger group for which data are insufficient to allow us to homologize with any confidence. The question then arises: Can we be sure even for genes in the first group that they all owe their resemblances to descent from a common ancestor possessing the gene concerned, i.e., that they really are homologous? Haldane considered the possibility that particular genes might be "independently evolved on several occasions." He thought that the production by mutation of "homologous dominant genes (other than deficiencies)" might indicate this evolution and would raise a problem "which strikes at the very root of the conception of homology." There is good evidence for homology of various dominant black mutations in different species, and although mutations to dominant alleles are much rarer than mutations to recessive ones we no longer consider that they present a special problem.

36

Recent developments in genetic studies on microorganisms, however, once again make it necessary to question the concept of homology. Through such processes as transduction and lysogeny (or virogeny) genetic information can be transferred from one organism to another without the intervention of any sexual process. Although no proof has yet been forthcoming that heritable changes have been produced in the mammalian germ-line by such processes, Bailey (1966) has suggested that a number of inherited histocompatibility changes in mice, which occurred with higher frequency on the control than the experimental side of a radiation experiment and which involved antigenic gains, were really the result of the incorporation of viral genomes. Krooth (1965) also has discussed the possible existence of virogeny in mammalian cells and has pointed out that confirmation of this would inevitably raise the question of its possible role in evolution. Tatum (1965) has discussed the possible future use of episomes, transducers, etc. for the control of human heredity. It would be in line with past experience in other spheres if the processes which may be used consciously in the future to change the mammalian genome also had been operative in nature in the past.

The possibility might be worth considering, therefore, that certain very similar or identical genes in different species do not exist because of possession of the gene by a common ancestor but because of some process of genetic transfer, followed by fixation of the transferred genetic material in the genome of the recipient species. The consequences can be envisaged in the light of Vavilov's (1922) law of homologous series in variation. Vavilov stated that closely related species are characterized by similar series of variations, similarities being more complete the more nearly allied are the forms. This is what we could expect with similarity by descent from a common ancestor. If, on the other hand, two species which are distantly related but are nevertheless associated in some way (e.g., because one preys on the other) present more frequent examples of apparent gene homology than groups of more closely related species, then the transfer of genetic information from A to B might be suspected.

No adequate genetic comparisons of this type yet can be done with respect to mammalian coat color, since only the mouse has been studied at all thoroughly. It is interesting to note, however, that the cat and mouse resemble each other more closely in coat color variation than one would expect in view of their very distant phylogenetic relationships. Both cat and mouse have mutations to chinchilla and acromelanism at the albino locus, as well as to recessive non-agouti, brown, and dilution at other loci. Other similar mutations have been reported (for instance to dominant black and pink-eyed dilution), but homologies are more doubtful. The

37

only coat-color mutations in the cat which have not yet been found in the mouse seem to be those of the tabby series, dominant white with associated deafness and sex-linked yellow. However, the last is found in another rodent, the Syrian hamster. Species fairly closely related to the cat, such as the mink and dog, have produced no sex-linked coat color mutations and generally tend to be rather different from the cat in their coat color genetics. Until some other mammalian species have been studied as thoroughly as the mouse, we cannot expect any decisive evidence on this problem from coat color genetics. Such evidence is more likely to come from antigenic studies, since antigenic loci seem much more likely to be subjected to processes of genetic transfer.

From his analysis of coat color variation, Haldane concluded that there were real differences among the genes concerned in their tendencies to mutate. Support of this conclusion has come from work by Schlager and Dickie (1966) on spontaneous mutation at five coat-color loci in mice, which showed differences among these loci in mutation frequencies. Haldane also concluded that there was no special tendency for a gene to mutate preferentially in one particular species or group of species. This still seems to hold generally for the major color genes, although mutations giving patterns of regular depigmentation, similar to belted in the mouse and Dutch in the rabbit, seem unknown in Carnivora. Conversely, the cat tabby locus, which undoubtedly exists in many other Carnivora, is unknown in rodents.

Haldane considered that these data on coat color mutations were of particular interest in the light they threw on evolutionary processes. We have seen from Tables IV-1, IV-2, and IV-3 that in all the three main multiple allelomorphic series the wild type of allele varies in different races or species. The absence of clear-cut Mendelian segregation in many interracial and interspecific crosses had led some biologists to deny the importance of Mendelian factors in evolution. Haldane pointed out, however, that if (as he believed) evolution had occurred partly by "slight changes in the intensity of action of genes," as from light-bellied agouti A^w to gray-bellied agouti A, the nature of these differences might be very difficult to determine in species crosses unless mutant alleles with larger effects also were available.

Many coat color morphisms now have been reported in mammals, in most of which there is a clear-cut difference between the normal and the mutant morph, although the mode of inheritance of the difference is seldom known for certain. Huxley (1955) has stressed the evolutionary significance of these morphisms, especially when different secondary monomorphisms have become established in some parts of the species range, since this may well be a first step in speciation. Secondary mono-morphism occurs in the Arctic fox *Alopex lagopus*, for only the white phase is found in Kamchatka and only the blue phase, in Alaska. A single incompletely recessive gene determines the difference between blue and white phases, according to Johansson (1960). Similarly, the deer mouse *Peromyscus polionotus* has a monomorphic island race *leucocephalus* with a very light coat color on a white sand reef off the Florida coast. There is on the mainland a cline for increasing pigmentation as one proceeds inland from the sandy beaches, the difference between pigmented and depigmented forms being partly under the control of the dominant gene for white cheek *Wc*. Haldane (1948) analyzed Sumner's data on this cline to estimate the magnitude of the selective forces involved. He was able to show that a selective advantage of only about 0.1 per cent on each side of the boundary between light and dark habitats would be sufficient to account for the cline.

Haldane pointed out that clines may result from the favoring of one form in one part of the species range and another elsewhere, as in *Pero-myscus polionotus*, or from the outward migration of a gene from its center of origin. Several possible examples of the latter process occur among melanic coat color morphisms in mammals. For instance, a melanic form of the wild rabbit has spread in Tasmania with remarkable rapidity over the last 50 years (Barber, 1954), reaching a frequency of about 30 per cent in the cleared rain forest. Barber believes that the recessive gene for non-agouti is responsible for the melanism; if so, the intensity of selection must be very high.

A similar cline seems to exist even in a mammal usually regarded as domesticated, namely, the cat. Haldane realized its value for population genetic studies because (1) the genetic basis of its color polymorphism had been worked out and (2) the gene for yellow was sex linked and had heterozygous expression in the form of tortoiseshell. Gene frequencies, therefore, could be calculated and observed phenotype frequencies com-pared with those expected on the basis of random mating. After "the Prof." had given me tutorials on cat genetics in London's back streets, I was able to show by examination of a large sample that there was, indeed, good agreement with the random mating hypothesis (Searle, 1949). The estimated frequency of the recessive blotched tabby allele was very high in London, but it is low or very low in a number of places outside Europe (Searle, 1964). Thus, there seems to be a cline in the frequency of the t^b gene as one proceeds outward from western Europe, which may well mean that this allele is still spreading from its center of origin. Esaki *et al.* (1962) have reported a similar example of what seems to be transient polymorphism in the Kiso native horses of Japan, in which the frequency of agouti (bay) is steadily increasing at the expense of non-agouti (black).

Haldane showed how much information of evolutionary and genetic value could be extracted from a study of coat color differences in mammals. Plenty of intriguing examples of coat color polymorphism or rare variation still await a more thorough investigation. If this were done, greater use could be made of the analytic methods devised by Haldane, and we would understand evolutionary processes better than we do now.

REFERENCES

BAILEY, D. W. 1966. Heritable histocompatibility changes: lysogeny in mice? *Transplantation*, 4:482–88.

BARBER, H. N. 1954. Genetic polymorphism in the rabbit in Tasmania. *Nature*, 173:1227.

BATEMAN, N. 1961. Sombre, a viable dominant mutant in the house mouse. *J. Hered.*, 52:186–89.

BILLINGHAM, R. E., AND W. K. SILVERS. 1960. The melanocytes of mammals. *Quart. Rev. Biol.*, 35:1–40.

CLEFFMANN, G. 1963. Die Bedeutung von Äusseren einflüssen auf die Pigmentzelle für die rhythmische Musterbildung im Haar. *Roux' Archiv.*, 154:239–71.

ESAKI, K., J. HAYAKAWA, T. TOMITA, J. BITO, K. NOZAWA, AND K. KONDO. 1962. Changes in frequency of occurrence of various colours in Kiso native horses. *Jap. J. Zootech. Sci.*, 33:218–25.

FOSTER, M. 1965. Mammalian pigment genetics. *Advances Genet.*, 13:311–39.

HALDANE, J. B. S. 1927. The comparative genetics of colour in Rodents and Carnivora. *Biol. Rev.*, 2:199–212.

———. 1948. The theory of a cline. *J. Genet.*, 48:277–84.

HUXLEY, J. S. 1955. Morphism and evolution. *Heredity*, 9:1–52.

JOHANSSON, I. 1947. The inheritance of the platinum and the white face characters in the fox. *Hereditas*, 33:152–74.

———. 1960. Inheritance of the colour phases in ranch bred blue foxes. *Hereditas*, 46:753–66.

KOMAI, T. 1951. On mosaic inheritance in mammals. *Amer. Natur.*, 85:333–34.

KROOTH, R. S. 1965. The future of mammalian cell genetics. *Birth Defects: Original Article Series of National Foundation*, New York, 1(2):21–56.

LYON, M. F. 1961. Gene action in the X-chromosome of the mouse (*Mus musculus* L.). *Nature*, 190:372–73.

———. 1962. Sex chromatin and gene action in the mammalian X-chromosome. *Amer. J. Hum. Genet.*, 14:135–48.

McCULLOCH, E. A., L. SIMINOVITCH, AND J. E. TILL. 1964. Spleen-colony formation in anemic mice of genotype WW^v. *Science*, 144: 844–46.

McCULLOCH, E. A., L. SIMINOVITCH, J. E. TILL, E. S. RUSSELL, AND S. BERNSTEIN. 1965. The cellular basis of the genetically determined hemopoietic defect in anemic mice of genotype Sl/Sl^d. *Blood*, 26:399–410.

MAGALHAES, H. 1954. Mottled-white, a sex-linked lethal mutation in the golden hamster, *Mesocricetus auratus*. *Anat. Rec.*, 120:752.

MARKERT, C. L., AND W. K. SILVERS. 1956. The effects of genotype and cell environment on melanoblast differentiation in the house mouse. *Genetics*, 41: 429–50.

MATHAI, C. K., S. OHNO, AND E. BEUTLER. 1966. Sex-linkage of the glucose-6-phosphate gene in Equidae. *Nature*, 210: 115–16.

MOYER, F. H. 1966. Genetic variations in the fine structure and ontogeny of mouse melanin granules. *Amer. Zool.*, 6:43–66.

OHNO, S., J. POOLE, and I. GUSTAVSSON. 1965. Sex-linkage of erythrocyte glucose-6-phosphate dehydrogenase in two species of wild hares. *Science*, 150:1737–38.

ONSLOW, H. 1915. A contribution to our knowledge of the chemistry of coat colour in animals and of dominant and recessive whiteness. *Proc. Roy. Soc. Lond., B.*, 89:36–58.

PHILLIPS, R. J. S. 1966. A cis-trans position effect at the *A*-locus of the house mouse. *Genetics*, 54:485–95.

ROBINSON, R. 1966. Sex-linked yellow in the Syrian hamster. *Nature*, 212:824–25.

RUSSELL, L. B., M. N. C. McDANIEL, AND F. N. WODDIEL. 1963. Crossing-over within the a "locus" in the mouse. *Genetics*, 48:907.

SCHLAGER, G., AND M. M. DICKIE. 1966. Spontaneous mutation rates at five coat-color loci in mice. *Science*, 151:205–6.

SEARLE, A. G. 1949. Gene frequencies in London's cats. *J. Genet.*, 49:214–20.

———. 1964. The gene-geography of cats. *J. Cat Genet.*, 1(5):18–24.

SILVERS, W. K. 1965. Agouti locus: homology of its method of operation in rats and mice. *Science*, 149:651–52.

STURTEVANT, A. H. 1929. The genetics of *Drosophila simulans. Carnegie Inst. Wash. Pub.*, 399:1–62.

TATUM, E. L. 1965. Perspectives from phsyiological genetics, pp. 20–34. *In* T. M. Sonneborn (ed.), *The Control of Human Heredity and Evolution*. Macmillan, New York.

TRUJILLO, J. M., B. WALDEN, P. O'NEIL, AND H. B. ANSTALL. 1965. Sex-linkage of glucose-6-phosphate dehydrogenase in the horse and donkey. *Science*, 148: 1603–4.

VAVILOV, N. I. 1922. The law of homologous series in variation. *J. Genet.*, 12:47–89.

ZUCKERKANDL, E., AND L. PAULING. 1965. Divergence and convergence in proteins, pp. 97–166. *In* V. Bryson and H. J. Vogel (eds.)., *Evolving Genes and Proteins*. Academic Press, New York and London.

ERNST CASPARI
Department of Biology, University of Rochester,
Rochester, New York

V. HALDANE'S PLACE IN THE GROWTH OF BIOCHEMICAL GENETICS

Haldane is known and admired primarily for his fundamental contributions to the genetic theory of evolution. He was, in addition, deeply interested in the biochemistry of gene action and made numerous contributions in this field. It is, therefore, fitting that in the present book a chapter be devoted to this aspect of his scientific activities.

His interest in biochemistry was a natural development, since he spent his early years as a scientist in the laboratory of his father who was a mammalian physiologist at a time when biochemistry—or physiological chemistry as it was called then—was still considered a branch of physiology, and later in the laboratory of Frederick Gowland Hopkins. He was professionally identified until 1932 as a biochemist, and referred to himself later as "a 'classical' biochemist (which means, in fact, one who has accepted the point of view of Hopkins)" (Haldane, 1954, p. 45). Both in his writings and in conversation, he would often express his admiration for Hopkins and acknowledge the great impact Hopkins had on his own intellectual development. As a result of this influence, it was axiomatic with Haldane at an early time that genic action has to be interpreted in terms of biochemical reactions, and that biochemical interpretations are basic to the morphological and embryological interpretations of gene action, which prevailed in the 1920's and 1930's. As he states in *New Paths in Genetics* (1942): ". . . for if I gained nothing else from ten years' work under so great a biochemist as Hopkins, I gained the conviction that biochemical explanations are more fundamental than morphological."

As were most of his contributions to genetics, Haldane's work in biochemical genetics was primarily theoretical. It is significant that three of his books (*Enzymes* [1930a], *New Paths in Genetics* [1942], and *The Biochemistry of Genetics* [1954]) deal partly or exclusively with topics of the biochemistry of gene action. When he joined the John Innes Horticultural Institute, he intended to initiate an experimental research program dealing with plant pigments. Even though this plan could not be carried out,

Haldane stimulated the research in plant pigments carried out in the 1930's by Robinson, Beale, Scott-Moncrieff, Lawrence, and others. He participated actively in this work by demonstrating that anthocyanin pigments assume a bluer hue in increasingly alkaline solutions and that the pH of the cell sap is controlled genetically.

More important than his experimental contributions to the field of the genetics of plant pigments was, however, his intellectual contribution in designing the program of the experiments. In order to appreciate the uniqueness of his approach, it may be compared with the simultaneous work with insect eye pigments (Caspari [1933]; Beadle and Ephrussi [1936]) which led ultimately to similar biochemical concepts. In the latter work, the original ideas and particularly the techniques used were patterned after embryological methods; the procedure consisted in transplantation experiments. It was the results of these transplantation experiments which forced the workers to the recognition of the biochemical basis of gene action and led, thus, to the search for the substances involved in the synthesis of eye pigments and, finally, to the elucidation of the complex biochemical problems in terms of enzyme chemistry in the classical *Neurospora* work of Beadle, Tatum, and their collaborators.

The work of Haldane and his collaborators was, in contrast, from the very beginning intended to elucidate the biochemical basis of gene action in a systematic manner. The colors of the petals of plants were chosen as objects of the study because a large array of genetically determined variation was available in a number of different species and because the pigments, contrary to the melanin pigments of vertebrates, are easily soluble and obtainable in relatively large quantities, which makes them amenable to the preparative methods of organic chemistry. By the middle and late 1930's, the structure and variations of the main classes of pigments had been established, and genes controlling the relative amounts of the different pigments, the formation and inhibition of copigments, the state of oxidation and methylation of the pigments, and the pH of the cell sap had been identified in several species. The petal pigments had become the best-investigated system from the chemical point of view. The effects on the pigments of combination with different carbohydrates were studied, but this aspect of the work had not been completed when the research project was stopped by World War II.

Although the first step of the projected analysis met with great success, the further steps of the project could not be carried out. It was apparently intended to identify the synthetic pathways by which the different substances are related to each other. Indirect hints actually had been obtained for some of these biochemical connections, but they were not investigated systematically. Finally, it was intended to investigate and identify the enzymes and catalytic agents involved in the formation of the plant pigments. These plans were not carried out because the whole area of research was not taken up again after World War II. The reason seems to be that in the meantime the extended investigations of Beadle, Tatum, and their collaborators on the synthesis of amino acids and vitamins in *Neurospora* had succeeded in establishing the relevant pathways and their interrelations and that these investigators had already started the analysis of the enzymes involved.

Looking at the situation in biochemical genetics from the present vantage point, it appears that the *Neurospora* work had given general answers to many of the questions raised in the work with plant pigments. Accordingly, Haldane devoted the longest chapter in his 1954 book to a discussion of the biochemical work on fungi.

While the work on plant pigments initiated by Haldane remained limited to the description of a final phenotype in chemically exact terms, his theoretical interest became concentrated quite early on the problem of the primary gene product. In a paper published in 1920 he first proposed a form of the gene-enzyme theory. (This paper is hard to obtain, and I have not been able to see it; its contents can be reconstructed from later references, particularly in his 1954 book.)

Haldane did not lay claim to being the first proponent of the gene-enzyme idea. Garrod and Hagedoorn had expressed this hypothesis earlier, and S. Wright and R. Goldschmidt arrived at the same conclusion for similar reasons at about the same time as did Haldane. Haldane gives credit for his stimulation to a paper by Cuénot (1903), who first investigated the genetic basis of the pigmentation of the mouse and came to the conclusion that the interaction of three gene-controlled substances must be involved in forming the gray coat of the wild mouse. From a historical point of view, it is even more important that Haldane called the attention of geneticists to Garrod's book *Inborn Errors of Metabolism* (1909) which proposed the theory of the biochemical block essentially in its modern form and had been forgotten and was unknown to most workers in the field of biochemical genetics in the middle and late 1930's. The reason for this neglect is not easy to understand, since many of the reasons adduced for the neglect of Mendel's work do not apply to Garrod. He was not a scientific outsider, but a highly respected medical scientist, and his book, as well as his Croonian Lecture to the Royal Society, were easily available. Schultz, in a recent article suggests that his work consisted of a number of special and isolated cases which at that time did not appear to have any close relation to the problems of interest to geneticists.

45

Haldane considered genes organs of the cell, and the question of the functions of these organs was, therefore, legitimate. He suggested in his 1920 paper that genes are catalysts with properties similar to enzymes and that they produce definite quantities of specific enzymes, multiple alleles differing in the amounts of the same specific enzyme they produce. This theory is similar to the theory of gene action proposed by Goldschmidt and elaborated in his book (1927) insofar as it assumes that gene and gene product are identical and that mutations are quantitative changes in the amounts of enzyme produced. Haldane continued his interest in the gene-enzyme relation, and in a paper which appeared in 1935 collected the evidence which was available at the time for the genetic control of specific enzymes.

Haldane was, however, not dogmatic about his original form of the gene-enzyme theory but made numerous suggestions in the course of time for changes in, and improvements of, the theory. Most important of these was his recognition that the primary gene product must differ from the gene itself and his rejection of his earlier notion that the differences between alleles of the same gene are quantitative in nature. The reason for this latter change was the recognition that when several pleiotropic effects of the multiple alleles of one gene are considered, it becomes impossible to arrange alleles in a series of quantitatively decreasing effects valid for all characters. Haldane concluded, therefore, that the differences between the gene products and the genes of different alleles at the same locus must be qualitative rather than quantitative.

The assumption of qualitative differences between the primary gene products at one locus led Haldane to propose that with suitable techniques the two gene products of a heterozygote should be demonstrable in the same cell. Accordingly, he pointed out (Haldane, 1937) that the antigens of the red blood cells of man and animals show exactly this feature, which has in the meantime come to be known as codominance. Haldane was the first to draw attention to this direct relation between antigens and their determining genes, and he used it to argue that these antigens may constitute primary gene products. He was not worried by cases in which antigens did not show codominance, since possibilities to account for this situation could be proposed and in some cases (e.g., Lewis factors) even demonstrated. He found, however, great difficulty in accounting for the appearance of hybrid antigens which had been discovered by Irwin (1932) in species hybrids of pigeons. Haldane wrote in 1954: "This observation is a conclusive disproof of the hypothesis that a particular type of gene always makes a particular type of antigen, and that no antigens are made otherwise." Nevertheless, in view of the fact that a

46

direct relation between genes and antigens was frequent, he did not reject the theory completely but continued to be bothered by this apparent exception. His last paper in biochemical genetics (1956) contains a proposed experimental design to test the frequency of the occurrence of hybrid antigens in heterozygous mice.

In addition to enzymes and antigens, Haldane entertained the idea that small molecules, such as vitamins and hormones, might be primary gene products. The general notion appears to have been that it is not the structure of the macromolecules themselves which is under direct genic control but their specificities, chemically identified as specific active groups. Nevertheless, it is very hard to develop a consistent point of view. Haldane was always extremely skeptical about his own formulations of the theory of gene action and considered them only as suggestions and approximations, valuable because they stimulated additional research, but to be abandoned whenever contradictory evidence was found. As a result, his theoretical ideas concerning primary gene action kept changing, and he was reluctant to accept any of his suggestions as final statements.

While the ideas concerning the relations of genes to enzymes and antigens and the stimulation of the extensive work on the pigments of flower petals form the major part of Haldane's contribution to biochemical genetics, numerous suggestions of his concerning other topics may be mentioned; for example, the interpretation of the results of mammalian tumor transplantation experiments of Little by assuming the activity of genetically controlled antigens, an interpretation which was and still is generally accepted (Haldane, 1933), and a proposal to explain the reproduction of genes by a template mechanism involving DNA and protein (Haldane, 1954). These will not be discussed further, but some remarks should be made on the impact which Haldane's ideas on the biochemistry of gene action had on his views on the processes of evolution. When R. A. Fisher (1931) first proposed his theory of the evolution of dominance, Haldane (1930b) made an alternate suggestion based on his theory of gene-enzyme relations. Fisher proposed that selection will act in such a way that modifiers accumulate which shift the curve relating gene dosage to phenotypic effect so that the heterozygote has the same phenotypic effect as has the homozygote. Haldane pointed out that it is not necessary to assume an influence of the modifiers on the shape of the curve, but that it is sufficient that the modifiers shift the position of the wild type of homozygote along the horizontal part of the curve some distance so that the heterozygote will also come to lie on the horizontal part of the curve. It is, therefore, not necessary to make any assumptions about the genetic control of the shape of the dose-effect curve.

The work on anthocyanins and other petal pigments had evolutionary implications to which Haldane called attention. The work was carried out on about ten different species of higher plants, and in addition to great similarities a number of differences were found. Comparisons among the different species were discussed by Haldane (1942, pp. 68–73), but the material available was not sufficient to permit firm conclusions on the evolution of the pigments.

Finally, mention must be made of Haldane's contribution to the theory of the origin of life (1929, 1932, 1938). This question was regarded as insoluble at that time, and it was Haldane's suggestion which proved to be the starting point of all modern developments in this field. Previously, it had been assumed that the first organisms must have been able to obtain their building materials and particularly their energy from inorganic sources; in other words, the original forms of life must have been complete prototrophs, possibly able to carry out even photosynthesis. Haldane, however, suggested that the first organisms may have been auxotrophs and that they may have obtained their energy from organic compounds. These organic compounds could have been formed by the action of ultraviolet light derived from the sun in an atmosphere devoid of molecular oxygen. This set of suggestions forms the basis of the modern theory of biochemical evolution. It was further elaborated by Oparin and was established later on a firm experimental basis.

It is apparent that Haldane's work in biochemical genetics constituted an important part of his scientific work. Trained as a biochemist, he held, from the beginning, the opinion that the nature of the gene and of gene action had to be explained in exact biochemical terms. This goal now has been accomplished to a large degree through the explosive development of the field of molecular biology. When Haldane's *The Biochemistry of Genetics* appeared in 1954, many of the problems raised in the book had been answered in the interval between the writing of the book and its publication. This is the typical fate of books in a field in which development is as rapid as it was in molecular genetics in the 1950's.

Because of external circumstances, mainly the lack of laboratory facilities, Haldane could not participate extensively in the developing experimental work in this field of biochemical genetics. He participated in the process of this field of his interest by reading widely and by communicating his knowledge and his speculations concerning the literature to the scientific world. In this way he became one of its prime stimulators and catalysts, and several of his ideas have been highly influential in directing the general trends of work in the field of biochemical genetics. Some have become accepted into the general framework of our knowledge of genetics, such as the codominance of the primary gene products and the qualitative difference between the primary gene products of alleles at the same locus. In the long run, his most fruitful and important contribution in the field of biochemical genetics may have been his insight that the primitive forms of life have been auxotrophs. This idea broke the impasse which had previously made it impossible to study the problem of the origin of life and enabled biochemists to consider this question in terms of chemistry and physics.

Haldane's most important contribution to the development of biochemical genetics, however, was his early appreciation of the need to describe the nature of the gene and of gene action in biochemical terms. While, as mentioned earlier, ideas of the relation of genes and enzymes were frequently proposed in the 1920's and 1930's, Haldane, with his biochemical background, was the only author in those days who took the suggestion seriously from a biochemical point of view, demanding that gene-controlled enzymes be found and identified and that the reactions they control be described in exact biochemical terms. He, in this way, prepared the ground for the fusion of genetics and biochemistry which, in the last twenty years, has borne such abundant fruit.

REFERENCES

BEADLE, G. W., AND B. EPHRUSSI. 1936. The differentiation of eye pigments in Drosophila as studied by transplantation. *Genetics*, 21:225–47.

CASPARI, E. 1933. Über die Wirkung eines pleiotropen Gens bei der Mehlmotte Ephestia Kühniella. *Z. Arch. Entw. mech.*, 130:353–81.

CUÉNOT, L. 1903. Hypothèse sur l'hérédité des couleurs dans les croisements des souris noires, grises et blanches. *C. R. Soc. Biol.*, 55:301–2.

FISHER, R. A. 1931. The evolution of dominance. *Biol. Rev.*, 6:345–68.

GARROD, A. E. 1909. *Inborn Errors of Metabolism*. Oxford University Press, Oxford. 216 pp.

GOLDSCHMIDT, R. 1916. Genetic factors and enzyme reaction. *Science*, 43:98–100.

———. 1927. *Physiologische Theorie der Vererbung*. Springs, Berlin. 247 pp.

HALDANE, J. B. S. 1920. *Some Recent Work on Heredity*. Trans. Oxford Univ. Junior Scientific Club Ser. 3, pp. I, 3.

———. 1929. The origin of life, p. 3. *In The Rationalist Annual*.

———. 1930a. *Enzymes*. Longmans, Green and Co., London, New York. 235 pp.

———. 1930b. A note on Fisher's theory of the origin of dominance. *Amer. Natur.*, 64:560–66.

———. 1933. The genetics of cancer. *Nature*, 132:265–67.

———. 1935. Contribution de la génétique à la solution de quelques problèmes physiologiques. *C. R. Soc. Biol.*, 119:1481–96.

———. 1937. The biochemistry of the individual. *In* J. Needham and D. E. Green (eds.), *Perspectives in Biochemistry*. Cambridge Univ. Press, Cambridge.

———. 1942. *New Paths in Genetics*. Harper, New York and London. 206 pp.

———. 1954. *The Biochemistry of Genetics*. G. Allen and Unwin, London. 144 pp.

————. 1956. The detection of antigens with an abnormal genetic determination. *J. Genet.*, 54:54–5.

IRWIN, M. R. 1932. Dissimilarities between antigenic properties of dove hybrids and parental genera. *Proc. Soc. Exp. Biol. Med.*, 29:850–51.

SCHULTZ, J. 1967. Review of The gene: a critical history, by E. A. Carlson. *Science*, 157:296–301.

WRIGHT, S. 1916. An intensive study of the inheritance of color and other coat characters in guinea pigs, with special reference to graded series. *Carnegie Inst. Wash. Pub.*, 241:59–160.

I. MICHAEL LERNER and NOBUO INOUYE
University of California,
Berkeley, California

VI. BEHAVIOR GENETICS, WITH SPECIAL REFERENCE TO MAZE-RUNNING OF *TRIBOLIUM*

"Sometimes I have had a problem in mind. If so I have generally discovered something for which I was not looking. . . . " (Haldane, 1962, *J. Genet.*, 58:141)

Among Haldane's versatile interests, animal behavior (or misbehavior as he sometimes called it) occupied a central place. Though not an active participant in experiments, he contributed numerous ideas, discussions, and biometrical analyses which have influenced the work of others to an extent that is not widely known. He regarded the discovery of bee "language" by Karl von Frisch (1923) as the most important advance in twentieth-century biology. In one of his early books, *Possible Worlds* (1928), Haldane wrote, "others . . . have been tackling the problem of how much one bee can tell another, and how it does it. Tomorrow it looks as if we should be overhearing the conversation of bees, and the day after tomorrow joining it. We may be able to tell our bees that there is a tin of treacle for them if they will fertilize those apple trees five minutes' fly to the south-east; Mr. Johnson's tree over the wall can wait!" The problem of communication in social insects fascinated him so much that he returned to the topic repeatedly in subsequent years. In his classic work *The Causes of Evolution*, he discussed the consequences of selection of a gene for altruistic behavior in a colony of bees. He argued that genes causing unduly altruistic behavior in the queens would tend to be eliminated. When the number of individuals in the colony is small, selection is at once effective, but in large colonies the initial stages of the evolution of altruism depend not on selection but on random survival. Problems of instinct and other aspects of behavior were discussed in later publications (Haldane, 1951, 1953; Haldane and Spurway, 1956). Haldane and Spurway (1954) dealt with the statistical analysis of von Frisch's observations of communication in *Apis mellifera*, summarized by them as follows:

The dance conveys about 5 cybernetic units of information concerning direction, of which the average recipient receives at least 2.5.

Between 100 and 3,000 metres the number of turns made in a given time fall off linearly with the logarithm of the distance. At greater distances it

51

falls off more slowly. The number of abdominal waggles made per straight run increases by 1 per 75 metres between 100 and 700 metres. It is suggested that this is the principal means by which distance is communicated.—K.R.D.

In a recent paper, written in honor of Bernhard Rensch, Haldane (1960) summarized his views on mind in evolution and dealt especially with behavior in lower animals. Some of our own recent work has been concerned with the behavior and population genetic aspects of the flour beetle, *Tribolium*, and these experiments will be described briefly here.

The experiments originated from an attempt to find a metric character in *Tribolium* for which automatic selection could be practiced. After a lifetime of working on selection with traits which required either extensive counting or laborious measuring, a device which would select phenotypes automatically or permit the experimental animals to sort themselves appealed considerably. Such a device for studying geotaxis and various other properties was constructed for *Drosophila* by Hirsch (1959). Modifications of this maze for *Tribolium* were built by Inouye (1965), and experiments on selection for right- or left-hand turning and for positive or negative geotaxis were initiated.

It soon became obvious that the best of the mazes constructed (straight T, illustrated by Inouye [1965] in the note on p. 170) was not an adequate apparatus for *Tribolium*, largely because we could find no reward to induce the beetles to complete the run. Beetles tended to wander apparently aimlessly through the maze, turning around or blocking a passageway for hours without budging. The thought then occurred to us that, before selecting for geotaxis or another property of this type, perhaps a strain of *Tribolium* could be developed which would be characterized by speed of completing the run through the maze. Hence, the experiments reported here.

Selection for Speed of Maze-running

The foundation stock consisted of samples of the synthetic strains of *T. castaneum* (marked with the sooty body color gene) and *T. confusum*, described by Lerner and Ho (1961). The general procedure was to separate males and females in the pupal stage. About a month after eclosion, the beetles were semi-starved for 72 hours: approximately one-quarter teaspoonful of flour was provided for each group of 300–400 beetles in that period. They were then placed in the initial tube with the maze in horizontal position (the first run was made in a vertical position, since geotaxis was also being tested). At the end of each of four successive half-hour periods, the beetles found in the final tubes were removed and counted. From the beetles of the foundation population which had com-

52

pleted the run within a two-hour period, ten pairs were chosen to become the parents of each of three mass matings of the two species.

The procedure followed in the succeeding generations was generally similar, though some variations were introduced. Thus, in selection from the F_1 and F_2 of both species as well as the F_3 of $T.$ $castaneum$, the beetles completing the run in the first two hours were run through the maze once more, so that selection was sequential and more rigorous. When the proportion of beetles completing the run within two hours increased markedly, the criterion of selection was changed and to one based on the outcome of the first half-hour only (F_3 and subsequent selection of $T.$ $confusum$ and F_4 of $T.$ $castaneum$). The results of selection reported in Tables VI-1 and VI-2, however, are based on the proportion of beetles completing the run in two hours.

It can be seen readily that selection intensity was not maintained constant throughout the experiment. Since our original purpose was merely to develop fast-running strains, neither this fact nor the variations used in the mating system were considered of consequence.

Tables VI-1 and VI-2 and Figs. VI-1 and VI-2 show the outcome of selection. The ease with which the performance of beetles of both species

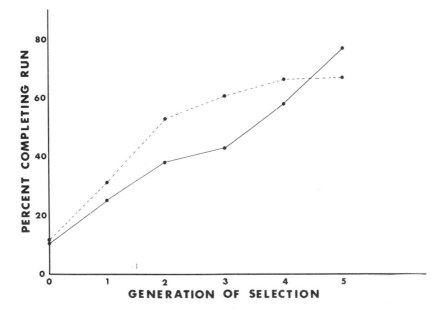

Fig. VI-1. Percentage of $T.$ $castaneum$ tested completing run in 2 hours. Solid lines = males; dashed lines = females.

TABLE VI-1

SELECTION RESULTS WITH *T. castaneum*[a]

GENERATION OF SELECTION	MATING NUMBER	PARENTAL MATING NUMBER	Males No.	Males %	Females No.	Females %
0	0–1	Stock	1084	10.1	928	11.6
1	1–1	0–1	1106	25.0	1148	31.5
	1–2	0–1	718	16.6	934	38.8
	1–3	0–1	820	33.2	963	23.2
Total	—	—	2644	25.2	3045	31.1
2	2–1	1–1	375	48.0	370	38.9
	2–2	1–1	400	26.3	401	54.9
	2–3	1–1	461	39.7	434	62.2
Total	—	—	1236	37.9	1205	52.6
3	3–1	2–1	348	76.7	380	75.3
	3–2	2–1	328	26.5	424	45.8
	3–3	2–1	411	47.7	354	65.4
	3–4[b]	2–2	195	36.4	208	43.8
	3–5	2–3	336	17.9	419	65.6
Total	—	—	1618	42.6	1785	60.2
4	4–1	3–1	428	61.2	459	89.5
	4–2	3–1	433	75.5	425	76.5
	4–3	3–2	460	28.0	337	59.6
	4–4	3–3	476	72.7	324	43.5
	4–5	3–3	188	38.3	262	42.4
	4–6	3–4	277	78.3	316	85.8
	4–7	3–5	343	42.6	297	45.5
Total	—	—	2605	57.5	2420	65.9
5	5–1	4–1	270	73.0	282	68.4
	5–2	4–1	472	72.2	248	33.1
	5–3	4–6	382	84.0	272	94.9
Total	—	—	1124	76.4	802	66.5
5	Crosses		292	66.4	243	72.0
	between		444	47.1	437	83.5
	lines		397	70.3	460	87.2
Total	—		1133	61.8	1140	82.5

[a] Each mating originated from ten pairs of parents.
[b] Only seven sires.

54

TABLE VI-2

Selection Results with *T. confusum*[a]

Generation of Selection	Mating Number	Parental Mating Number	Percentage Completing Run in 2-Hour Period			
			Males		Females	
			No.	%	No.	%
0	0–1	Stock	1057	18.2	922	32.2
1	1–1	0–1	410	44.1	472	58.9
	1–2	0–1	414	22.5	380	40.3
	1–3	0–1	189	53.4	287	29.3
Total	—	—	1013	37.0	1139	45.2
2	2–1	1–1	460	48.0	534	62.7
	2–2	1–2	326	54.3	320	77.8
	2–3	1–3	372	68.8	364	51.9
	2–4	1–4	430	75.6	405	77.8
Total	—	—	1588	61.6	1623	67.0
3	3–1	2 1	388	63.4	349	62.8
	3–2	2–1	269	63.2	472	56.3
	3–3	2–2	450	19.6	347	38.6
	3–4	2–2	467	54.4	411	46.2
	3–5	2–3	432	39.1	377	43.5
	3–6	2–4	477	71.1	472	64.6
Total	—	—	2483	51.0	2428	52.7
4	4–1	3–1	441	50.1	452	67.7
	4–2	3–1	239	31.8	231	58.4
	4–3	3–2	436	34.4	349	91.7
	4–4	3–3	394	62.7	410	54.4
	4–5	3–4	360	49.7	411	70.1
	4–6	3–5	320	61.9	373	45.8
Total	—	—	2190	48.9	2226	64.8
5	5–1	4–1	412	73.5	396	64.6
	5–2	4–4	283	73.8	418	82.8
	5–3	4–6	365	51.2	392	80.4
Total	—	—	1060	65.9	1206	76.0

[a] Each mating originated from ten pairs of parents.

can be improved is dramatic. This is particularly so because, as is obvious, there is so much erratic variation in the speed of maze running between matings. We have not identified the sources of variability, but, as Tables VI-1, VI-2, and subsequent tables demonstrate, there can be startling reverses of form between sexes, between parents and offspring, and

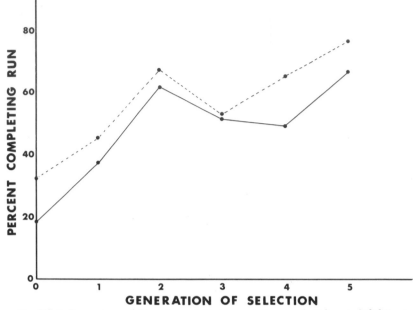

Fig. VI-2. Percentage of *T. confusum* tested completing run in 2 hours. Solid lines = males; dashed lines = females.

between repeat runs of the same beetles in the same and in different mazes. In spite of these phenomena, an unquestioned rapid change has occurred in the performance of successive generations.

Tests of Selected Lines against Controls

Because of the great variability in performance just noted, it could be held that the improvement may have a temporal basis and not be genetic in nature. In order to check this hypothesis, the F_3 generation was tested against control lines. To avoid the possibility of bias because of variation in the mazes themselves, several techniques were used. When the selected strains were tested separately from the controls, the runs were performed in duplicate in two separate, but similar, mazes: first, the selected line was run through maze 1, while the control ran maze 2; on rerun, the procedure was reversed.

For *T. castaneum*, the control used was the synthetic strain A2 (*see Tribolium Information Bulletin*, Vol. 8 [1965], p. 3). Lacking the sooty marker, it is described as the wild line in Table VI-3. Its particular advantage lies in the fact that, in addition to testing the selected and control lines separately, mixed runs could be held in the same maze and the comparative performance of the two scored on the basis of the body color difference between the beetles. As shown in Table VI-3, the selected line outperformed the controls in every possible comparison. The only conclusion possible is that the changes observed over the generations have, indeed, a genetic basis.

TABLE VI-3

INTER-STRAIN TESTS OF SPEED OF MAZE-RUNNING

SPECIES				MAZE 1		MAZE 2	
				No.	%	No.	%
T. castaneum	Strains tested separately	Males	Wild	205	24.9	204	4.9
			Selected	186	42.5	214	57.9
		Females	Wild	213	50.7	213	22.5
			Selected	229	76.0	229	87.3
	Strains tested together	Males	Wild	204	8.8	—	—
			Selected	186	25.8	—	—
		Females	Wild	—	—	213	24.9
			Selected	—	—	220	60.5
T. confusum	Strains tested separately	Males	Synthetic	241	7.5	240	27.9
			Selected	236	65.7	236	48.3
		Females	Synthetic	208	26.9	*208*	*47.6*
			Selected	*211*	*31.3*	217	54.8

Note: Percentages indicate proportion of beetles tested completing run in a 2-hour period. In both species the third selected generation was used. See text for explanation of italics.

The situation in *T. confusum* was rendered somewhat more complicated because the selected line had no markers. Hence, mixed runs were not possible, and even in separate runs an element of confusion was introduced by what later proved to be an experimental error. The control used was the original synthetic line which provided the foundation of the selected line. As presented in Table VI-3, the outcome of the tests of males was clearly the same as in *T. castaneum*. The tendency in the females was in the same direction if the performances in the same maze are compared. If, instead, the comparison is made between the simultaneous runs by the two lines (synthetic in maze 1 and the selected line in maze 2, and vice-versa), only in the first of these is the selected line superior (54.8 vs. 26.9 per cent). In the second comparison (shown in italics in Table VI-3), the selected line appeared to be inferior to the synthetic.

Because the beetles of the two lines cannot be distinguished by sight, the possibility that in the course of the experiments the labels of the two cultures became switched could not be excluded. Hence, a supplementary test was undertaken. Females of the selected and the synthetic lines were divided into two groups each and mated, respectively, to selected and synthetic line males. The offspring of the four sets of matings were then tested for maze running. Table VI-4 shows the expected ranking of the beetles on the basis of the labels in Table VI-3 together with the outcome of the test. It is clear that the results strongly favor the hypothesis that in fact there was a labelling error in the original test. It is, therefore, concluded that the results of selection in $T.$ $confusum$ do not differ basically from those in $T.$ $castaneum$.

TABLE VI-4

PERCENTAGE OF BEETLES COMPLETING RUN IN A 2-HOUR PERIOD

MATING	1	2	3	4
Male parent	Selected	Synthetic	Selected	Synthetic
Female parent as shown in Table VI-3.	Selected	Selected	Synthetic	Synthetic
Expected F_1 ranking on this basis.	1	2–3	2–3	4
Male F_1: number	813	694	566	442
percentage	58.7%	42.5%	75.3%	64.9%
Female F_1: number	844	752	559	426
percentage	76.4%	53.2%	81.6%	49.3%
F_1 combined percentage	67.7%	48.1%	78.4%	57.3%
Actual F_1 ranking	2	4	1	3
Real genotype of female parent.	Synthetic	Synthetic	Selected	Selected

Note: F_1 test of anomalous results with $T.$ $confusum$ shown in Table VI-3.

REPEATABILITY OF PERFORMANCE

It has been noted already that reruns of the fastest beetles were made in all but the initial generation. The results, shown in Table VI-5, once more, illustrate the vagaries of maze running by $Tribolium$. The beetles used for the second run are those which had completed the first run in the specified period. Had repeatability of performance been 100 per cent, all of the beetles tested on the rerun should have completed it in the same period of time. This is obviously very far from the results obtained. Indeed, in a number of instances the second run was poorer than the first. Thus only 5.6 per cent of the males of the F_4 of $T.$ $castaneum$ tested for the half-hour run completed the rerun in this time. The success of selection in spite of such erratic behavior is very impressive. Although no marked trend can be observed in the table, the startling improvement in the rerun performance of the F_5 of *T. castaneum* should be noted. It may indicate that selection can lead to increased genetic control over performance and, hence, to increased repeatability.

TABLE VI-5

PERFORMANCE OF FASTEST BEETLES ON RERUN

			PERCENTAGE COMPLETING RUN							
			Males				Females			
		LENGTH OF TEST RUN	First Run		Second Run		First Run		Second Run	
SPECIES	GENER-ATION		No.	%	No.	%	No.	%	No.	%
T. castaneum	1	2 hrs.	1106	25.0	268	36.2	1148	31.5	359	19.8
	2	2 hrs.	1236	37.9	455	38.7	1205	52.6	614	63.2
	3	2 hrs.	1618	42.1	680	45.6	1785	59.2	943	80.4
	4	1 hr.	1852	38.8	709	43.9	1767	46.0	767	67.8
	4	½ hr.	277	26.7	71	5.6	337	33.8	114	42.1
	5	½ hr.	1797	42.6	749	78.9	1457	57.7	828	76.0
T. confusum	0	2 hrs.	1057	18.2	193	43.2	922	32.2	292	51.5
	1	2 hrs.	1013	37.0	370	32.4	1139	45.2	514	57.0
	2	2 hrs.	1588	61.6	974	42.0	1623	66.9	1084	65.8
	3	2 hrs.	2483	51.0	1177	65.5	2432	52.6	1187	69.5
	4	½ hr.	2190	33.1	722	45.2	2226	51.6	1114	43.7
	5	½ hr.	1060	50.3	530	63.6	1206	57.3	684	71.1

In addition to reruns of the fastest beetles, complete samples of males and females in the fifth selected generation of *T. castaneum* were given a second run. The results, which appear in Table VI-6, give pause for reflection. In the males repeat performance improved on the rerun, a result which not only lends confirmation to the suggestion that selection can lead to increased genetic control over performance but also raises the possibility of selecting for ability to learn, as well as for speed. In the females there was no improvement. Once again, no clear-cut reasons for the difference between the behavior of the two sexes can be given. The line of investigation opened by these questions, however, may be a profitable one to explore.

TABLE VI-6

LEARNING ABILITY OF *T. castaneum* (FIFTH GENERATION)

	MALES		FEMALES	
	First Run	Second Run	First Run	Second Run
Number tested	397	390	437	430
Percentage completing run in				
½ hr.	49.4	62.3	69.1	51.9
1 hr.	64.5	74.4	81.2	74.9
2 hrs.	70.3	77.2	83.5	85.8

PHYSIOLOGICAL BASIS FOR SPEED OF RUNNING

Reasonably early in the course of these experiments, we began to wonder just exactly what we were selecting for. Observations on dispersal patterns in both *T. confusum* and *T. castaneum* (Naylor, 1959, 1961) have indicated that the beetles are sensitive to quinone secretions of their odoriferous glands (*see* Engelhardt *et al.*, 1965, for literature sources). It has occurred to us that selection may have been directed toward increased sensitivity to such secretions. It is known that under conditions of crowding, starvation, or, generally, "excitement," the stored fluid product of the glands is discharged by the beetles. The semi-starvation and crowding in the initial tube undoubtedly provided such conditions. The hypothesis suggested regarding sensitivity (and its complement that selection has been for an increased amount of secretion) seemed worthy of test.

Unfortunately, the specific kinds of the ethyl and methyl benzoquinones produced by *Tribolium* are not available in synthetic form, making conclusive tests of the hypothesis difficult. Several indirect tests, however, were possible. In the first one, a related substance was tested. The results of this experiment (in which the reaction of selected and control beetles to bromoquinone were tested) were inconclusive, particularly because the smell of the material used, at least to human nostrils, was rather different from that of the products of the beetles themselves.

The second approach involved the use, as a tester, of flour in which other beetles had lived (conditioned flour) and which, therefore, contained the noxious substances. Results of a test in which the initial tube of the maze contained flour of this kind, shown in Table VI-7, at first sight seem to favor the hypothesis proposed. The complication lies in the fact that the differences between the results with conditioned flour and without

TABLE VI-7
T. castaneum TESTED WITH CONDITIONED FLOUR

	MALES				FEMALES			
	Selected (F₃)		Synthetic		Selected (F₃)		Synthetic	
DISTRIBUTION OF BEETLES	No.	%	No.	%	No.	%	No.	%
Completed run in ½ hr.	19	10.3	0	0	128	57.7	6	2.8
in 1 hr.	35	19.0	0	0	152	68.5	34	15.8
in 1½ hrs.	46	25.0	0	0	165	74.3	43	20.0
in 2 hrs.	47	25.5	0	0	166	74.8	50	23.3
Failed to complete run	72	39.1	12	5.9	24	10.8	40	18.6
Failed to leave initial tube	65	35.3	191	94.1	32	14.4	125	58.1
Total	184	—	203	—	222	—	215	—

(*see* Table VI-3) are difficult to assess. Further work along these lines is obviously worthwhile.

The third possibility, still in prospect, is to use a direct biological assay. The *Tribolium* stock center at Berkeley has mutant strains of both species (*see Tribolium Information Bulletin*, vol. 8) in which the odoriferous glands are modified so as to cut down the amount of secretion considerably (in *T. confusum* by 95 per cent, according to Engelhardt *et al.*, 1965). We propose to observe the speed of running of selected individuals in the presence of different numerical combinations of normal and mutant beetles in the initial tube as a test of the sensitivity of the selected lines to the quinone secretions.

At this stage of our experiments, few formal conclusions, except that speed of maze-running is readily selected for in *Tribolium*, are possible, but the prospect of combining leads from population, ecological behavior, and physiological genetics by investigating the traits described is an exciting one. The fact that the catholic interests of Haldane included all of these areas seems to us to make this contribution to his memory, inadequate as it is, an appropriate one.

Acknowledgments

We wish to express our appreciation for the technical help rendered by Mrs. Barbara Strong and Jon W. Wolfard in carrying out these experiments. The work was supported in part by USPHS grant GM-08942.

References

Engelhardt, M., H. Rapoport, and A. Sokoloff. 1965. Odorous secretion of normal and mutant *Tribolium confusum*. *Science*, 150:632–33.

Frisch, K. von. 1923. Über die "Sprache" der Bienen. *Zool. Jahresker. Physiol. Abt.*, 40:1–186.

Haldane, J. B. S. 1928. *Possible Worlds*. Chatto and Windus, London.

———. 1932. *The Causes of Evolution*. Longmans, Green and Co., London.

———. 1951. *Everything Has a History*. G. Allen and Unwin, London.

———. 1953. Animal ritual and human language. *Diogenes*, no. 4, pp. 3–15.

———. 1960. Mind in evolution. *Zool. Jb.*, 88:117–24.

———. 1962. A parade of ignorance. Review of Darwinism and the study of society. *J. Genet.*, 58:138–42.

Haldane, J. B. S., and H. Spurway. 1954. A statistical analysis of communication in *Apis mellifera* and a comparison with communication in other animals. *Insectes Sociaux*, 1:247–83.

———. 1956. Imprinting and the evolution of instincts. *Nature*, 178:85–6.

Hirsch, J. 1959. Studies in experimental behavior genetics: II. Individual differences in geotaxis as a function of chromosome variations in synthesized *Drosophila* populations. *J. Comp. Physiol. Psychol.*, 52:304–8.

INOUYE, N. 1965. Mazes for *Tribolium*. *Tribolium Information Bull.*, 8:165–70.
LERNER, I. M., AND F. K. Ho. 1961. Genotype and competitive ability of *Tribolium* species. *Amer. Natur.*, 95:329–43.
NAYLOR, A. F. 1959. An experimental analysis of dispersal in the flour beetle, *Tribolium confusum*. *Ecology*, 40:453–65.
————. 1961. Dispersal in the red flour beetle, *Tribolium castaneum* (Tenebrionidae). *Ecology*, 42:231–37.

N. A. MITCHISON
National Institute for Medical Research,
Mill Hill, London, England

VII. ANTIGENS

In 1932 Haldane visited Dunn, in Columbia, and C. C. Little in his private mouse laboratory at Bar Harbor. When he returned to London on the "Mauritania" he took back three inbred lines of mice. At that time the idea of inbreeding mice was still new, and this was the first time I know of that they had been brought into Great Britain. Twenty-four years later I made the same crossing with more mice and was delighted to hear from the old sailor in charge of the pet deck that mine was only the second lot of mice that he had looked after. The mice must have been some of the first occupants of Haldane's new department of eugenics at University College.

The reason Haldane became interested in inbred mice and their antigens is quite clear. The geneticist, especially the student of mammalian genetics, has available today a wide variety of characters controlled by single genes. Most of these fall into the general category of biochemical mutants, and they require sophisticated techniques for recognition. During the 1930's these techniques were not known, and attention was focused for the most part either on physical characteristics such as stature or physique, which are controlled by a large number of genes acting in concert, or on rare pathological conditions. The red cell antigens are the outstanding exception. They display a remarkably simple pattern of inheritance in which interaction between genes is detected only very rarely. An individual belongs to blood group A, for example, only if one of his parents does. Not only do the genes for these antigens present a simple pattern for study but they also segregate at high frequency in all the populations of vertebrates that have been studied. Above all, human populations are highly polymorphic, which must at the time have offered an irresistible attraction to the human geneticist.

When Haldane began to take an interest in the inbred mice, it was already clear, mainly from the work of Little and his colleagues at Bar Harbor, that the factors governing tumor transplantation displayed the same simple pattern of inheritance as did the red cell antigens.

These topics were reviewed in two lectures which Haldane delivered to the Royal Institution (Haldane, 1933). In retrospect, two aspects of these two lectures are remarkable: the way in which Haldane picked his way through the jungle of empiricism that had beset transplantation work on tumors, and his success in concentrating on that part of the work which was amenable to simple explanation. A great deal was already known about the biology of transplantation, partly through the Bar Harbor work, but also through the pioneer studies of Bashford and his colleagues, at the Imperial Cancer Research Fund in London, and of W. H. Woglom, in Columbia. Woglom had already arrived at the conclusion that the rejection of transplanted tumors in rats is brought about by an immunological reaction on the part of the host against antigens in the tumors. Unfortunately the lack of inbred stocks prevented him from deciding whether the antigens were specific to the donor or to the tumor. His ideas do not seem to have been accepted by the Bar Harbor group at the time. Indeed, for many years, Little, and later Snell, preferred to talk of transplantation factors for tumors rather than antigens. The term "histocompatibility factor" which Snell finally adopted is notably conservative. In the 1933 lectures Haldane put forward for the first time the hypothesis that the factors identified at Bar Harbor were simply antigens controlled by genes also present and active in normal tissues.

From this point, Haldane's interest in antigens seems to have followed two paths. His subsequent publications on antigens are concerned preponderantly with the population genetics of human blood groups. His contribution to this field has been summarized admirably by Penrose (cited by Pirie, 1966). The problem to which he devoted most attention was an analysis of the available measurements of the A B O blood group frequencies. His most important contribution to this topic (Haldane, 1940) is concerned chiefly with the statistics of measurement and a systematic review of the data available at the time. From this, certain conclusions about the degree of isolation and movement of human populations were drawn. These conclusions were tentative and have now been largely submerged in the much more extensive data collected subsequently (*see*, for example, Mourant, 1954). For the general reader, perhaps the most enjoyable part of this work is the criteria according to which Haldane accepts or rejects data. One sympathizes with Babacan who is rejected because he found that of 100 Turks examined in Ankara 9.3 per cent belonged to group B. The data of Gauch, on the other hand, probably deserved their fate.

The maintenance of heterozygosis for genes controlling antigens was of lasting interest to Haldane. He examined in considerable detail the expected rate of approach to homozygosis in inbreeding (Haldane, 1936) and during back-crossing of the type devised by Snell to produce co-isogenic strains of mice (Haldane, 1948). His warning that inbreeding will not produce complete genetic uniformity has been borne out by later work on skin grafts among inbred mice.

The maintenance of polymorphism of blood groups still lacks complete explanation. Perhaps no general theory can be expected, but rather the situation will remain a confused one in which many kinds of minor selective advantage play a part in disease susceptibility. The idea Haldane put forward in 1949, that selection for resistance to parasites plays an important role in maintenance of polymorphism, almost certainly is correct. An example of the danger of homozygosis that Haldane particularly liked to quote is the fate of the Gran Michel clone of bananas, wiped out by a single epidemic.

Haldane (1944) drew attention to the lack of any satisfactory mechanism to account for Rhesus polymorphism and suggested that it, therefore, must be of recent origin. The idea seems to me an attractive one because it affords an explanation of the variation in frequency of hemolytic disease after heterospecific pregnancy for different blood groups. It is tempting to believe that groups such as M N S or P apparently can cross the placenta without causing hemolytic disease because the origin of their polymorphism is remote.

He returned to a consideration of rhesus immunization from time to time. He suggested to me that I should examine the breeding records of zoos to find examples of perinatal death in interspecific hybrids with an increasing incidence in birth order. In this suggestion one can detect a combination of three of his interests—blood groups, mammalian hybridization (1932), and ethology. He was well aware that interspecific mating is a perversion and that zoological curators tend to exploit it.

The second path taken by Haldane led into mechanisms of immunology, especially into what we would now call the molecular biology of antigens. Before following his thoughts in this direction, perhaps we should note what happened to the mice. He does not appear to have done any work on them himself. Some of them were distributed among colleagues, and one way or another they formed the nuclei from which many inbred stocks in use in Great Britain today are derived. For example, most of the inbred mice used at the National Institute for Medical Research belong to the CBA line, and are derived from the stock originally brought over by Haldane.

The most important thing that happened to them at the time, however, was that a newly qualified doctor, Peter Gorer, joined Haldane in 1933.

In the biometry department at University College, Gorer started a study of mouse blood groups. He began by discovering three blood groups among the strains of mice, one of which he named "antigen II." This became, in due course, that landmark of transplantation biology, the H-2 locus.

Gorer then turned his attention to the mechanism of rejection of tumor grafts, and by 1935 he had succeeded in identifying the circulating antibodies that are elicited by transplanted tissue, and thus verified the hypothesis that grafts are rejected because they possess antigens which the host lacks. A formal demonstration that the transplantation factors originally identified in Bar Harbor segregated together with the hemagglutinin antigens had to wait until Gorer was able to collaborate with Snell (Gorer *et al.*, 1948).

The hope that a study of antigens might tell something much more direct about gene action stems from the simplicity of inheritance. This is the point made by Haldane in his contribution to the *Festschrift* for Gowland Hopkins (1937). The argument runs as follows. If a number of genes operate in sequence in order to make a final product, we are likely to find evidence of gene interaction, i.e., multifactorial inheritance of the product. For example, a failure early in the sequence will deprive enzymes controlled by later genes of their substrates. Early genes thus tend to be epistatic in relation to late ones. This and other types of gene interaction do not often occur in the inheritance of blood groups. It is this simplicity which also underlies the laws of transplantation. Furthermore, with only a few exceptions, expression of isoantigens does not depend on environmental influence, age, or sex. It must be a matter of some satisfaction that the first clear exception to this generalization was discovered by Gorer himself when he observed that the mouse erythrocyte isoagglutinins cannot be detected until shortly after birth.

Haldane, therefore, suggested that the isoantigens are primary gene products. How well has this suggestion stood up to later tests?

An up-to-date discussion of the one-gene-one-antigen hypothesis must start with a clear distinction between carbohydrate and protein antigens. Modern dogma holds that information flows from DNA to RNA to protein; carbohydrates are down the line from the enzymes that arrange their structure and cannot therefore be regarded as primary gene products. The question is whether the antigens that interest us, particularly the isoantigens of mice and men, are protein or carbohydrate in their determinant groups. Most of us hope that they will turn out to be carbohydrates, because this will make their analysis so much easier. The fact that the antigens which have been analyzed most fully are carbohydrates provides the strongest ground for hope that others will turn out to be similar in arrangement.

Let us consider a well-analyzed example of carbohydrate structure. In searching for an example, one turns either to the somatic antigens of *Salmonella* or to the Lewis-ABO blood groups of man. Both have been the subject of admirable recent reviews written from a structural standpoint (Lüderitz *et al.*, 1966; Watkins, 1966). One might well select as an example the substitution of tyvelose for adequose in groups D and B of *Salmonella* which Mäkelä (1965) has shown to be controlled by a single genetic locus. This substitution of a single sugar is known to cause a variety of changes in O factors depending on the other sugars adjacent to the site at which the dideoxysugar attaches. I choose instead the human blood group system because it attracted Haldane's particular interest (1954, 1956).

A summary of the information available about blood group mucoid is given in Fig. VII-1. The summary combines the genetic theory of Grubb and Ceppellini with the chemistry of Morgan and Watkins (Race and Sanger, 1965) but is in part my own interpretation. The genetics here is extremely simple. The genes Le (Lewis) and Se (secretor) are responsible for the addition of fucoses by means of distinct linkages. Three unlinked genetic loci are responsible for the addition of sugars to polysaccharide backbone, which is in turn linked to peptide. In each case the active and inactive alleles are present in man at fairly high frequencies, and the part played by the H gene, present at very high frequency, need not detain us. The alleles A and B add one of the two sugars shown, or a third allele O does nothing. A or B can act only if Fuc_2 has already been added to the structure, but Se and Le act independently of one another. A and B act on only a fraction of the available side chains and when they do so they apparently block access of anti-H antibody to Fuc_2 and of anti-Le[a] antibody to Fuc_1.

In the first instance, apparently the mucoid is secreted into body fluids and is then passively adsorbed onto red cells. This accounts for the ability of anti-Le antibodies to agglutinate red cells. Antibodies look at this simple pentasaccharide from at least six different angles which I display in the manner suggested by Lüderitz *et al.* (1966). The antibody combining sites probably extend over three to six saccharides, but the antibodies known at present can be defined by their reaction with pairs of saccharides. The most remarkable interactions are given by the two fucose branches. Antisera are known which bind either one of the two fucoses singly, with or without interference from the neighboring fucose, and other antisera are known that bind the two fucoses jointly, although

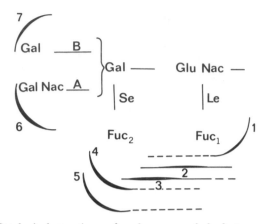

Fig. VII-1. Serological reactions of a human carbohydrate prosthetic group. (Adapted from papers by Morgan, Watkins, Ceppellini, and Grubb [cited by Race and Sanger, 1965].)

(*1*) Anti-Le^a. Reacts with Fuc$_1$, and presence of Fuc$_2$ interferes sterically. Interference is weak for reaction in solution (saliva from nonsecretors more active than saliva from secretors), strong in reaction after adsorption onto red cells (sera contain weak anti-Le^b). Relatively high concentration of salivary antigen probably permits weak affinities to operate.

(*2*) Anti-Le^{bL}. Fuc$_1$ and Fuc$_2$ contribute to binding site. Needs both Fuc's for reaction in solution and after adsorption onto red cells.

(*3*) Anti-Le^{bH}. Fuc$_1$ and Fuc$_2$ contribute to binding site. Needs both Fuc's for detectable reaction after adsorption onto red cells, but only Fuc$_2$ needed for reaction in solution. Difference in apparent reactivity after adsorption probably for same reason as in (*1*) above.

(*4*) Anti-Le^c. Reacts with Fuc$_2$, and presence of Fuc$_1$ interferes (bears same relation to Fuc$_2$ as anti-Le^c does to Fuc$_1$).

(*5*) Anti-H. Reacts with Fuc$_2$, but Fuc$_1$ contributes to binding sites of some sera.

(*6*) Anti-A.

(*7*) Anti-B.

Abbreviations: Gal, galactose; Gal Nac, N-acetylgalactoseamine; Glu Nac, N-acetylglucoseamine; Fuc, fucose; A, B, Se, and Le are A, B, secretor, and Lewis genes.

some of these display a preference for one over the other. With the exception of anti-Le^c, which is made in rabbits, these antibodies have been found in individual humans. The site toward which a man directs his response appears to depend partly on that part of the antigen which he produces himself, to which he is therefore tolerant, and partly on luck. Absorption of antisera is not required, although anti-Le^a apparently has to be used at a dilution high enough to render a minor component directed partly toward Fuc$_2$ inoperative.

When a carbohydrate structure of this nature is examined in such detail, the one-antigen-one-gene theory collapses. All the antibodies directed primarily toward fucose display some degree of interaction between Fuc_1 and Fuc_2, which are in turn controlled by different genes. The most striking interaction is displayed in the reaction with Le^b antisera. An individual may possess the antigen $Le(a- b+)$ ($=Fuc_1 + Fuc_2$), although neither parent does, i.e., one has Fuc_1 and the other Fuc_2. The discovery of a child of this type by Sanger and Race (1958) provided decisive confirmation of the theory of Grubb and Ceppellini.

What we know about this blood group system indicates that single genes control the addition of carbohydrates close to one another, and that the binding sites of antibodies directed against the carbohydrates inevitably tend to overlap from one sugar residue to another, thus making interactions the rule rather than the exception.

Does this imply that the transplantation antigens, which still appear to obey the one-antigen-one-gene rule, are not carbohydrates? In other words, is the discrepancy betweeen the simple pattern of inheritance displayed in transplantation experiments and the more complex pattern that appears here and elsewhere due to a real molecular difference or is it a result of the methods used?

This problem has been discussed by Fox (1958), who has shown in some detail that the simple criterion of rejection that is normally used in transplantation experiments results in misleading simplicity. It is clear, for example, that transplantation experiments would be unlikely to detect an antigen of the $Le(a- b+)$ variety in which the products of two genes contribute to the binding site. Another limitation of the transplantation experiments has been pointed out by Fox. Animals to which most attention has been devoted are inbred mice, and most of the strains have a good deal of genetic material in common. This restricts the interaction antigens that can be found. In the example just discussed, the antigen defined by anti-Le^b sera could not have been recognized as an interaction product in a race that did not segregate for the Le gene. It would not then have been distinguishable from the H antigen. Hence, it is not unlikely that some of the mouse transplantation antigens which at present behave as single gene products may be subdivided in the future when genes are introduced from distant mouse strains. Haldane (1954) made this point, and suggested a method to identify hybrid antigens. Mice of one strain would be rendered immunologically tolerant of a second strain and then grafted with tissue from the F_1 hybrid. Rejection of the graft would indicate the presence of hybrid antigens. This suggestion has not, so far as I know, been implemented.

Irwin (1966) found a clear example of an interaction antigen present in normal doves that could not have been detected without a reagent obtained by making interspecific hybrids. A single-locus ch-4 controls the antigenic specificities *abc* in *Streptopelia chinensis*, and *abcdef* in *S. humilis*, *S. orientalis*, and *S. senegalensis*. When the ch-4 gene from *chinensis* is brought into the presence of a second gene (ch-8) from *humilis* or *senega-lensis* the gene then produces the specificities *abcdef*. It follows, therefore, that the *def* specificities found in *humilis*, *orientalis*, and *senegalensis* are interaction products, even though, in genetic experiments, *abc* and *def* behave as a single character.

Finally, the admission has to be made that exceptions to the simple laws of transplantation crop up fairly frequently now that the genetics of skin graft rejection in mice has become a subject of intensive work. The Y antigen, for example, apparently is able to cause graft rejection in females of some genetic constitutions, while in others it cannot do so. An interesting list of exceptions has been compiled by Bailey (1965), who also has uncovered some remarkable kinds of interaction.

Let us now consider the problem of hybrid antigens for proteins. This problem is altogether more obscure because the antigens of proteins are often, though not always, determined by tertiary structure rather than amino-acid composition. Hence, the chemistry is a good deal more in-accessible than is the case for carbohydrates, for antigenic character itself is often the only information available about tertiary structure. In general, the question we have to ask is whether the tertiary structure of a protein can be controlled by factors other than amino-acid sequence, and, in particular, whether gene substitution in another part of the genome can alter the product of a cistron.

Evidently, we are concerned with a phenomenon that Haldane's father encountered in his work on the uptake of oxygen by hemoglobin, and the effect on this of carbon dioxide. Hybrid protein antigens are an example of the category defined by Monod *et al.* (1963) as allosteric effects, in which a substance influences the properties of a particular site on a protein molecule by reaction with a spatially distinct site. The binding of a molecule of oxygen by hemoglobin is known to produce a change in conformation detectable serologically as well as crystallographi-cally. In this sense, then, environmental changes can alter antigens (Reichlin *et al.*, 1966). One could probably find out whether a man had died of carbon monoxide poisoning by a serological test of his hemoglobin for deficiency of the deoxyhemoglobin determinant. This particular exception to the one-antigen-one-gene law is not, as Haldane would say, compatible with life.

Another example of an allosteric effect that is a little closer to what we are looking for is found in the work of Pollock (1964) on penicillinase.

He found that binding by antibody can alter the efficiency of the enzyme as a catalyst and can, in particular, enhance it. This strongly suggests that the effect of interaction with antibody is not simply steric interference with access to the substrate but is due to conformational change.

I cannot find an example of genetic variation in one cistron causing a conformational change in the product of a non-allele. It is not at all unlikely, for instance, that allotypic variation in the gamma globulin H-chain, particularly in the Fc region, may produce conformational changes in the L-chain, but an effect of this kind has not yet been discovered. Interaction between the products of alleles, on the other hand, occurs frequently; it is known as complementation and may occur in a positive or, less frequently, in a negative sense. In negative complementation, which comes closest to what we are looking for, two defective molecules, each with residual activity and medially overlapping defects, interact in a negative way so as to decrease residual activity (Bernstein *et al.*, 1965). Examples of negative interaction have been found by Bernstein and his colleagues in phage T4D, where it has the effect of decreasing burst size in certain combinations of temperature-sensitive mutants. Presumably negative complementation of this type could be detected serologically as a new antigen.

Information about genetic control should provide prima facie evidence about the chemistry of hybrid antigens. The most likely source of hybrid protein antigens is multi-chain proteins, where the chains are products of alleles. No corresponding mechanism is known to operate for carbohydrates, and there is no reason to expect carbohydrate interaction antigens to be controlled by alleles. Hybrid antigens produced by allelic interaction are likely, therefore, to be proteins. Most of the hybrid antigens that have been detected in genetic studies, but not yet subjected to chemical analysis, turn out to be controlled by alleles (Miller, 1954; Chovnick and Fox, 1953; Fox, 1958). We must expect, therefore, that these antigens will turn out to be proteins. This is a disappointment insofar as the prospects of analysis are concerned.

References

Bailey, D. W. 1965. *Transplantation*, 3:531.
Bernstein, H., R. S. Edgar, and G. H. Denhardt. 1965. *Genetics*, 51:987.
Chovnick, A., and A. S. Fox. 1953. *Proc. Nat. Acad. Sci., Wash.*, 39:1035.
Fox, A. S. 1958. *Ann. N.Y. Acad. Sci.*, 73:611.
Gorer, P. A., S. Lyman, and G. D. Snell. 1948. *Proc. Roy. Soc. Lond., B.*, 135:499.
Haldane, J. B. S. 1932. *Nature*, 129:906.
———. 1933. *Nature*, 132:265.
———. 1936. *J. Genet.*, 32:375.

————. 1937. *In* J. Needham and D. E. Green (eds.), *Perspectives in Biochemistry*, p. 1. Cambridge Univ. Press, Cambridge.

————. 1940. *Human Biol.*, 12:457.

————. 1944. *Nature*, 153:106.

————. 1948. Appendix (p. 104) to G. D. Snell. *J. Genet.*, 49:87.

————. 1949. *La recerca sci.*, 19 (Suppl.):68.

————. 1954. *The Biochemistry of Genetics*. G. Allen and Unwin, London.

————. 1956. *J. Genet.*, 54:54.

IRWIN, M. R. 1966. *Proc. Nat. Acad. Sci., Wash.*, 56:93.

LÜDERITZ, O., A. M. STAUB, AND O. WESTPHAL. 1966. *Bacteriol. Rev.*, 30:192.

MÄKELÄ, P. H. 1965. *J. Gen. Microbiol.*, 41:57.

MILLER, W. J. 1954. *Genetics*, 39:983.

MONOD, J., J.-P. CHANGEUX, AND F. JACOB. 1963. *J. Mol. Biol.*, 6:306.

MOURANT, A. E. 1954. *The Distribution of the Human Blood Groups*. Blackwell, Oxford.

PENROSE, L. S. 1966. Cited by N. W. Pirie. *Roy. Soc. Biog. Mem.*, 12:231.

POLLOCK, M. R. 1964. *Immunology*, 7:707.

RACE, R. R., AND RUTH SANGER. 1965. *Blood Groups in Man*. Blackwell, Oxford.

REICHLIN, M., E. BUCCI, C. FRONTICELLI, J. WYMAN, E. ANTONINI, C. IOPPOLO, AND A. ROSSI-FANELLI. 1966. *J. Mol. Biol.*, 17:18.

SANGER, RUTH, AND R. R. RACE. 1958. *Heredity*, 12:513.

WATKINS, W. 1966. *In* A. Gottschalk (ed.), *Glycoproteins*. Elsevier, Amsterdam.

JEAN SUTTER
Institut National d'Études Démographiques,
Paris, France

VIII. HALDANE AND DEMOGRAPHIC GENETICS

When the development of human population genetics (or demographic genetics) is studied at the present time, J. B. S. Haldane is acknowledged as the first scientist who laid its basic principles.

In his well-known series of articles "A Mathematical Theory of Natural and Artificial Selection" published from 1924 to 1934, Haldane: (1) set the rules necessary for accurately observing the phenomena; (2) pointed out selective processes which had not been considered formerly; and lastly (3) tried to integrate Mendelian genetics into demographic structures.

Reviewing the various types of sexual reproduction and all the possible character transmission types, he pointed out that before appraising—in the whole population—the long- or short-term effects of a slow or rapid selection process, the following had to be ascertained: (1) the mode of inheritance of the character considered; (2) the systems of breeding in the groups of organisms studied; (3) the intensity of selection; (4) its incidence (e.g., in both sexes or only one); and (5) the rate at which the proportion of organisms showing the character increases or diminishes. It should then be possible to obtain an equation connecting (3) and (5).

Later on, his evaluation of the consequences of his "k" coefficient indicated the magnitude of the selection operating in a population. Then he appraised the various types of selection.

FAMILIAL SELECTION

When selection is thought of, it is always the Darwinian concept of struggle for life which comes to the mind. This struggle is to be noted in any species as a whole, at least among its members who live in a given area. Haldane even suggested the case where such a struggle was limited to the members of one family only. It is what he called "familial selection." At the outset, he demonstrated the importance of this new concept.

Haldane had been studying two cases. In one, a couple produced so many embryos that their environment could support them and they had not even enough room to live; finally, the surviving offspring had to fight members of other families. b) some embryo deaths are selective—Haldane pointed out the example of the agouti gene in yellow mice. It is well known that in the yellow $\times$ yellow crossing a quarter of the embryos die at the blastula stage. Durham (1911) demonstrated that the size of the litter is not smaller in such a case, since the death of the homozygous embryos allows the other embryos to survive by giving them more room. There, a complete selection process is to be noted, but the lethality can be incomplete and the embryo may suffer only a partial disadvantage. Such conditions determine selection and its rhythm: selection will be more or less effective and its rhythm slower or quicker.

Obviously, such a selection process can be broken down into merely "effective" or "very effective" in the mixed litters. Haldane studied three litters of twenty embryos each. The first one consisted wholly of the strong type; the second contained ten strong and ten weak; and the third litter, only weak embryos. The hypothesis supposes that in each case there is only enough food and room for ten embryos and that the strong type has an advantage over the weak so that, out of equal numbers, 50 per cent more of the strong will survive than of the weak. The numbers of embryos were even at the beginning, but ten strong embryos from the first litter, six strong ones and four weak ones from the second litter, and ten weak ones from the third litter survived. In other words, sixteen strong embryos and fourteen weak ones will be obtained. If the competition had been as free as with pelagic larvae, eighteen strong ones and twelve weak ones would have survived. Clearly, in familial selection, the same advantage acts more slowly than in normal selection, since it is only effective in mixed families.

"The survival of many of the embryonic characters of viviparous animals and seed plants must have been due to familial selection," stressed Haldane (1924). He generalized his concepts on this point when he determined the impact of familial selection on simple Mendelian characters. When he built his model in conformity with the Hardy-Weinberg law, he showed that the composition of the species changed at a rate 50 per cent smaller than would have been observed had the selection applied to the whole of the species, as was thought to be the case before his research.

As easily inferred, the mechanism of familial selection plays a most important part in human population. By now, we know to what extent selection may vary with the mother's age, the rank of birth, and the size of the family. We know, too, that some families suffering from hereditary defects lose many fetuses, produce stillborn babies, and experience neonatal deaths. We can avail ourselves of intra-uterine mortality tables. We know that 80 per cent of the fetuses examined after early miscarriages have morphological anomalies and that 50 per cent of such embryonic miscarriages suffer from chromosomal anomalies.

OVERLAPPING GENERATIONS

Another important contribution by Haldane to the edification of demographic genetics began when, after having studied the mathematical theory of natural or artificial selection and having shown the evolution of populations in the case of entirely separated generations, he considered the case of their overlap.

When the generations do not overlap, the composition of a generation can be calculated from the composition of another and the resulting finite difference equation investigated. One knows from Norton (1910, personal communication from Haldane) that if the generations overlap the finite difference equation is then represented by an integral equation.

In dealing with generations which do not overlap, where he considered that the intensity of selection was independent from the size of the population, Haldane met the problem of measuring population growth. His calculation was made for a death rate and a birth rate in the population which are not functions of its density. He showed that the oscillations of the population number around an exponential function of the time "are either damped or at least increase less rapidly than the population itself." If population is in equilibrium, oscillations are damped and a stable equilibrium occurs. Haldane emphasized that his demonstration was a new proof of the great value of Lotka's research (1922) concerning the stability of normal age distribution in populations.

Moving from this standpoint of the Lotka theorem, Haldane considered the mode of selection of a dominant autosomal factor in the population, only for female zygotes. The following assumptions were made: the sex ratio at birth is taken as fixed; the number of dominant and recessive female zygotes is fixed; random mating occurs; and, as a whole, selection and population growth are slow. Then Haldane computed the reproduction rates of the three female phenotypes at a time t, and he defined selection as the probability for a female zygote to reach age x.

In doing so, he integrated the mode of selection in demographic structures and finally showed that selection, when generations overlap, produces an effect analogous to that obtained when generations are separated. He also showed that the mode of selection was the same for the sex-linked factor.

75

Haldane also integrated his work with the population model of Dublin and Lotka (1925) related to the real structure of the United States population in the 1920 census.

Finally, he also computed, according to certain assumptions, the differential reproduction rate of the three female phenotypes at time t. These assumptions were: when recessives are rare; when dominants are rare; when the death rate and the reproduction rate are the same in the two sexes, etc. Thus his work was very complete.

Haldane's attempt was the first to find the solution to genetic problems by integrating them into demographic structures. Evidently, he was the first to conceive that a synthesis was necessary between demography and genetics in order to establish the real mode of selection and its processes in a human population. From this point of view, it is now rather extraordinary to be able to judge how Haldane has, up to a certain point, a share in the generalization of the Lotka theorem. In this field he was, again, one of the first to have appreciated the importance of the work of the famous demographer. His own genius did the rest.

MENDELIAN POPULATION GENETICS

Soon after the accession to Mendelian genetics, scientists dealing with population problems tried to ascertain the consequences of Mendelian mechanisms observed at the level of the individual. The works of Pearson, Hardy, and Weinberg before 1910 gave birth to Mendelian population genetics and, simultaneously, originated important concepts, such as gene equilibrium, to characterize populations. World War I stopped this research. It was only after 1920 that, moving from the specific problems of populations to those of evolution, neo-Darwinism was built up which attempted to explain evolution in a Mendelian way. The concept of selective mechanisms, therefore, came about as a result of integrating Mendelism into Darwinism. After 1920 the work of the famous neo-Darwinians, Sewall Wright, Haldane, and Fisher, was slowly built up. In Sweden, after 1928, Wahlund and Dahlberg, who specialized more in human population problems than did the aforementioned investigators, created the notion of isolate which, by splitting large populations into partial populations, proved to be of great value in the field of research. For human species many difficulties arise when we try to apply the facts of general biology to the study of real evolutionary phenomena. We recognize that the demographic aspect of the problem has been more or less coped with by each of these authors. Sewall Wright was not aware of that particular aspect of human problems, and, if Fisher was fully conscious of it, his views are liable to criticism. Wahlund's position was similar to Wright's, and Dahlberg's demographic concepts were poor. Haldane had the sharpest views by far.

Yet it must be emphasized that Haldane's brilliant interpretation met practically no following at the time. Involved in other fields, he himself did not push his concepts after the aforementioned work on a demographic model, he never participated in any other practical genetic investigation at the population level.

Integration of genetic problems into demographic structures progressed very slowly during the past forty years, because of the domination of the determinist models. The evolution of probabilities was the instrument which made it possible to launch these studies again. Among others, Malécot (1966) made use of the chain processes of modern probabilities which enabled him to set up stochastic models of very prominent interest.

On the other hand, the creation at the same time of stochastic models in demography facilitated the integration of the two modes of thinking. The intrinsic problems of fertility measurement, as seen, for instance, from the cohort viewpoint, offer a new possibility for integrating genetics into demography. In 1961 Haldane enthusiastically supported our use of this technique at the Institut National d'Études Démographiques.

We must admit that the intellectual step of integrating the genetic phenomena into the demographic structures opens the path to progress for the metrics of human sciences. The crises of some of them, such as physical anthropology, can find no solution but by integration into demography. Furthermore, let us insist on the necessity of interdisciplinary studies in human sciences, in order to know the parental structures and the demographic factors which underly the gene flow and the genetic drift. In the future we shall be able to solve human problems only in this manner. Fundamental science will clearly profit from it as will the acute problems in the field of public health.

REFERENCES

DUBLIN, L. I., AND A. J. LOTKA. 1925. On the true rate of natural increase. *J. Amer. Statist. Ass.*, 20:305–39.

DURHAM, FLORENCE M. 1911. Further experiments on the inheritance of coat color in mice. *J. Genet.*, 1:159–78.

HALDANE, J. B. S. 1924–34. A mathematical theory of natural and artificial selection. Part I. *Trans. Camb. Phil. Soc.*, 23:19–41. Parts II–IX. *Proc. Camb. Phil. Soc.*, 1:158–63; 23:363–72; 23:607–15; 23:838–44; 26:220–30; 27:131–36; 27:137–42; 28:244–48. Part X. *Genetics*, 19:412–29.

LOTKA, A. J. 1922. The stability of the normal age distribution. *Proc. Nat. Acad. Sci., Wash.*, 8:339–45.

MALECOT, G. 1966. Probabilités et Hérédité. P.U.F. et I.N.E.D., Pub. No. 34, 357 pp. Paris.

WILLIAM J. SCHULL and JEAN W. MAC CLUER
Department of Human Genetics,
University of Michigan School of Medicine,
Ann Arbor, Michigan

IX. INBREEDING IN HUMAN POPULATIONS, WITH SPECIAL REFERENCE TO TAKUSHIMA, JAPAN[1]

INTRODUCTION

Throughout a career distinguished by its originality and breadth, J. B. S. Haldane maintained a lively interest in the consequences of inbreeding. Numerous instances of this can be adduced, but one of his earlier, now classic, papers appeared in 1939 in the Annals of Eugenics, and was entitled "Inbreeding in Mendelian Populations with Special Reference to Human Cousin Marriage" (with Pearl Moshinsky). Attention was centered upon the expected frequencies of rare recessive phenotypes under different systems of mating, a matter which had concerned others before Haldane. As was so frequently the case, he brought to the problem new insights and, for the first time, explored the consequences of these systems upon the spread of sex-linked genes. He returned briefly to this general theme in 1947 in an evaluation of "The Dysgenic Effect of Induced Recessive Mutations," to demonstrate that the number of recessive homozygotes expected per generation from a single induced recessive mutation is half the mean coefficient of inbreeding of the population concerned.

His move to India in the later years of his life and encounter with the wealth of mating types arising from a caste culture provided renewed stimulation to thoughts and work in this direction. One of the more interesting products of this time involved "An Enumeration of Some Human Relationships" (Haldane and Jayakar, 1962). This paper not only contained a discussion and specification of the logical structure of human relationships but, in a more general vein, constituted a deliberate effort to bridge the serious gap between genetics and anthropology. The latter aim bears further testimony, if such were needed, to Haldane's efforts to ensure that the ever-expanding bounds of human knowledge, to which he himself contributed so much, would serve to diminish rather than enlarge the barriers among different sciences.

[1] This work was supported by a grant to the University of Michigan from the U.S. Atomic Energy Commission (contract AT(11-1)-1552).

79

Takushima

Some four miles to the west of Kyushu in the neighborhood of the 33rd parallel, in a region which figured prominently in Japan's sixteenth and seventeenth century contacts with the western world, lies Takushima. At the time of interest to us, the summer of 1964, the inhabitants of this island numbered 1,321 (*see* Fig. IX-1 for a distribution of their ages and sex); they were aggregated in two villages of 149 and 93 households, respectively. As is true of many of the smaller islands of the Japanese archipelago, few of the events of historical consequence to this island have been recorded. We do know, however, that it has been a part of the Matsuura *han*, a minor fiefdom in western Japan, for possibly seven centuries, and archeological remains attest to the presence of individuals on the island of Yayoi (200 B.C.–200 A.D.). References to Takushima in the correspondence of those peripatetic chroniclers of sixteenth century Japan, the Jesuit missionaries, suggest a population at that time of 300–500 persons. Almost 300 years later in 1844, the *shūmon aratame*, a type of census instituted in 1623 and designed to enforce the proscription on Christianity promulgated by the Tokugawa, reported 814 men, women, and children living on the island. As judged by households, the

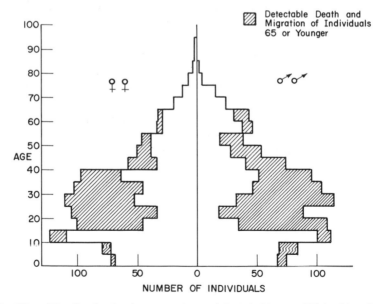

Fig. IX-1. The distribution by age and sex of the inhabitants of Takushima in the summer of 1964.

population changed little in the succeeding fifty years, since they numbered but 183 in 1897 as contrasted with 179 in 1844. This record of growth, though limited, is not conspicuously at variance with the changes in the total population of Japan over the same period of time (Taeuber, 1958). The number of inhabitants of Takushima is, of course, reliably known for recent years: in 1935, it was 1,240; in 1945, 1,399; in 1950, 1,483; and in 1958, 1,651. To the extent that past changes in the population can be discerned, the years prior to 1844 or so were characterized by a slow, natural increase; the next century (to 1955, say), by more rapid growth ascribable primarily to declining mortality rates; and the recent years, by a declining population, reflecting lower birth rates and increased migration to centers of greater economic opportunity.

Our interest centers not on the island itself but on the opportunities which its small, more or less closed population affords to appraise the contribution of certain routinely collected observations in Japan—particularly those associated with the household censuses, the *koseki*, required by law since 1871—to an investigation of the genetic demography of a much larger population of which this island is a portion, namely, Hirado-shi, an administrative unit of about 40,000 people. Since space does not permit a thorough exploration, we propose to consider the relevance of these observations to only two problems, namely, the specification of birth intervals and the determination of the probability of a consanguineous marriage in western Japan.

We begin the latter task by attempting to formulate a more realistic definition of random mating than the conventional, simple one which implicitly assumes that a fixed group of women exists, each of whom a man is equally likely to marry. Clearly, this does not correspond with experience where we recognize that at the least age and propinquity influence the likelihood of the marriage of two individuals. Let us suppose that these are, in fact, the *only* two important considerations in the selection of a spouse. We might assert, then, that random mating holds if the probability that two newly born individuals will marry depends solely upon the distances between their dates of birth and their places of residence. Intuitively, it follows that the probability of a particular consanguineous marriage will be a function of the age constraints imposed upon the selection of a spouse, of the marriage circle (the distance over which spouses are commonly drawn), and of the abundance of one's relatives of the appropriate kind and ages within the marriage circle. Of course, other attributes, e.g., socioeconomic status, influence the probability of marriage, and to these we shall return, but for the moment let us restrict our attention to this simplistic point of view.

Cavalli-Sforza and his colleagues (Barrai *et al.*, 1962; Cavalli-Sforza *et al.*, 1966) and Hajnal (1963) have developed models which attempt to subsume the age and residency constraints into a common equation of estimation. To do so, however, they are obliged to make numerous assumptions with respect to migrational patterns and the ages of one's relatives, since the relevant distributions are not obtainable from routine demographic data. Takushima permits one to evaluate the soundness of these assumptions within one specific culture. Through the *koseki* and the results of an *ad hoc* census, it is possible to describe the differences between ages of uncles and nieces, aunts and nephews, first cousins of various kinds, and so on. Of course, distributions of the age of wife at marriage and maternity and of the age of husband at marriage and paternity generally are available in published demographic data.

All of the models derived to date are applicable, *in sensu strictu*, only to stable populations, that is, to populations whose relevant demographic parameters are constant over time. Actual applications generally have assumed also that the populations in question are stationary, that is, not increasing in size. The arguments all proceed from theory based on large samples, and, though usually applied to small groups of individuals, the stochastic element is ignored. Failure to consider random fluctuations in the estimates of the parameters of interest, when based upon small samples, reflects both "the state of the art" and the formidableness of rigorous analysis. Monte Carlo simulation may provide some insight into the loss of precision in prediction when the stochastic element is disregarded. Be this as it may, with present knowledge there appears to be no satisfactory alternative to the stability assumption, but this is not true with regard to some of the other assumptions in the models. Specifically, for example, the assumption that no correlations exist between vital rates experienced by relatives is subject to test. That is to say, we can, or should be able to, ascertain whether there are significant correlations between parents and offspring or between siblings in frequencies of survival, of marriage and age at marriage, of having various numbers of children and the intervals between such, of migration and the distance, and others. Similarly, we can evaluate the assumption, central to the arguments of Hajnal and Cavalli-Sforza, that the distribution of the difference between the dates of birth of a boy and girl between whom a specified relationship holds is expressible as some linear function of three independent distributions, namely, ages at maternity and paternity and the difference between the dates of birth of the sibling pair through whom relationship stems. Let us turn, now, to the data from Takushima, and what they disclose about these various assumptions and distributions.

Figs. IX-2 to IX-4 reveal the ages of men and women at first marriage and the difference between age of husband and wife for each marriage. Superimposed upon each histogram is a Gaussian curve with the sample mean and variance. Note that this population, though rural, is not characterized by particularly early ages at marriage; the means correspond closely, in fact, to those for the United States. It should be pointed out, perhaps, that in much of Japan, particularly the rural areas, most marriages are not freely contracted by the individuals involved but are generally arranged by their parents or the heads of the households if different from their parents. Many considerations—physical, social, and economic—enter into the arrangement of a marriage, and the importance of specific considerations undoubtedly changes with the passage of time and the ages of the prospective bride and groom. In rural Japan, an unmarried daughter of twenty-five or so is something of a source of embarrassment to the family, and, as a consequence, characteristics once thought to be desirable in a young woman's spouse-to-be are apt to be viewed as less important as she nears this age.

We observed that the distribution of the difference between ages of husband and wife, though reasonably symmetrical, is leptokurtic; this may stem from the fact, as noted, that many marriages are arranged.

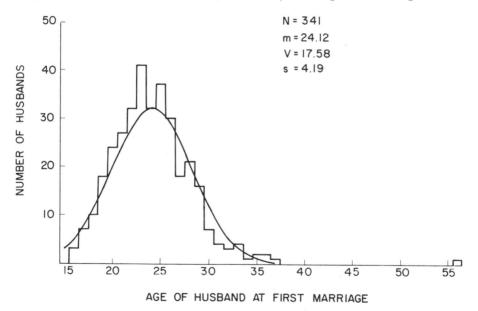

Fig. IX-2. The distribution of ages at first marriage of husbands residing in Takushima in 1964. Superimposed is a Gaussian curve with the sample mean and variance.

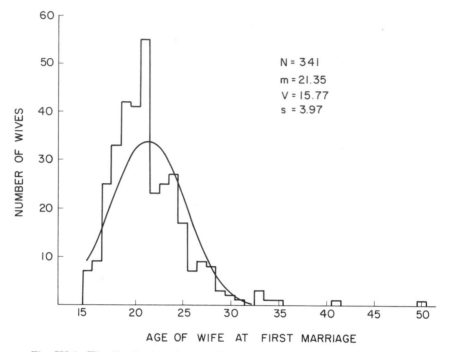

Fig. IX-3. The distribution of ages at first marriage of wives residing on Takushima in 1964. A Gaussian curve with the sample mean and variance is superimposed on the observed distribution.

Clearly, the ages of both husband and wife at marriage would be more nearly Gaussian if the outliers were excluded. It is worth noting that the observed array of differences is reasonably well represented by a distribution based upon the difference between the distribution of the ages of the husband and wife at first marriage and the correlation between them (the broken line in Fig. IX-4). Figs. IX-5 and IX-6 present the distribution of age at paternity and age at maternity, and both, though not bell-like, appear adequately approximated by normal distributions. Conceivably, these distributions, as well as those discussed earlier, might be rendered more nearly Gaussian by some transformation; Cavalli-Sforza and his colleagues, in fact, represent ages at marriage for husbands and wives as the logarithm of the difference between the actual age and the minimum age at marriage for the sex in question. This is a nicety, however, which may be wasted in view of certain other assumptions implicit in the models.

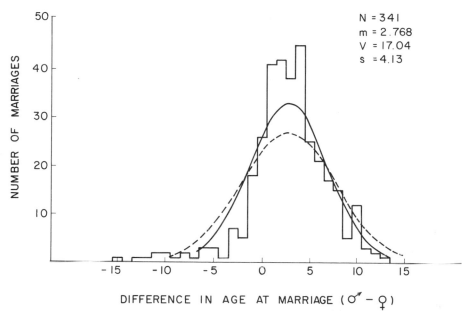

Fig. IX-4. The distribution of differences in ages at first marriage of husbands and wives residing on Takushima in 1964. Superimposed upon the observed distribution is a Gaussian curve with the same mean and variance.

Now, both the Cavalli-Sforza and the Hajnal models assume that the distribution of age differences between any specified class of relatives can be expressed satisfactorily as a linear function of the differences in ages between siblings and a weighted sum of the mean age at paternity and the mean age at maternity. The weights correspond to the number of male and female ancestors interposed between the relatives in question and the siblings through whom relationship passes. More specifically, it is assumed that the mean and variance of the distribution, which is taken to be normal, of the intervals between birth dates of unlike-sexed pairs of live-born relatives of type z are

$$\mu(a_z) = (\alpha_2 - \alpha_1)\mu_p + (\beta_2 - \beta_1)\mu_m$$

$$V(a_z) = (\alpha_2 + \alpha_1)V_p + (\beta_2 + \beta_1)V_m + V(a_s)$$

where μ_p, V_p, μ_m, and V_m are, respectively, the mean age at paternity, the variance in ages at paternity, the mean age at maternity, and the variance in ages at maternity; $V(a_s)$ is the variance of the distribution of intervals

85

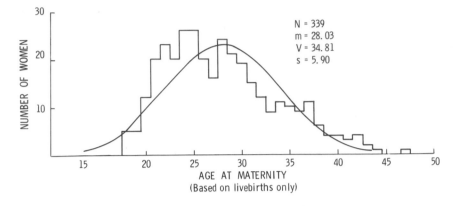

Fig. IX-5. The distribution of ages at maternity of women residing on Takushima in 1964. A Gaussian curve with the same mean and variance as those observed is superimposed.

between dates of birth of live-born siblings (the mean of this distribution is assumed to be zero, for if all possible sib-pairs are considered each sibling pair will appear twice); once the difference will be positive, and once negative; and, finally, α_2, α_1, β_2, and β_1 are the number, respectively, of male ancestors in the female line and in the male line and of female ancestors in the female line and in the male line. Table IX-1 sets out the observed means and variances for certain types of relationships, as well as the means and variances expected on the basis of the foregoing argument.

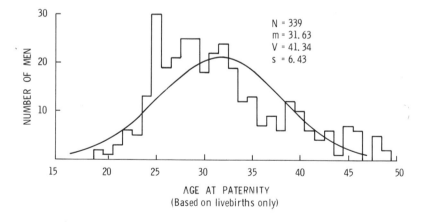

Fig. IX-6. The distribution of ages at paternity of men residing on Takushima in 1964. A Gaussian curve with the same mean and variance as those observed is superimposed.

The correspondences between observed and expected values are, in general, good—usually within 10 per cent of one another. Ideally, of course, the observed distributions would be based upon a cohort of marriages contracted at some fixed period and followed through time. Our distributions were compiled retrospectively and tend to underestimate means and/or variances because the longer intervals are underrepresented. In Fig. IX-7 we have superimposed upon the observed array of differences in dates of birth of live-born maternal parallel cousins a normal curve with parameters equal to those specified by the model under consideration. Again, the fit looks respectable, albeit not perfect.

Thus far, we have concerned ourselves solely with the effect of age upon the probability of marriage. Possibly insofar as Takushima is concerned this is sufficient, and migration need not trouble us. We know, for example, that among some 374 marriages involving individuals whose current legal residence is Takushima, there are 51 immigrant spouses (16 males, 35 females), 27 of whom were born within 25 kilometers of Takushima. Insofar as emigration is concerned, it is apparent from Fig. IX-1 that in the recent past substantially more males than females

TABLE IX-1

The Means and Variances of the Distributions of Differences between Dates of Birth of Boys and Girls between Whom the Specified Relationship Holds on Takushima

Nature of Relationship	$\mu(a_z)$		$V(a_z)$	
	Observed	Expected[a]	Observed	Expected[b]
Uncle-Niece				
Bro Da	29.60 ± 0.82	31.63	121	119
Sis Da	24.80 ± 0.55	28.03	109	112
Aunt-Nephew				
Sis So	-23.40 ± 0.50	-28.03	87	112
Bro So	-29.42 ± 1.01	-31.63	122	119
First Cousins				
Bro-Bro	0.94 ± 0.92	0	125	160
Bro So-Sis Da	-5.47 ± 0.86	-3.60	137	154
Sis-Sis	2.09 ± 0.78	0	136	147
Bro Da-Sis So	8.66 ± 1.05	3.60	128	154

Note: We assume: $\mu_p = 31.63$ $\mu_m = 28.03$ $V_i = 77.60$
$V_p = 41$ $V_m = 35$
[a] $E[\mu(a_z)] = (\alpha_2 - \alpha_1)\mu_p + (\beta_2 - \beta_1)\mu_m.$
[b] $E[V(a_z)] = V_i + \alpha V_p + \beta V_m.$

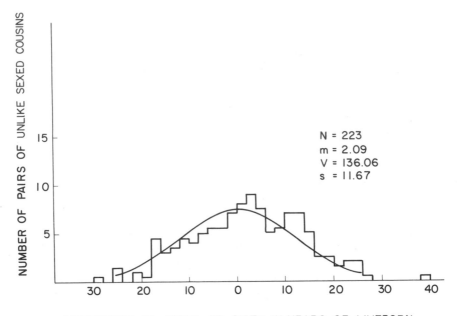

N = 223
m = 2.09
V = 136.06
s = 11.67

DIFFERENCE IN DATES OF BIRTH IN YEARS OF LIVEBORN
MATERNAL PARALLEL COUSINS (♂ AGE − ♀ AGE)

Fig. IX-7. The observed array of differences in ages of liveborn maternal parallel
cousins for Takushima in 1964. A normal curve with parameters equal to those specified
by the model described in the text is superimposed.

have migrated from the island. The net migrational effect would appear
to be a greater loss of males than of females. Cavalli-Sforza and his colleagues found that the model just described must be modified to recognize
differential migration, if the observed frequencies of the various classes
of consanguineous marriages in Parma are to be suitably approximated.
When modified, the model does appear to account for the observed distribution of types of first-cousin, first-cousin-once-removed, and second-
cousin marriages. This is not true for Takushima, nor, more importantly
perhaps, for the southwestern portion of Hiradojima with its much larger
population. In Table IX-2 are given the observed numbers of the various
kinds of cousin marriages for Takushima and the southwesternmost four
administrative areas, *machi*, of the city of Hirado. Observe that not only
does the model fail to predict with the requisite accuracy the frequency
of the various types of relationship within a specified class of consanguineous marriages for the several classes of marriages recorded but it also
fails to predict the relative frequencies of the three classes of consanguineous marriage. Thus, where we observe the ratio of first-cousin to
first-cousin-once-removed to second-cousin marriages on Takushima to be

42:11:19, we expect 16:3.4:52.6; on Hirado the comparable figures are 201:49:92 and 76:16:250. It should be noted, however, that the predicted ratio of marriages of first cousins to marriages of first cousins once removed agrees moderately well with that observed, whereas the observed and expected frequencies of second-cousin marriages differ by a factor of three. The latter unions are, of course, more apt to go unrecognized, but this fact alone will not account for the discrepancy. Relationship in these data is not based upon interviews which admit of systematic under-reporting because of ignorance of one's second cousins but upon a careful check of household records over approximately the last 100 years. Furthermore, the departures of observation from expectation cannot be solely an outgrowth of our failure to adjust for migration, since an obvious consequence of the greater mobility of the male is the more frequent marriage of first cousins related through sisters, but this would lead to a poorer fit, for even now the expected number of such marriages exceeds the observed. If migration were taken into account, however, presumably the fit of the expected numbers of the various classes of consanguineous marriages would be improved, since migration would diminish the frequency of second-cousin marriages as a class. Despite this assertion, it is clear that factors other than age and migration must be operative.

Traditionally, Japanese society has been oriented toward the family rather than the individual, and within the family authority has been vested in one person, the *tōshu*, the designated head. Succession to this latter position normally passes from eldest son to eldest son. Until quite recently, the authority wielded by the head was substantial indeed. He could, for example, deny to his younger brothers the right to establish a branch household. He also could deny *koseki* entry to an individual, and since legal marriage in Japan involves the entry of the wife's name in the *koseki* of which her husband is a member, approval of the head was the *sine qua non* of a legal marriage. Under these circumstances, as the prospective head, the eldest son's life and marriage were matters of great moment to the family. They were, in fact, of such importance that the family could not suffer mutual inclination on the part of the son and some young woman to interfere with the requirements of the family. In short, the eldest son operated under a different set of constraints than those which governed the lives of his younger siblings. We ask, therefore, do the types of consinguineous marriages associated with eldest sons differ from those of other sons? If so, the failure of the model may conceivably stem from the fact that the population under consideration is inhomogeneous. Since the numbers of marriages on Takushima are patently too small to afford much insight into this possibility, we have turned to the

TABLE IX-2

THE DISTRIBUTION OF TYPES OF FIRST COUSIN, FIRST COUSIN ONCE REMOVED, AND SECOND COUSIN MARRIAGES ON TAKUSHIMA AND IN THE FOUR SOUTHWESTERNMOST MACHI OF HIRADO. THE EXPECTED NUMBERS ARE BASED UPON THE ASSUMPTION THAT THE PROBABILITY OF A CONSANGUINEOUS MARRIAGE DEPENDS SOLELY UPON THE INTERVAL BETWEEN THE DATES OF BIRTH OF THE SPOUSES.

	TAKUSHIMA		HIRADO	
TYPE	Observed	Expected	Observed	Expected
First Cousins[a]				
Bro—Bro	8	10.42	41	49.87
Sis—Sis	12	10.79	44	51.62
Bro Da—Sis So	12	10.79	69	51.62
Bro So—Sis Da	10	10.00	47	47.89
Total	42		201	
First Cousins Once Removed[b]				
Bro So So—Bro Da	1	0.12	1	0.52
Bro Da So—Bro Da	—	0.28	1	1.26
Bro So Da—Bro So	1	0.80	7	3.57
Bro Da Da—Bro So	1	1.52	4	6.78
Sis So So—Sis Da	—	0.07	—	0.30
Sis Da So—Sis Da	1	0.22	—	0.97
Sis So Da—Sis So	1	0.65	1	2.91
Sis Da Da—Sis So	—	1.30	4	5.81
Sis So So—Bro Da	2	0.02	2	0.07
Sis Da So—Bro Da	1	0.07	2	0.30
Sis So Da—Sis So	—	0.28	1	1.26
Sis Da Da—Sis So	—	0.65	2	2.91
Bro So So—Sis Da	—	0.28	1	1.26
Bro Da So—Sis Da	1	0.65	2	2.91
Bro So Da—Sis So	—	1.52	8	6.78
Bro Da Da—Sis So	2	2.56	13	11.39
Total	11		49	
Second Cousins[c]				
Bro So So—Bro So Da	1	1.17	10	5.69
Bro So So—Bro Da Da	1	1.15	4	5.55
Bro Da So—Bro So Da	4	1.20	4	5.82
Bro Da So—Bro Da Da	—	1.20	7	5.82
Sis So So—Sis So Da	1	1.20	12	5.82
Sis So So—Sis Da Da	—	1.17	2	5.66
Sis Da So—Sis So Da	2	1.23	4	5.97
Sis Da So—Sis Da Da	—	1.23	3	5.97
Sis So So—Bro So Da	1	1.15	8	5.55
Sis So So—Bro Da Da	2	1.08	6	5.23
Sis Da So—Bro So Da	2	1.20	1	5.82
Sis Da So—Bro Da Da	2	1.17	12	5.66

TABLE IX-2 Continued

TYPE	TAKUSHIMA		HIRADO	
	Observed	Expected	Observed	Expected
		Second Cousins[c]		
Bro So So—Sis So Da	2	1.20	4	5.82
Bro So So—Sis Da Da	—	1.20	6	5.82
Bro Da So—Sis So Da	1	1.20	4	5.82
Bro Da So—Sis Da Da	—	1.23	5	5.97
Total	19		92	

[a] $\chi^2 = 0.83$ $\chi^2_3 = 8.57$.
[b] $\chi^2_{15} = 71.99$.
[c] $\chi^2_{15} = 29.15$.

southwestern end of Hirado for data pertinent to this point. Table IX-3 presents the distributions of types of first-cousin marriages for both Takushima and the region just mentioned. It is interesting that eldest sons appear to exhibit no preferences in their choice of a first cousin. Possibly this could have been anticipated, for upon the head of the family falls the burden of support of his parents in the later stages of their life. More properly, perhaps, this burden falls upon the wife of the head who may grudgingly or ungrudgingly minister to the wants of her in-laws.

Needless to say, the parents strive to ensure the latter attitude insofar as this is possible; they accomplish this in proportion to their knowledge of the graces and foibles of the young woman whom they select for their son. It seems logical to presume that, in general, they know the daughters of their siblings (their son's cousins) better, on the average, than they know other young women. Among their nieces, however, the paragon they seek may equally often be the daughter of a brother as of a sister

TABLE IX-3

TYPES OF FIRST COUSIN MARRIAGES INVOLVING ELDEST SONS AS CONTRASTED WITH OTHER SONS ON TAKUSHIMA AND IN THE SOUTHWESTERN END OF HIRADO

TYPE OF FIRST COUSIN MARRIAGE	ELDEST SON	OTHER SON		RANK UNKNOWN		TOTAL
		Not Yōshi	Yōshi	Not Yōshi	Yōshi	
Bro—Bro	19	11	3	8	0	41
Sis—Sis	19	8	1	13	3	44
Bro Da—Sis So	26	13	10	19	1	69
Bro So—Sis Da	22	11	6	7	1	47
Total	86	43	20	47	5	201

and of a sibling of the father as of the mother. This line of reasoning would account for the more frequent occurrence of consanguineous marriages reported among eldest sons (Yanase, 1951) and also their apparent randomness with respect to type. But what about the other sons? We observe that the four types of first-cousin marriages depart significantly from expectation. The causes of this, if real, may be complex. One possible factor is the occurrence of "adoptive son marriages," the *muko-yōshi*. This is a legal act which combines adoption and marriage in that the adopted son is married to a daughter of the adoptive parents at the time of adoption. Among the sixty-three other sons enumerated in Table IX-3, no less than twenty first-cousin marriages involved a *yōshi*, and the distribution of these latter marriages by type is nonrandom ($\chi^2 = 9.03$, df $= 3$). An argument with its roots in Japanese culture can be adduced to account for this, but it is profitless to pursue it at this time. It should be apparent, nonetheless, that the incorporation of socioeconomic and traditional elements into the model of random mating is patently more difficult than the incorporation of variables such as age and migration. The former variates are difficult to specify, and no less difficult to quantify, but, if our model is to be realistic in the sense that it recognizes the effects of these variables upon mate selection, clearly efforts to specify and quantitate these variates must continue.

We turn now to the second problem area previously mentioned, namely, the estimation of the distribution of intervals between successive live births. From personal interviews and the *koseki*, a complete reproductive history has been obtained for each married couple, at least one of whom was alive and residing on Takushima in 1964. These data afford an opportunity to investigate birth intervals in a population with ostensibly little or no birth control and to make comparisons with published results for several other populations.

Since 1948 induced abortion has been legal in Japan, but, in many rural areas, including Takushima, the artificial interruption of pregnancy is not condoned. Of 242 couples questioned, only ten indicated approval; three had no opinion, and the remaining 229 disapproved. Of 391 women, only 17 had had one or more induced abortions. It seems unlikely, therefore, that abortions appreciably affect mean birth intervals or completed family sizes in this population.

Table IX-4 presents the mean intervals in months between successive live births for completed families of sizes two through ten. For the purposes of this analysis, a family was included only if the wife had been married just once, and her marriage had lasted at least until she was forty-five. We have not recorded the interval between the beginning of cohabitation and the first birth because it was often difficult to determine precisely when cohabitation began. While a given husband and wife generally were disposed to indicate when they began to live together, often they did not remember the precise month, and the *koseki* was of no value for it is common practice, particularly in rural Japan, not to legalize a union until the birth of the first child. Finally, family sizes not represented by at least two families were not tabulated.

Although the total number of families is small, certain trends are apparent. The length of the reproductive period, as approximated by the interval between the first and the last birth, extends with increasing family size. Within birth orders, there is a general decrease in length of interval with rising family size. Within family sizes, there is an overall pattern of increasing length of interval with ascending birth order, with some tendency for the last interval to be lengthened; however, analysis of variance on sixteen completed families of size eight and on thirteen completed families of size five gave no indication of a birth-order effect. Moreover, there was no evidence for heterogeneity between families within families of sizes five and eight.

The trends apparent in these data also have been pointed out by Sheps in the Hutterites (1965), but, whereas the Hutterite mean birth intervals

TABLE IX-4

MEAN INTERVALS IN MONTHS BETWEEN SUCCESSIVE LIVE-BIRTHS ON TAKUSHIMA

Completed Family Size	2	3	4	5	6	7	8	9	10
No. of families	10	7	12	17	19	22	24	13	9

Birth No.	Interval in Months								
2	47.60	43.86	46.50	31.24	35.53	33.57	31.46	33.23	29.33
3	—	55.00	47.25	34.94	37.26	32.14	34.50	31.54	27.11
4	—	—	52.92	34.88	35.74	28.14	30.42	30.62	29.67
5	—	—	—	50.35	40.32	32.43	32.25	27.00	28.56
6	—	—	—	—	38.26	35.43	33.42	31.00	26.00
7	—	—	—	—	—	38.24	36.42	27.92	30.89
8	—	—	—	—	—	—	38.08	29.54	29.00
9	—	—	—	—	—	—	—	28.31	28.67
10	—	—	—	—	—	—	—	—	41.22

| Interval, 1st to last | 47.60 | 98.86 | 146.67 | 151.41 | 187.11 | 199.90 | 235.21 | 239.15 | 266.67 |

| Mean interval | 47.60 | 49.43 | 48.89 | 37.85 | 37.42 | 33.32 | 33.60 | 29.89 | 29.63 |

are of the order of two years or less, the Japanese intervals are approximately one-third longer. For families of a given size, there is a much shorter interval between first and last births in the Hutterites than in the Japanese. This is interesting in view of the fact that Hutterite marriages tend to occur earlier than do Japanese and that both mean family size and the range in family sizes are larger in the Hutterites than in the Japanese. It would appear, therefore, that for fixed family sizes, relatively less of the potential reproductive span is utilized in the Hutterites than in the Japanese. The implications of this are numerous; it could, for example, be testimony to reproductive exhaustion, or to differences in approach to family planning.

Although a direct comparison is not possible, the Takushima birth intervals also appear to be longer than those calculated by Henry (1958) from parish records in a village in Normandy for couples married between 1674 and 1742 (Table IX-5). For families of size six, excluding intervals following an infant death, Henry found the mean length of intervals between live births to be 24.3, 26.7, 27.3, and 29.3 months for birth orders two through five. In a similar analysis of a set of Indian women, Dandekar (1959) calculated mean intervals at 24.6, 26.8, 27.4, and 30.0 months for families of size six. These figures correspond to the Takushima intervals of 35.5, 37.3, 35.7, and 40.3 months. Thus, there appear to be real differences between populations, not only in the average size of families, but also in patterns of reproduction, particularly in the spacing of children. In the "average" family of a given size, the intervals between successive children and the total reproductive span can be quite different from population to population. Whether these differences reflect differences in fecundability, in the length of the period of *post partum* sterility, in the frequency of non-live births, or in cultural factors cannot be determined readily from the available data.

TABLE IX-5

THE MEAN BIRTH INTERVALS IN MONTHS FOR FAMILIES OF
SIX IN THREE DIFFERENT POPULATIONS

BIRTH ORDER	POPULATION		
	French (1674–1742)	Indian	Japanese
2	24.3	24.6	35.5
3	26.7	26.8	37.3
4	27.3	27.4	35.7
5	29.3	30.0	40.3

Evidence exists in other populations for an association between increased *post partum* sterility and breast feeding. This should not be an important factor in lengthening Japanese birth intervals, since infants usually are weaned before they are one year old. The existence of such a correlation can be investigated, however, by looking at the birth intervals following infant deaths, that is deaths in the first year of life. In cases in which an infant has died, it would be informative to classify birth intervals according to the age in months at which the preceding death occurred. This type of analysis is planned for the larger population of Hirado, but the small number of infant deaths recorded on Takushima makes this approach impractical. Instead, we have shown in Table IX-6 the mean birth intervals classified by presence or absence of a preceding infant death, by consanguinity of the parents, and by decade of marriage. For all time periods and for both consanguineous and non-consanguineous marriages, the mean interval following an infant death is shorter than the corresponding interval with no infant death. On the average, the death of an infant shortens the interval to the next birth by about twelve months. A decrease of this magnitude is difficult to explain solely on the basis of cessation of breast feeding. It is possible that there is a conscious attempt to replace a dead child. If so, it might be expected that, because of the importance of sons, the interval following the death of a male child would be shorter than that following a female death. There was no evidence for a sex difference in these data, however, and no explanation is obvious for the very short birth intervals associated with infant deaths.

TABLE IX-6

THE EFFECT OF AN INFANT DEATH ON THE INTERVAL IN MONTHS TO THE BIRTH OF THE NEXT CHILD

MARRIAGE CONTRACTED	F = 0		F > 0		TOTAL	
	No Infant Death	Infant Death	No Infant Death	Infant Death	No Infant Death	Infant Death
Before 1930	35.78	21.11	35.91	23.00	35.81	21.74
	(392)	(38)	(164)	(19)	(556)	(57)
1930–39	34.99	31.42	32.19	29.33	34.65	31.00
	(221)	(12)	(31)	(3)	(252)	(15)
1940–49	35.04	24.33	38.32	21.80	36.53	23.43
	(141)	(9)	(117)	(5)	(258)	(14)
1950–59	35.37	22.25	35.09	23.40	35.25	22.89
	(62)	(4)	(45)	(5)	(107)	(9)
Total	35.40	23.60	36.27	23.47	35.67	23.56
	(816)	(63)	(357)	(32)	(1173)	(95)

Note: Figures in parentheses are the numbers of intervals in each category.

Among the cases in which there is no preceding infant death, a remarkable constancy occurs in average birth interval length over a period of more than forty years. There is a noticeable, but unexplained, rise in the mean interval with infant death for marriages contracted in the decade 1930 to 1939.

Returning now to the distribution of completed family sizes (Fig. IX-8), 155 families have been included in all. Of these, thirteen (8.4 per cent) are childless, a figure somewhat higher than the 6.4 per cent observed for rural Japan as a whole and much higher than the two per cent found in the Hutterites. Excluding the childless marriages, the distribution is slightly skewed to the left. Superimposed on the observed distribution is a truncated negative binomial distribution, fitted by the method described by Brass (1958). A fitted truncated Poisson distribution is nearly identical to the negative binomial. The observed distribution differs significantly from the truncated Poisson and the negative binomial ($\chi^2 = 21.90$, df = 10, p $\doteq$ .01). Thus, the negative binomial and Poisson distributions, which traditionally are used to describe the distribution of human family sizes, do not appear to be good models for this population. In a population with long intervals between offspring, the finite length of the reproductive period becomes an important factor. Furthermore, the requirement of independence of successive trials is not met, since every conception is

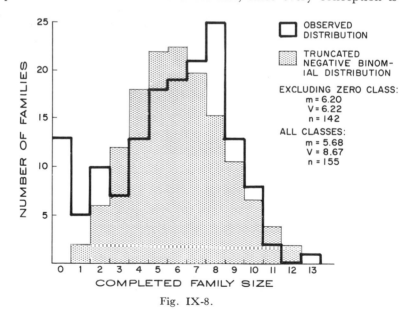

Fig. IX-8.

followed by a rather long period during which the woman cannot conceive again. Some aspects of this problem have been investigated by Dandekar (1955), but further consideration of the distribution of human family sizes is clearly needed.

The data presented here, both with respect to birth intervals and expected numbers of consanguineous marriages, clearly raise more issues than they resolve. It will be recalled, however, that they were collected, not with a view toward their contribution to specific biological hypotheses but rather to determine whether the household censuses of Japan could be used to illumine a number of problem areas which require extensive bodies of family-linked observations. It appears that the *koseki* in their numbers and time depth can be so used and provide, moreover, a unique resource. Certainly, data of the kind which can be gleaned from the *koseki* are available in the United States only for exceptional groups or at the expense of substantial effort through automated record linking.

Satisfied that the data are worth the mining, our interests have turned to Hirado proper. On this larger island with its larger population, it will be possible to come to grips with the influence of such diverse factors as religion, migration, socioeconomic class, and inbreeding on both the intervals between births and the frequencies of consanguineous marriages. It should be possible also to begin to develop some notion of the stability of certain of the parameters associated with population structure. We believe these studies, in concert with those in Italy of Cavalli-Sforza and his colleagues and in the United States of Lederberg and Bodmer, hold promise for a depth of insight not previously possible into the dynamics and statics of human population growth.

(This study represents the efforts of members of five universities, namely, Juntendo University, Kyoto Prefectural University of Medicine, Kyushu University, Tokyo Medical and Dental University, and the University of Michigan. We are also greatly indebted to many individuals at many levels of local government without whose support this study would not have been possible; though circumstances do not permit mention of everyone, our gratitude is no less real.)

REFERENCES

BARRAI, I., L. L. CAVALLI-SFORZA, AND A. MORONI. 1962. Frequencies of pedigrees of consanguineous marriages and mating structure of the population. *Ann. Human Genet.*, 25:347–77.

BRASS, W. 1958. Simplified method of fitting the truncated negative binomial distribution. *Biometrika*, 45:59–68.

CAVALLI-SFORZA, L. L., M. KIMURA, AND I. BARRAI. 1966. The probability of consanguineous marriages. *Genetics*, 54:37–60.

DANDEKAR, K. 1959. Intervals between confinements. *Eugen. Quart.*, 6:180–86.

DANDEKAR, V. M. 1955. Certain modified forms of binomial and Poisson distributions. *Sankhya*, 15:237–52.

HALDANE, J. B. S. 1947. The dysgenic effect of induced recessive mutations. *Ann. Eugen.*, 14:35–43.

HALDANE, J. B. S., AND S. D. JAYAKAR. 1962. An enumeration of some human relationships. *J. Genet.*, 58:81–107.

HALDANE, J. B. S., AND PEARL MOSHINSKY. 1939. Inbreeding in Mendelian populations, with special reference to human cousin marriage. *Ann. Eugen.*, 9:321–40.

HAJNAL, J. 1963. Random mating and the frequency of consanguineous marriages. *Proc. Roy. Soc., Lond., B.*, 159:125–77.

HENRY, L. 1958. Intervals between confinements in the absence of birth control. *Eugen. Quart.*, 5:200–11.

SHEPS, M. C. 1965. An analysis of reproductive patterns in an American isolate. *Pop. Studies*, 19:65–79.

TAEUBER, I. 1958. *The Population of Japan.* Princeton University Press, Princeton. 461 pp.

YANASE, T. 1951. Heredo-clinical investigation concerning the highly inbred villages in western Japan, especially Shiiba-mura, Miyazaki-ken. *Igaku Kenkyū*, 21:183–209.

CEDRIC A. B. SMITH
Galton Laboratory,
University College,
London, England

X. TESTING SEGREGATION RATIOS

SUMMARY

There are a number of classical papers by Haldane and others on the apparently simple problem of estimating and testing segregation ratios in family data. Here some new approaches are explored. The problem of the effects of disturbances such as family limitation and heterogeneity are discussed, and it is shown how they can be tackled in simple situations. Multiple alleles are also considered. It becomes clear that there are still many problems to solve.

THE RELEVANCE OF SEGREGATION RATIOS

Mendelian genetics began with the study of segregation ratios. Mendel discovered that if a hybrid plant carrying yellow peas (Yy) is crossed with a plant carrying green peas (yy), nearly half the progeny carry yellow peas and nearly half, green. In addition, the two types of progeny occur in random order. That is, each time one of the progeny comes into existence it is as if someone tosses a coin; when the coin falls heads, the new plant bears yellow peas, and when tails, green peas. In such a case in a reasonably large sample, the numbers of "yellow" and "green" plants will be nearly equal, just as the numbers of heads and tails tend to be equal in a large number of tosses of a coin. With more statistical sophistication, one can apply a χ^2 or similar test to see if the deviations from equality are no bigger than expected from random fluctuation.

In more complicated cases, however, many statistical problems still remain. These are partly matters of finding a solution to yet unsolved problems and partly of making known solutions simpler and easier to apply.

Consider a character determined by genes at a single locus in man or in some other diploid organism. Suppose we know the genotypes of a married couple. Then Mendel's laws in the most literal form would state the following: Before each child is born, it has a known probability (e.g., $\frac{1}{2}$ or $\frac{1}{4}$) of having any given phenotype. What is more, each child

99

has the same probability, independently of the phenotypes of the previous children. And each probability is always an exact multiple of $\frac{1}{4}$. For example, each child of a mating between parents with blood groups $A_1B \times A_1B$ has probabilities $\frac{1}{4}A_1A_1 + \frac{1}{2}A_1B + \frac{1}{4}BB$ (i.e., $\frac{1}{4}$ of being A_1A_1, etc.). (We will use the convention that genotypes are written in italics, phenotypes in roman letters, so that as regards phenotypes, or blood groups, the children would have probabilities $\frac{1}{4}A_1 + \frac{1}{2}A_1B + \frac{1}{4}B$.)

Such rules will hold approximately for many characters, such as the ABO blood groups, but absolute agreement cannot be expected for a number of reasons, singly or in combination:

a) Heterogeneity in the material. That is, what appears to be a single character sometimes may result from a gene at one locus, sometimes at another locus, and sometimes from environmental effects. Some individuals may be diploid at the locus in question, others triploid or haploid.

b) Unreliability of classification. For example, a borderline case may be called "normal" on the basis of its observed characters, when genetically it more appropriately would be called "abnormal."

c) Statistical bias. The sample recorded may not be representative of the complete population. Thus, when affected cases die young, they may not be included.

d) Alterated segregation ratios, as a consequence of selection, mutation, family limitation, meiotic drive, or chromosome abnormalities. If the locus in question is very near another one on the same chromosome, which is subject to selection or meiotic drive, its own segregation will also be affected.

Some of these influences may change the segregation ratios considerably. Mutation is a very rare event, and for that reason one might think that it could be ignored without appreciable loss, but this is not necessarily so. Let us consider hemophilia as an example. This is a severe disease and strongly selected against. It arises from time to time by mutation: in most cases it will be completely eliminated within two or three generations as a result of selection. Thus, quite an appreciable fraction of hemophilia cases will be new mutations. When a male hemophilic arises directly by mutation, usually none of his brothers carry the abnormal gene, and so none of his brothers will be affected. This will result in an appreciably altered segregation ratio. Haldane used essentially this fact to study the mutation rates for hemophilia and sex-linked muscular dystrophy in the two sexes (Haldane, 1947, 1956).

The appropriate question to ask is not, therefore, if observed segregation ratios agree absolutely exactly with the theoretical Mendelian expectations, but whether they agree within some tolerance limit. How wide should the limits be? This depends on the object of our investigation. One may want to study the general pattern of inheritance of a character, e.g., whether it can be regarded as resulting from a single nonrecessive gene or a single recessive gene. It is then sufficient to show that the ratios agree with the Mendelian ones with fair accuracy: small deviations can be attributed to some of the effects mentioned above and are not very important. On the other hand, one may be interested in determining the exact amount of selection operating on genes and genotypes. The general pattern of inheritance then can be considered well established and attention concentrated on the deviations from the Mendelian values. A great deal of work on the pattern of inheritance through the study of segregation ratios is ascribable to Newton Morton and his colleagues. Their method of analyzing genetic data is of great importance, but I do not consider it further in this paper. Here I restrict discussion to the simpler problem of finding out from observational data just what segregation ratios actually occur and whether they agree reasonably well with those expected under Mendelian theory.

THE GENERAL PRINCIPLES OF STATISTICAL ESTIMATION

If we consider one single locus, only a limited number (four or fewer) phenotypes of offspring Φ_r, Φ_s, . . . are possible in any one family. In each family each child will have a certain probability, φ_r, say, of having phenotype Φ_r. If the Mendelian ratios held exactly, φ_r would take one of the values 0, $\frac{1}{4}$, $\frac{1}{2}$, $\frac{3}{4}$, 1, and usually we expect φ_r not to be very different from one of these values. The probabilities for φ_r can be estimated by standard procedures. For example, suppose that we have a number of matings of the type $A_1B \times A_1B$ in our sample, and that these matings have in all 22 A_1 + 51 A_1B + 27 B children ($n = 100$ children in all). Let φ_1, φ_2, and φ_0 stand for the respective probabilities of obtaining an A_1, A_1B, or B child. The most obvious estimates of φ_1, φ_2, and φ_0 are $22/100 = .22$, $51/100 = .51$, and $27/100 = .27$, respectively. Consider first the simplest type of situation. Suppose that we know for certain the genotypes of the parents (e.g., $A_1B \times A_1B$). There will be certain possible genotypes Γ_1, Γ_2, . . . of the offspring. Each such genotype Γ_r we suppose to have its own probability γ_r of occurring. This γ_r we take to be a constant, though not necessarily exactly that expected under simple Mendelian theory, and successive children are assumed to be mutually independent. In general, only phenotypes Φ_s will be recognizable, not individual genotypes. We suppose that each genotype Γ_r has a known phenotype Φ_s without any uncertainty or error of classification. Under these conditions, φ_1 = the probability of Φ_1 (— group A_1, in our example) and is clearly estimated by the observed proportion $22/100 = .22$ of A_1 children, with standard error

$$\sqrt{[\varphi_1(1 - \varphi_1)/n]} = \sqrt{[.22 \times .78/100]} = .041 \qquad (2.1)$$

Similarly, φ_2 has the estimate $.51 \pm .050$.

There is at present much ferment in statistics over the problem of statistical inference. Because of this, statisticians are very concerned with the question of how statistics are to be interpreted. Even in the very simple problems of estimation ratios and proportions, such considerations are relevant.

In this connection we must first remark that if we assume any particular mathematical model to be true, then the information provided by any given sample can be expressed conveniently in the form of the likelihood function. Thus, if we have a multinomial distribution divided into $(k + 1)$ classes Φ_r with respective probabilities φ_r, and if in a sample of n objects, the number of objects falling in class Φ_r is x_r, the (natural) log likelihood for that sample is $\Sigma x_r \ln \varphi_r$. Here we must remember that the sum of the probabilities φ_r for all classes Φ_r is necessarily 1. We have only k independent probabilities, $\varphi_1, \varphi_2, \ldots \varphi_k$, the remaining one, φ_0, say, being given by

$$\varphi_0 = 1 - \varphi_1 - \varphi_2 - \ldots - \varphi_k \qquad (2.2)$$

For example, if we have just two classes, Φ_1 and Φ_0 (i.e., normal and affected), the probability φ_0 of being affected is simply $1 - \varphi_1$. In such a case, we can regard our task as simply the estimation of φ_1, for whatever conclusion we come to about the value of φ_1 will imply a corresponding conclusion about the value of $\varphi_0 = 1 - \varphi_1$. We can write the log likelihood function L in terms of φ_1 as

$$\begin{aligned} L(\varphi_1) &= x_1 \ln \varphi_1 + x_0 \ln \varphi_0 \\ &= x_1 \ln \varphi_1 + x_0 \ln (1 - \varphi_1) \end{aligned} \qquad (2.3)$$

We can plot this graphically against the value of φ_1 or tabulate it numerically. Even in more complicated situations than this, so long as we have only two complementary probabilities to deal with, φ_1 and $\varphi_0 = 1 - \varphi_1$, it will still be possible and useful to draw the graph of the log likelihood function $L(\varphi_1)$. As an example of such a curve, suppose that we have a sample containing, let us say, six normals and 24 affected out of 40 individuals. The log likelihood curve for φ_1, the proportion of normals, is shown in Fig. X-1, and its natural antilogarithm, the curve for the likelihood itself, in Fig. X-2. This is a bell-shaped curve, with peak at $\varphi_1 = .40$, which is the "maximum likelihood point," usually called $\hat{\varphi}_1$.

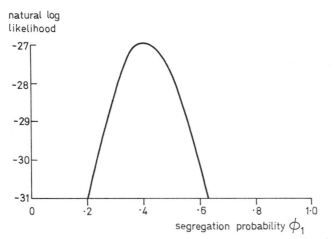

Fig. X-1. The log likelihood values for a family with sixteen normal and twenty-four affected children.

It decreases rapidly on either side of the peak, becoming negligible for values of φ_1 below about .2 or above about .6. This would seeem to suggest that it is very probable that φ_1 does, in fact, lie somewhere within this range.

A slight warning is needed here. It is tempting to interpret the likelihood curve as if it was a probability distribution. Thus, the curve in Fig. X-2 looks very like a Gaussian or normal curve. If we have a sample of 16 normals out of 40, it is conventional to estimate the proportion of normals

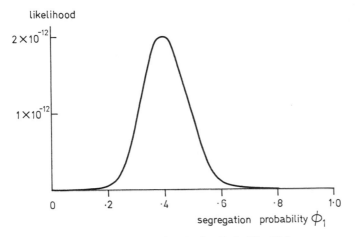

Fig. X-2. The likelihood values for the family in Fig. X-1.

as $16/40 = .40$ with standard error $\sqrt{(.4 \times .6/40)} = .077$. Now the likelihood curve in Fig. X-2 does agree quite well with a Gaussian curve with mean .40 and standard deviation .077 (or more accurately, with some constant multiple of this, since the vertical scale may need regraduating to make the total area under the curve equal to one). It is natural to leap to conclusions and treat the likelihood curve as if it were a Gaussian distribution. We would then argue that, since about 95 per cent of the area under the curve lies within the range of values differing by not more than 2 s.d. from the mean, we can say that φ_1 has a 95 per cent probability of lying between $.40 - 2 \times .077 = .25$ and $.40 + 2 \times .077 = .55$. This argument is not technically correct. The likelihood curve is not a distribution curve and, strictly speaking, cannot correctly be treated as one.

The question of just how we should interpret the curve is controversial. Different schools of statisticians answer it differently, but any self-consistent method of interpretation must be in agreement with the rules of personal probability, as demonstrated by L. J. Savage (1954). This paper is not the appropriate place to discuss the point in detail. We remark only that, besides being self-consistent, the method of interpretation using personal probability is simple and in general agreement with common sense. It proceeds as follows: We first specify an "initial distribution" intended to represent our initial opinions as to the relative probability of various possible values of φ_1; that is, what we think before the observational data has been brought to our notice. Three conceivable initial distributions are shown in (a), (b), and (c) of Fig. X-3. The distribution (a) is uniform, that is, it means that we think that any value of φ_1 between 0 and 1 is equally likely. This is not a very plausible initial distribution, since experience with segregation ratios shows that φ_1 usually lies somewhere near one of the Mendelian values $\frac{1}{4}$, $\frac{1}{2}$, or $\frac{3}{4}$. Distribution (b) means that we expect φ_1 to take one of these values exactly. No other value is regarded as having an appreciable probability of occurrence. This is leaning too far toward the other extreme. Distribution (c) shows a plausible kind of initial distribution, intermediate between (a) and (b); values near the Mendelian ones have high probability, but other values are not completely excluded. The next step is to multiply the chosen initial distribution by the likelihood function to get the final distribution. (This is Bayes's theorem for personal probability.) The vertical scale is supposed to be adjusted so that the total area under this distribution curve, or total probability, is equal to one. Thus, if we multiply the initial distribution (a) of Fig. X-3 by the likelihood curve of Fig. X-2, we obtain the final distribution (a) of Fig. X-4. This closely

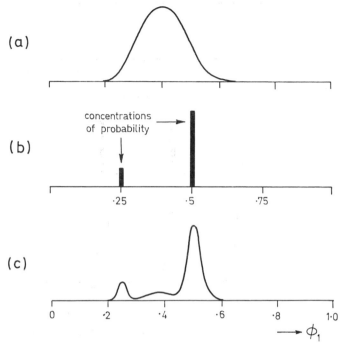

Fig. X-3. Possible choices of initial distribution for φ_1.

approximates a Gaussian distribution with mean .4 and standard deviation .077. Thus, we can say that there is a .95 probability that φ_1 lies within two standard deviations of the mean, i.e., between .25 and .55. The interpretation is that it would be reasonable to bet at odds 19 to 1 that φ_1 lies in this range. (This is the result we got when we treated the likelihood function as if it were a distribution function which, as we can now see, is equivalent to assuming that the initial distribution is uniform.) If we take the initial distribution (*b*) of Fig. X-3, however, the final distribution (*b*) of Fig. X-4 then gives a high probability to the value $\frac{1}{2}$ for φ_1 and much lower probabilities to the values $\frac{1}{4}$ and $\frac{3}{4}$. This is as expected. If we suppose that the only possible values for φ_1 are $\frac{1}{4}$, $\frac{1}{2}$, or $\frac{3}{4}$ and then find in a sample 16 normal out of 40 children, it is only natural to conclude that φ_1 is much more likely to be $\frac{1}{2}$ than $\frac{1}{4}$ or $\frac{3}{4}$. If we use initial distribution (*c*), the final distribution shown in Fig. X-4 (*c*) rather resembles a mixture of (*a*) and (*b*). The values of φ_1 in the immediate neighborhood of $\frac{1}{2}$ have high probabilities, but the probability is not concentrated completely on the single value $\varphi_1 = \frac{1}{2}$. This seems a

105

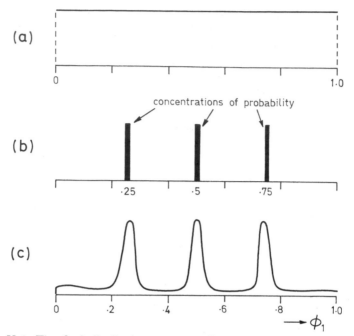

Fig. X-4. The final distributions corresponding to the initial distributions in Fig. X-3.

reasonable conclusion, taking into account both the evidence of the sample itself and previous experience with segregation ratios.

Several problems arise in applying this approach, in spite of its theoretical simplicity. In the first place, some choice of initial distribution has to be made. This choice is not always easy; it requires careful consideration. Which values of φ_1 seem probable and which improbable? Different people will give at least slightly different answers to this question, so no two people will give precisely the same interpretation to the data. This statement looks at first sight quite alarming. It apparently would threaten statistics, and indeed science in general, with a multitude of differing, and possibly contradictory, conclusions, but this danger is more apparent than real. It really reflects no more than common observation; no two people do look on the same piece of evidence in quite the same way. The extent of disagreement is likely to be small, if enough evidence is available. In mathematical terms, if the sample is sufficiently large, then the final distribution representing the conclusions drawn from it usually will be nearly independent of the choice of initial distribution, so long as any reasonable and plausible initial distribution is used. For example, it would be of negligible practical importance whether we judged the probability that φ_1 lies between .25 and .55 to be .95 or .97. In either case, it would be very high.

In practice, what causes rather more trouble than this problem is the complication of the calculation. If there is only one independent parameter φ_1 involved, no great difficulty arises. One can draw the curves for the initial distribution and likelihood, multiply the corresponding heights to get the curve for the final distribution, and examine it visually or calculate it numerically just as we did above. If we have several independent parameters, however, φ_1, φ_2, φ_3, . . . , the curves become replaced by multidimensional surfaces which cannot be represented graphically and would require immense efforts to tabulate. One, therefore, looks for some convenient way to compress the results into a more easily appreciated form.

One useful result states that in a reasonably large sample the likelihood function will (usually) approximate quite closely a Gaussian form. Suppose that we have k independent parameters φ_1, φ_2, . . . , φ_k to estimate. Let $(\hat{\varphi}_1, \hat{\varphi}_2, \ldots, \hat{\varphi}_k) = (\mu_1, \mu_2, \ldots, \mu_k)$ be the values which maximize the likelihood, and let

$$\mathcal{J}_{rs} = -[(\partial/\partial\varphi_r)(\partial/\partial\varphi_s) \, L(\varphi)]_{\varphi=\mu} \qquad (2.4)$$

be the (r, s) element of the Fisher information matrix $\mathbf{J}$. Let $\mathbf{v}$ denote the inverse matrix $\mathbf{J}^{-1}$. Then apart from a constant factor, the likelihood function is approximately the same as the probability density function of a Gaussian distribution with mean $\mathbf{\mu}$ and variance $\mathbf{v}$; or, in other words, the log likelihood has the form

$$L(\varphi) = \text{const} - \tfrac{1}{2}(\varphi - \mathbf{\mu})^{\mathrm{T}}\mathbf{J}(\varphi - \mathbf{\mu}) \qquad (2.5)$$

(where ^{T} denotes matrix transposition).

If the initial distribution is nearly uniform, or at any rate varies not too much in the neighborhood of the maximum likelihood point μ, the final distribution will be approximately the likelihood multiplied by a constant. This means that, on taking the observed data into account, we can think of φ as having a multivariate Gaussian distribution with mean vector $\mathbf{\mu}$ and variance matrix $\mathbf{v}$. Now this is effectively the conventional maximum likelihood theory, only in slightly different terms; $\mathbf{\mu} = \hat{\varphi}$ is there called the "maximum likelihood estimate" of φ, and $\mathbf{v}$ is its "error variance matrix."

Suppose, however, that the initial distribution is not uniform; what then? Of course, we can proceed formally by setting up a suitable initial distribution and multiplying it by the likelihood to get the appropriate final distribution, but quite often an informal approach is good enough. One looks at the likelihood function and then judges with care what conclusion to draw from it. Thus, suppose we expect a 1:1 segregation to hold, i.e., that φ_1 is not very different from .5, and we find the sample proportion $16/40 = .40$ with standard error .08. Since the observed proportion .40 differs from the expected .50 by only 1.2 standard errors, the two are clearly compatible: we would conclude that the expected 1:1 ratio is quite a likely one. If we had an observed proportion $6/40 = .15$ with standard error $\sqrt{(.15 \times .85/40)} = .053$, we see that the difference between observed and expected is more than six standard errors. Hence, clearly we can regard the 1:1 segregation as highly unlikely. If in a very large sample of a segregation we found, let us say, 5147 dominants out of 10,000 individuals, this would give an observed proportion .5147 with standard error $\sqrt{(.51 \times .49/10,000)} = .005$; hence, this would deviate from the Mendelian value .5000 by about 3.0 standard errors, normally considered a highly significant deviation. If the recessive, however, had, say, a 3 per cent disadvantage compared with the dominant, the expected segregation ratio would then be .5075:.4925 instead of the Mendelian .5000:.5000. The deviation observed from this is only about 1.5 standard errors, which is quite reasonable. We know that recessives often have some disadvantage. If we were to admit as plausible a disadvantage of the order of 3 per cent, then the observed data would be quite compatible with a 1:1 ratio modified slightly by selection. Some ways of doing these calculations more formally are suggested by Smith (1965). The informal approach, however, seems adequate for most occasions.

We, therefore, will regard it as sufficient answer to any question about segregation ratios to give the estimates $\hat{\varphi}_r = \mu_r$ of the frequencies φ_r, together with their respective variances v_{rr} and covariances v_{rs}. If possible, we will use maximum likelihood estimates, but, where this would require tedious calculations, inefficient estimates may be used instead.

In particular, if we find in a sample of n that there are x_r individuals of phenotype Φ_r, then the maximum likelihood value for φ is

$$\mu_r = \hat{\varphi}_r = x_r/n. \tag{2.6}$$

The variance of φ_r is

$$v_{rr} = \mu_r(1 - \mu_r)/n. \tag{2.7}$$

The covariance of φ_r and φ_s is

$$v_{rs} = -\mu_r\mu_s/n. \tag{2.8}$$

These are the usual estimates and their error variances and covariances derived either from the multinomial distribution or from the maximum likelihood theory.

Significance tests, such as χ^2, traditionally are used in the analysis of segregations. There are several objections to this in principle. Such tests answer only the question of whether the observed data conform to one particular null hypothesis, such as that $\varphi_1 = .5$. They do not take into account possible deviations from this hypothetical value because of selection or similar influences. They do not show how wide a range of values of φ_1 reasonably agree with observation. They do not fit in well with the theory of personal probability given above, which means that reliance on them can lead to inconsistency. Nevertheless, a complete refusal to use or to consider them would be pedantic. Used with sufficient care and judgment, they can be quite effective. They also have the advantage that they are generally understood by those who use ordinary statistical methods. If a test gives a highly significant discrepancy from a null hypothesis, this can be stated in a publication without further amplification. Unconventional forms of statement, even when theoretically superior, may be unfamiliar and require detailed explanation.

FACTORS OF SUPPORT

More precise and numerical ways of expressing the conclusions drawn from a given sample can be achieved by using factors of support, which can be defined as follows: Suppose we wish to compare a number of possible hypotheses H_1, H_2, H_3, . . . , concerning the parameters φ_r. Initially, we judge that the probabilities of these hypotheses are in the ratios $P_1 : P_2 : P_3 :$ . . . . After the data have been taken into account let the (final) probabilities be in the ratios $P_1\Lambda_1 : P_2\Lambda_2 : P_3\Lambda_3$ . . . . Then the numbers Λ_1, Λ_2, Λ_3 are called "factors of support" or "Bayes factors" for the hypotheses H_1, H_2, H_3, . . . respectively. They represent the extent to which the evidence changes one's opinions of the relative probabilities of the hypotheses. This is a modification, due to I. J. Good (1950), of an idea of H. Jeffreys. Its importance is that it often turns out that the numerical values of these factors Λ_h do not depend to any important extent on the exact form of the initial distributions. Even if they are not absolutely objective in the sense of being completely independent of differences in personal judgment, they are nearly enough so for practical purposes (Smith, 1965). Their values can be found by using Bayes's theorem. Incidentally, it follows at once from the definition that only the ratios $\Lambda_1 : \Lambda_2 : \Lambda_3$ . . . are relevant.

109

In particular, consider the following situation. For convenience, let the set of parameters φ_r be denoted by a (column) vector φ. Suppose that hypothesis H_h is associated with an initial distribution of Gaussian form for the parameters φ, with mean $\mathbf{m}_h$ and variance matrix $\mathbf{v}_h$. Take the example above, where we have observed 16 normal in a sample of 40 children. We may consider the three following hypotheses: H_1, the segregation ratio is nearly $1:1$, i.e., φ_1 is near .5; H_2, the ratio is nearly $1:3$, i.e., φ_1 is near .25; H_3, the segregation is not a simple Mendelian one, so that φ_1 might take any value between 0 and 1. To be more precise, we might think that under hypothesis H_1 it is very unlikely that φ_1 would differ by more than .05 from its Mendelian value .5. We could represent this nearly enough by a Gaussian initial distribution with mean $m_{11} = .5$ and standard deviation $\sigma_{11} = .02$, i.e., variance $v_{111} = .02^2 = .0004$. Hypothesis H_2 could similarly be represented approximately by a Gaussian distribution with mean $m_{21} = .25$ and variance $v_{211} = .02^2 = .0004$. Hypothesis H_3 is not so easily represented by a Gaussian distribution, since φ_1 is restricted necessarily to lie between 0 and 1, whereas a Gaussian distribution has no absolute limits like these. One may feel that for the sake of simplicity of calculation, however, that no great harm would be done by approximating to it by, say, a Gaussian distribution with mean .5 and standard deviation .5; i.e., $m_{31} = .5$ and $v_{311} = .25$. (In any case, any reasonable choice of v_{311} would give much the same answer. See below.) In addition, let $\mathbf{j}_n$ be the inverse $\mathbf{v}_h$ of the variance matrix $\mathbf{v}_h$. When we have only one parameter φ_1, $\mathbf{j}_h$ consists of the single element $j_{h11} = v_{h11}^{-1}$. Thus, for hypotheses H_1 and H_2 we have $j_{111} = j_{211} = .0004^{-1} = 2500$, and for hypothesis H_3, $j_{311} = .25^{-1} = 4$.

Suppose also that the sample is reasonably large, so that the likelihood function also has a nearly Gaussian form. The peak occurs at $\mathbf{u}$, and the Fisher information matrix is $\mathbf{J}$. Let us write

$$\mathbf{A}_h = \mathbf{j}_h(\mathbf{j}_h + \mathbf{J})^{-1}\mathbf{J}. \qquad (3.1)$$

Then the factor of support for hypothesis H_h is

$$\Lambda_h = \sqrt{\det \mathbf{A}_h} \exp - \frac{(\mathbf{m}_h - \mathbf{u})^T\mathbf{A}_h(\mathbf{m}_h - \mathbf{u})}{2}. \qquad (3.2)$$

When we have only one parameter φ_1 to consider, this amounts to writing

$$A_h = j_{h11}J_{11}/(j_{h11} + J_{11}) \qquad (3.3)$$

$$\Lambda_h = \sqrt{A_h} \exp [- \tfrac{1}{2}A_h(m_{h1} - \mu_1)^2]. \qquad (3.4)$$

In our example, we found the maximum likelihood value to be $\hat{\varphi}_1 = \mu_1 = .4$, with amount of information $\mathcal{J}_{11} = 166.7$. On substituting these values in (3.3) we get

$$A_1 = A_2 = 156.2, \qquad A_3 = 3.906.$$

A further substitution in (3.4) then gives

$$\Lambda_1 : \Lambda_2 : \Lambda_3 = 5.7 : 2.1 : 2.0$$
$$\simeq 3 : 1 : 1.$$

In other words, the data will increase our confidence in hypothesis H_1 (a $1:1$ ratio) by a factor of three times as compared with H_2 and H_3. If we begin with no very strong views as to which hypothesis is correct, we will tend to favor H_1 at the expense of H_2 and H_3. But the evidence is insufficient to override any strong reasons we may have for believing in one or other of the hypotheses. If we had initial opinions represented by the probability ratio $P_1 : P_2 : P_3 = 10 : 100 : 1$, say, favoring H_2, then the final probability ratio would be $P_1\Lambda_1 : P_2\Lambda_2 : P_3\Lambda_3 = 57 : 210 : 2$ still definitely favoring H_2. The sample is really too small to be at all decisive.

It is easy to verify that these conclusions do not depend at all critically on the assumed values of the variances v_{h11} of the initial distributions. If one took, say, $v_{111} = v_{211} = .00001$, $v_{311} = .05$, the conclusions would be very similar. We find that $\Lambda_1 : \Lambda_2 : \Lambda_3 = 5.7 : 1.9 : 3.9$ instead of $5.7 : 2.1 : 2.0$.

Difficulties in Estimating Segregation Ratios

Problems can arise in even what seems to be the most straightforward cases of segregation ratio estimation. In the first place, any estimation procedure depends on the assumption that the sample obtained is truly representative of the population. This holds if we have complete ascertainment of all relevant families in some district. When a rare or moderately rare abnormality is being investigated, however, it may not be easy to obtain a good sample. A family with several abnormals has usually a greater chance of being observed and recorded than one with only one affected. This can bias our results to an unknown extent, unless we are very careful, and one cannot accurately correct for an unknown bias. The only completely safe approach is to make sure that the survey is as nearly representative as possible, either by covering some area completely, or by a careful sampling procedure, such as a random sample.

Even when the sample is reliable, a possibility often remains of variation from one family to another in the probability of being affected, sometimes because what is apparently one and the same abnormality is due to different genes in different families. The customary procedure is to apply a χ^2 test of homogeneity. But the question this is designed to answer is "Is there heterogeneity?" rather than "How much heterogeneity is there?"

In other words, just as when we were considering Mendelian ratios, it seems better to give an estimate rather than a significance test, but this produces some complicated statistical problems. An efficient estimate of the heterogeneity can be obtained only by fitting some mathematical model, but an appropriate model can be specified only if we know in advance what kind of heterogeneity to expect. Let $\varphi_{1(1)}$ represent the probability of a child having phenotype Φ_1 in the first family $\varphi_{1(2)}$, the same probability in the second family, and so on. If the difference between families is merely that environmental influences or genetic background are somehow altering the segregation ratios slightly from family to family, the values of $\varphi_{1(1)}$, $\varphi_{1(2)}$, ... would be clustered together, often quite close to the expected Mendelian value. If, instead, the condition is sometimes due to a recessive gene, sometimes to a nonrecessive, then $\varphi_{1(f)}$ for different families f would sometimes be near .50 and sometimes near .25, a much wider range of variation.

In the argument which follows, we concentrate attention on one particular phenotype, say Φ_r, considered on its own. In order to simplify the appearance of the formulas, we drop, in general, the suffix r corresponding to this phenotype, speaking simply of phenotype Φ. Similarly we let $\varphi_{(f)}$, rather than $\varphi_{r(f)}$, denote the probability in family f that any one child will have phenotype $\Phi = \Phi_r$.

Suppose we have a sample containing F families altogether. We will let $n_{(f)}$ denote the total number of children in family f, and $x_{(f)}$ the number having phenotype Φ. Hence $\mu_{(f)} = x_{(f)}/n_{(f)}$ is the observed proportion of Φ children in family f, and is an estimate of $\varphi_{(f)}$. We will also let $y_{(f)} = n_{(f)} - x_{(f)}$ denote the number of children in family f not of phenotype Φ. If we sum over-all families, we will find $N = \Sigma n_{(f)} = $ the total number of children in the complete sample,

$$X = \Sigma x_{(f)} = \Sigma n_{(f)}\mu_{(f)} \qquad (4.1)$$

the number of Φ children, and

$$Y - \Sigma y_{(f)} = N - X \qquad (4.2)$$

the number of not-Φ children.

Usually we cannot say in advance which one of a wide variety of models is appropriate in detail. In order to get around this difficulty, we may try some less specific and detailed formulation of the problem. For example, we may try to study the general shape of distribution of the probabilities $\varphi_{(1)}$, $\varphi_{(2)}$, ... in the different families. This distribution will have a mean, M_φ, say, and a variance V_φ, and we may try to estimate these from the observed data.

The arithmetic mean of the observed proportions

$$\bar{\mu} = \Sigma\mu_{(f)}/F \qquad (4.3)$$

is an obvious estimate of M_φ, the mean expected proportion. It is certainly not the most accurate estimate, however, for it gives equal weights to the observed proportions $\mu_{(f)}$ in the different families, whereas one would expect that in a larger family $\mu_{(f)}$ would be a more accurate estimate of $\varphi_{(f)}$, and, therefore, should be given greater weight. It is quite a difficult problem to find the optimal weight, and we will not go into the question here. We will use simply the family size $n_{(f)}$ as weight; if this is not optimal, it is at least reasonable, and it gives the weighted mean

$$m = \frac{\Sigma n_{(f)}\mu_{(f)}}{\Sigma n_{(f)}} = \frac{X}{N} \qquad (4.4)$$

That is, we estimate the mean probability of a Φ child by the proportion of Φ children in the whole sample, which seems intuitively appealing.

TABLE X-1

No. of Children				No. of Boys $x_{(f)}$				Total
$n_{(f)}$	0	1	2	3	4	5	6	
1	9	15	—	—	—	—	—	24
2	9	20	10	—	—	—	—	39
3	4	5	7	6	—	—	—	22
4	1	1	3	2	2	—	—	9
5	0	2	0	1	0	0	—	3
6	0	0	0	0	1	1	1	3
Total	23	43	20	9	3	1	1	100

As an example, take the following data on the segregation of sex (where Φ denotes male sex). Table X-1 shows 24 families with one child, 39 with two children, 22 with three, and so on, so the total number of children is

$$N = 24 \times 1 + 39 \times 2 + 22 \times 3 + 9 \times 4 + 3 \times 5 + 3 \times 6 = 237.$$

There are 23 families with no boys, 43 with one, and so on, so the total number of boys is

$$X = 23 \times 0 + 43 \times 1 + 20 \times 2 + 9 \times 3$$
$$+ 3 \times 4 + 1 \times 5 + 1 \times 6 = 133$$

The estimate of M_φ, the mean expected proportion of boys, is

$$m = X/N = 133/237 = .561$$

How much does this proportion vary from family to family, i.e., what is its variance V_φ? Again the problem of finding an optimal estimate of V_φ is troublesome, and we will not attempt it here. A reasonable estimation procedure goes as follows. Calculate

$$H = \sum \frac{x_{(f)} y_{(f)}}{n_{(f)}}$$

$$K = \frac{-N(N-1)}{N-F}$$

$$N_2 = \sum n_{(f)}{}^2 \tag{4.5}$$

(where the summation is over all families f with at least one child). In general, we will use N_r to denote $\sum n_{(f)}{}^r$, so that $N_0 = F$, $N_1 = N$, and, using an inverted I to mean -1, $N_I = \sum n_{(f)}{}^I = \sum (1/n_{(f)})$. Then

$$v = \frac{XY + KH}{N^2 - N_2} \tag{4.6}$$

is an unbiased estimate of V_φ. To calculate this from Table X-1, proceed as follows: Consider first the nine families with $n_{(f)} = 1$ children in all, $x_{(f)} = 0$ of which are boys, and, hence, $y_{(f)} = n_{(f)} - x_{(f)} = 1$ are girls. Each such family contributes a term $x_{(f)}/n_{(f)} = 0 \times 1/1$ to H, and, therefore, the nine families of this type contribute $9 \times 0 \times 1/1 = 0$ to H. Similarly, the 15 families of one child, with one boy and no girls contribute $15 \times 1 \times 0/1 = 0$. In this way we find

$$H = 9 \times \frac{0 \times 1}{1} + 15 \times \frac{1 \times 0}{1} + 9 \times \frac{0 \times 2}{2} + 20 \times \frac{1 \times 1}{2} + \ldots = 28.217$$

$$K = -237 \times 236/137 = -408.263$$

$$N_2 = 24 \times 1^2 + 39 \times 2^2 + 22 \times 3^2 + 9 \times 4^2$$
$$+ 3 \times 5^2 + 3 \times 6^2 = 705$$

$$Y = N - X = 237 - 133 = 104$$

$$N^2 - N_2 = 55464$$

whence from (4.6) we find that $v = .042$. (It helps to keep about five or six significant figures in the first part of the calculation since some may be lost by subtraction when calculating $XY + KH$.)

We now wish to find the standard errors of the estimates m and v. The error variance of m is given by

$$\text{var}(m) = m(1 - m)/N + (N_2 - N)v/N^2 \qquad (4.7)$$

from which we find in our case

$$\text{var}(m) = .00139, \text{ S.E. } (m) = .037.$$

Thus m has a 95 per cent chance of lying between $.561 - 2 \times .037 = .49$ and $.561 + 2 \times .037 = .63$. This is evidently quite comparable with a $1:1$ ratio. The error variance of v is much more difficult to find. In the first place we note that

$$\text{var}(v) = \frac{\text{var}(XY) + 2K \text{ cov}(XY,H) + K^2 \text{ var}(H)}{(N^2 - N_2)^2} \qquad (4.8)$$

The exact expressions for these are somewhat complicated.

Let us denote the third and fourth moments of the distribution of φ by

$$M_{\varphi 3} = \mathcal{E}(\varphi - M_\varphi)^3; \qquad M_{\varphi 4} = \mathcal{E}(\varphi - M_\varphi)^4. \qquad (4.9)$$

Then, assuming that the sample sizes are fixed, we find after some algebraic manipulation

$$
\begin{aligned}
\text{var}(XY) = \ & (N_4 - 6N_3 + 11N_2 - 6N)M_{\varphi 4} \\
& + 2(N_2{}^2 - 2NN_2 + N^2 - N_4 + 2N_3 - N_2)\, V_\varphi{}^2 \\
& + 2(N - 3)(N_3 - 3N_2 + 2N)M_{\varphi 3}(2M_\varphi - 1) \\
& + (N_2 - N)[(N^2 - 6N + 3) \\
& \qquad - 4(N^2 - 7N + 9)M_\varphi(1 - M_\varphi)]\, V_\varphi \\
& + N(N - 1)[(N - 1) + \\
& \qquad (-4N + 6)M_\varphi(1 - M_\varphi)]M_\varphi(1 - M_\varphi) \qquad (4.10)
\end{aligned}
$$

$$
\begin{aligned}
\text{cov}(XY,H) = \ & (N_3 - 6N_2 + 11N - 6F)M_{\varphi 4} \\
& + (NN_2 - 3N^2 + 2NF + N_3 - 9N_2 \\
& \qquad + 20N - 12F)M_{\varphi 3}(2M_\varphi - 1) \\
& - (N_3 - 2N_2 + N)\, V_\varphi{}^2 \\
& - 4(NN_2 - 4N^2 + 3NN_0 - 4N_2 \\
& \qquad + 13N - 9F)V_\varphi M_\varphi(1 - M_\varphi) \\
& + (NN_2 - 4N^2 + 3NN_0 - 3N_2 + 3F)V_\varphi \\
& + (N - F)[N - 1 + \\
& \qquad (-4N + 6)\, M_\varphi(1 - M_\varphi)]M_\varphi(1 - M_\varphi) \qquad (4.11)
\end{aligned}
$$

$$\begin{aligned}\operatorname{var}(H) =\ & (N_2 - 6N + 11F - 6N_{\mathrm{I}})(M_{\varphi 4} + 2M_{\varphi 3}\,[2M_\varphi - 1])\\ & - (N_2 - 2N + F)\,V_\varphi{}^2\\ & + [(N_2 - 7N + 13F - 13N_{\mathrm{I}})\\ & - 4(N_2 - 8N + 16F - 9N_{\mathrm{I}})\,M_\varphi\,(1 - M_\varphi)]\,V_\varphi\\ & + [(- 4N + 10F - 6N_{\mathrm{I}})\,M_\varphi\,(1 - M_\varphi)\\ & \qquad + (N - 2F + N_{\mathrm{I}})]\,M_\varphi\,(1 - M_\varphi)\qquad (4.12)\end{aligned}$$

To use these expressions we need to know the higher moments $M_{\varphi 3}$ and $M_{\varphi 4}$ of the distribution of φ; or, at least, we require estimates of these moments. These would be troublesome to get. For many purposes, it will be adequate to use the error variances calculated on the hypothesis of homogeneity, $V_\varphi = 0$, which implies that $M_{\varphi 3} = M_{\varphi 4} = 0$ also. For we can reasonably expect the actual error variance to be greater when there is heterogeneity than when there is homogeneity; but if V_φ appears to be small, as is the case here, it will not be much greater and will give a reasonable guide. Now if we put $V_\varphi = M_{\varphi 3} = M_{\varphi 4} = 0$ in the formulas above, we get

$$\begin{aligned}\operatorname{var}(v) =\ & \frac{N(N-1)}{(N^2 - N_2)^2}\Bigg[\frac{N-1}{(N-F)^2}\Big\{2(NF + 2F^2 - 3NN_{\mathrm{I}})\,M_\varphi{}^2(1 - M_\varphi{}^2)\\ & + (NN_{\mathrm{I}} - F^2)M_\varphi(1 - M_\varphi)\Big\} - 2M_\varphi{}^2(1 - M_\varphi)^2\Bigg].\qquad (4.13)\end{aligned}$$

We will in practice replace M_φ by its estimate m. Since there are 24 families of size 1, 39 families of size 2, and so on, we find in our sample

$$N_{\mathrm{I}} = \frac{42}{1} + \frac{39}{2} + \frac{22}{3} + \frac{9}{4} + \frac{3}{5} + \frac{3}{6} = 54.183.$$

Substituting this in (4.13) and putting $m = .561$ in place of M_φ we get

$$\operatorname{var}(v) = .000301;\qquad \text{S.E. } (v) = .017.$$

Thus v rather exceeds twice its standard error; there is some suggestion of heterogeneity, though it is not very strong.

One question of interest which sometimes arises is this: Sometimes the estimate v of the variance V_φ may turn out negative. Since V_φ cannot be negative, how can we interpret this? If we take the phrase "v is an estimate of V_φ" to mean "v is a plausible value of V_φ," then such a negative value for v seems paradoxical and can cause puzzlement. It is usually suggested that it should be replaced by zero. We suggest, however, another interpretation, namely, that in large enough samples the likelihood curve is nearly Gaussian in form with peak at v and standard deviation equal to the standard error. If the peak occurs at a negative value v, this means that we have effectively the situation shown in Fig. X-5. The top curve represents the likelihood considered as a function of V_φ. We suppose that mathematically it has a Gaussian form, which means that it is a bell-shaped curve extending over both positive and negative values of V. The second curve represents some reasonable initial or prior probability distribution of different values of V_φ. Since negative values of V_φ cannot occur, this has zero height to the left of the origin. On multiplying these, we get the final or posterior probability distribution shown in the third curve. Again, this will be zero to the left of the origin, but it will have a peak at or very near the origin, showing that when v is negative there is a high probability that the actual heterogeneity is zero or very small. The precise conclusions will depend on the exact form assumed for the initial distribution, but a negative v is readily interpreted in this way. It would alter the interpretation to put it equal to zero.

Note, however, that in formula (4.7), we calculate the error variance of m in terms of m and v. In fact, the error variance, calculated in the conventional way, is

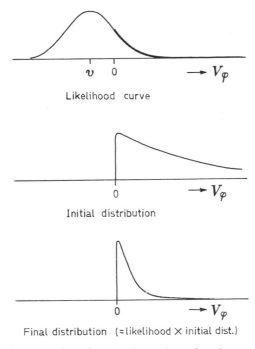

Likelihood curve

Initial distribution

Final distribution (=likelihood × initial dist.)

Fig. X-5. Interpretation of a negative estimated variance.

and we have replaced the unknown M_φ and V_φ by their estimates m and v to get (4.7). Since V_φ cannot in fact be negative, it is arguable that one should use 0 instead of v in this particular formula when v is negative, since that will certainly be nearer the true value V_φ.

FAMILY LIMITATION

Family limitation may sometimes occur. If several abnormals have already been born, the parents may fear that future children will be affected also, and, hence, be less willing to have another child. Alternatively, they may be more willing than otherwise, in the hope of having a normal one. Unfortunately, not much is known about the exact extent to which probabilities are affected, but the pattern of changes could presumably be quite complicated, and this is implied in the estimation of the amount of family limitation. We will not, therefore, discuss the estimation problem here in detail but only show how simple types of family limitation can be detected.

If the birth of an abnormal makes the parents less willing to continue the family, the result will be that the final children in the various families will be abnormal more often than one would expect from the segregation ratio. As long as the data are homogeneous, so that the expected segregation is the same in all families, the proportion of affected in all the families together will not be changed by family limitation. This is because before it is born each individual child has the same probability φ_1 of being affected, and so the proportion of affected in a large number of children will be nearly φ_1. Since the proportion of affected among last-born children is greater than φ_1, that among other children must be smaller than φ_1. We can, therefore, test for the presence of family limitation by comparing these two proportions.

Thus, if we wished to test whether the occurrence of a boy child encouraged or discouraged further reproduction, we could set out a table as follows:

TABLE X-2
TEST FOR FAMILY LIMITATION

SEX	LAST-BORN CHILDREN	OTHER CHILDREN	TOTAL
Male	50	83	133
Female	50	54	104
Total	100	137	237

The proportion of males in last-born children is $50/100 = .50$, with standard error .042. In other children, it is $83/133 = .62$ with standard error .042. The standard error of the difference .61 − .50 = .11 is .065; hence, this is not significant at the 5 per cent level, showing no strong evidence for family limitation. (A similar conclusion would result from using any other method of testing the 2 × 2 Table 5.1, e.g., using Woolf's (1957) we obtain $\chi^2 = 1.84$ with 1 degree of freedom.) This is not surprising; it is rather more likely that family limitation where the sex of children is concerned will take a more subtle form; many parents will prefer a family of mixed sexes; and the family is more likely to be terminated when the last two children have different sexes than when they have the same sex. A more complicated test then is required.

Note that, if the segregation proportion φ_1 is not homogeneous, but varies appreciably from family to family, family limitation can introduce some subtle biases and changes in the apparent ratios. We will not go into that here, but a good discussion is given by L. A. Goodman (1964). Note also that, where there is a parental age or birth order effect, as in Down's syndrome (mongolism), it may also happen that the last-born child will have a raised probability of being affected, so that such a parental age effect will not easily be distinguished from family limitation.

ANALYSIS OF SEGREGATIONS WITH RECESSIVITY

In very many cases the genotypes of parents may not be deducible with certainty from their phenotypes. The simplest case arises when we have a pair of alleles, say, G and g, with g recessive to G. Phenotypically, there are three possible matings, namely, g × g, G × g (and reciprocally, g × G) and G × G. The first mating should only give g children (apart from illegitimates). The second should be a mixture of $GG \times gg$, with only G offspring, and $Gg \times gg$, with Mendelian expectation $\frac{1}{2}G + \frac{1}{2}g$. The third can be genetically either $GG \times GG$ or $GG \times Gg$ (or reciprocally $Gg \times GG$: we will not distinguish between reciprocal crosses) or $Gg \times Gg$. Of these, the matings $GG \times GG$ and $GG \times Gg$ give only G children. The mating $Gg \times Gg$ has children according to a Mendelian expectation $\frac{3}{4}G + \frac{1}{4}g$. The analysis of these matings is a classical problem in statistical genetics. A great number of papers have been written on this, including some by Haldane (1932, 1938). In fact, most of these papers give virtually the same solution to the problem, although similarities are concealed by sometimes treating it as an estimation problem, sometimes as a significance test, and by presenting the arithmetical computations in different ways. (For references, see Smith, 1956, 1959.)

Consider the mating type G × g. Assume the following model: Each mating G × g has a probability α_1 of being $GG \times gg$ (giving only G offspring), and a probability $\alpha_0 = 1 - \alpha_1$ of being $Gg \times gg$. If the mating

CEDRIC A. B. SMITH

is in fact $Gg \times gg$, then any one child has a probability φ_1 of being G, and $\varphi_0 = 1 - \varphi_1$ of being g. The segregations are assumed to be homogeneous, so that for each pair of parents the values of $\alpha_1, \alpha_2, \varphi_1, \varphi_2$ are the same.

One possible way of analyzing the data would be to use the likelihood function, as follows: Let an observed family of n children contain x dominants G and y recessives g. We will assume, for the present, that there is no family limitation, so that the family size n is statistically independent of the types of children born. If $y > 0$, the mating type must have been genetically $Gg \times gg$, and hence the likelihood of occurrence of such a family is

$$L = \alpha_0 \varphi_1{}^x \varphi_0{}^y = (1 - \alpha_1)\varphi_1{}^x(1 - \varphi)^y \qquad [y > 0] \qquad (6.1)$$

On the other hand, if $y = 0$, the family could have arisen from a mating $GG \times gg$ with likelihood $\alpha_1 \times 1$ and from a mating $Gg \times gg$ with likelihood $\alpha_0 \times \varphi_1{}^x \varphi_0{}^y = \alpha_0 \varphi_1{}^n$ (since $x = n$ when $y = 0$).

Thus, the total likelihood in such a case is

$$L = \alpha_1 + \alpha_0 \varphi_1{}^n = \alpha_1 + (1 - \alpha_1)\varphi_1{}^n \qquad [y = 0]. \qquad (6.2)$$

The likelihood, therefore, is given in all cases by formulas (6.1) and (6.2). As we have said, in principle, any conclusions we wish to draw from the experiment should follow from these. There are certain inconveniences, however, in attacking the problem in this way. L is here a function of 2 variables. One is φ_1, the segregation probability we are studying. The other is α_1, the probability that a G $\times$ g mating is $GG \times gg$, or, in other words, that a dominant G individual is homozygote GG. This probability will depend on the gene frequencies and mating structure of the population. If the gene frequencies are $pG + qg$, and mating is at random without selection, the relative probabilities of GG and Gg are in the ratio $p^2:2pq$. Hence, on dividing by the total $(p^2 + 2pq)$, we find that the absolute probabilities are

$$\alpha_1 = p^2/(p^2 + 2pq) = p/(1 + q)$$
$$\alpha_0 = 2pq/(p^2 + 2pq) = 2q/(1 + q). \qquad (6.3)$$

A study of the likelihood function will give evidence jointly on a number of different points, such as segregations, gene frequencies, and mating structure. From the point of view of a scientific investigation, however, it seems simpler and in some ways better to try to disentangle the issues and to treat them separately as far as possible. If they are taken all together, any deviation from reality in one respect of the model can affect the correctness of the calculations about the other aspects. By taking the

120

issues as far as possible individually, we have more security than other-wise in the conclusions, although we may have to pay for this by a decrease in efficiency in the statistical sense.

In the present example, we can eliminate the influence of gene frequencies and mating structure by restricting ourselves entirely to families with at least one recessive *gg* offspring. The mating is then certainly *Gg* × *gg*. Because we exclude all families in which all children are dominant G, the segregation proportions in the sample will be biased. Various ways have been proposed of correcting for this bias. The one which follows is suggested by some of Li's work (1964, 1966).

The key to the analysis is the fact that as soon as one recessive child has been born we know that the mating is *Gg* × *gg*. Let us, therefore, consider first the set of all children born after the first recessive. For each child the probability of being dominant is φ_1, and the probability of being recessive is φ_0. We will assume homogeneity, i.e., equality of φ_1 in all segregating families. If there are altogether X dominants and Y recessives out of $N = X + Y$ children (following the first recessive) in all families taken together, we can estimate φ_1 as $\mu_1 = X/N$ with standard error $\sigma_1 = \sqrt{[\mu_1(1 - \mu_1)/N]}$.

In fact, if we assume that the segregation probability φ_1 is homogeneous, i.e., is the same in all G × g families which are capable of segregation, this will still be valid even when there is family limitation, and we can apply the method of Section 5 to test for family limitation. Unfortunately, however, the method of Section 4 for estimating heterogeneity will not hold accurately. The reason is this: Suppose that φ_1 varies from family to family, and consider all families of a given size n. The families in which only dominants occur will have to be excluded from the sample, which means that families with a high φ_1 will be more likely to be excluded than those with low φ_1.

Thus, when we consider our sample, in which only families with at least one recessive have been counted, the distribution of values of φ_1 will differ from that in the original population. An inspection of the mathematics of this shows it to be rather complicated, so that there is no obvious way of modifying the method of Section 4 to correct for the bias. One can use that method, however, to get an estimate of at least the order of magnitude of any heterogeneity.

As an example, suppose that we have the following 50 families shown in Table X-3 from a G × g mating with at least 1 g child.

Among the children which follow the first g child, we find the analysis presented in Table X-4.

121

TABLE X-3

DATA ON SEGREGATION WITH RECESSIVITY

OBSERVED SEQUENCE OF CHILDREN	gg	ggg	Gg	gG	Ggg	gGg	GGg	gGG	GgG	ggG	ggGG	gGgG	gGGG	GGgG	Ggggg	TOTAL
Observed frequency	9	6	9	9	2	1	3	1	3	1	2	1	1	1	1	50

TABLE X-4

ANALYSIS OF CHILDREN FOLLOWING FIRST RECESSIVE

CHILDREN	G	g	TOTAL
Last in family	10	19	29
Not last	6	7	13
Total	16	26	42

The estimated proportion of G is accordingly $16/42 = .38$ with standard error $\sqrt{(.38 \times .62/42)} = .075$. A range of two standard errors on either side of the estimate covers the value .50; hence, these data are quite consistent with a $1:1$ ratio. The observed numbers are rather small to test for family limitation, but, for Table X-4, the χ^2 for independence is 1.0 (by Woolf's method) with 1 degree of freedom, giving no suggestion of any appreciable limitation. Although the method of Section 4 is not strictly applicable, use of it gives an approximate estimate $v = .011$ for V_φ, the variance of φ_1. This is clearly negligible.

The remaining part of the information provided by the sample consists of the numbers, a, of G individuals preceding the first g in the various families. The observed distribution is summarized in Table X-5.

TABLE X-5

OBSERVED FREQUENCIES OF NUMBER OF G CHILDREN PRECEDING FIRST g

		a		
c	0	1	2	TOTAL
1	9	—	—	9
2	15	9	—	24
3	3	5	3	11
4	4	0	1	5
5	0	1	0	1
Total	31	15	4	50

Note: c = total numbers of children; a = number of G children preceding first g.

If we assume that there is no family limitation and no heterogeneity, this table also provides information about the value of φ_1, the probability of any child being G. For in all families of c children from a mating $Gg \times gg$ the family begins with a g child with probability φ_1; it begins with G, g, with probability $\varphi_1 \varphi_0$; it begins with G, G, g, with probability $\varphi_1^2 \varphi_0$; and so on, with probabilities in a geometric progression with ratio φ_1, except that the last case of all children G has probability φ_1^c. Families with only G children, however, are by definition excluded from the sample. The remaining probabilities of 0, 1, 2, . . . , $(c - 1)$ G children at the beginning of the family will still be in the ratio $\varphi_1 : \varphi_1 \varphi_0 : \varphi_1^2 \varphi_0 : \ldots \varphi_1^{c-1} \varphi_0$, but to turn these ratios into proportions one must divide by their total, $1 - \varphi_1^c$, to make them sum to 1. We conclude that the expected proportion of families beginning with a g children is $\varphi_1^a \varphi_0 / (1 - \varphi^c) = \varphi_1^a (1 - \varphi_1) / (1 - \varphi_1^c)$. By comparing these expected frequencies with the observed numbers (Table X-5), one should be able to estimate φ_1. (Note, however, that this estimate does depend in an important way on the absence of family limitation and also, to a lesser degree, on homogeneity in the values of φ_1.)

One simple, ingenious, and highly efficient way to perform this estimation is given by Li (1966). It may be worthwhile repeating here in a slightly modified and simplified form. Let $n(c,a)$ denote the observed number of families of c children beginning with a g's, i.e., $n(c,a)$ is the entry in columns c and a of Table X-5. Let $n(c)$ be the total number of families of c children, i.e., the c'th entry in the last column. Define as follows for all values of a less than $\frac{1}{2} c$:

$$
\begin{aligned}
\alpha(c,a) &= n(c,a + 1) + n(c,a + 2) + \ldots + n(c,c - a - 1) \\
\beta(c,a) &= n(c,a) + n(c,a + 1) + \ldots + n(c,c - a - 2) \\
\gamma(c,a) &= n(c,a) + n(c,c - a - 1) \\
\delta(c,a) &= n(c,a) - n(c,c - a - 1) \\
u(c,a) &= \alpha(c,a) \, \delta(c,a) / \gamma(c,a) \\
w(c,a) &= \beta(c,a) \, \delta(c,a) / \gamma(c,a)
\end{aligned}
\tag{6.4}
$$

(provided that $\gamma(c,a)$ is different from 0; otherwise, $u(c,a)$ and $w(c,a)$ become indeterminate). Thus, taking the families of $c = 3$ children in Table X-5, we obtain

$$
\begin{aligned}
\alpha(3,0) &= n(3,1) + n(3,2) = 5 + 3 = 8 \\
\beta(3,0) &= n(3,0) + n(3,1) = 3 + 5 = 8 \\
\gamma(3,0) &= n(3,0) + n(3,2) = 3 + 3 = 6 \\
\delta(3,0) &= n(3,0) - n(3,2) = 3 - 3 = 0 \\
u(3,0) &= 8 \times 0/6 = 0.00 \\
w(3,0) &= 8 \times 0/6 = 0.00.
\end{aligned}
$$

123

In all we obtain the following values, rejecting the indeterminate 0/0 cases:

$u(2,0) = 2.25$	$w(2,0) = 3.75$
$u(3,0) = 0.00$	$w(3,0) = 0.00$
$u(4,0) = 1.00$	$w(4,0) = 4.00$
$u(4,2) = 1.00$	$w(4,2) = 0.00$
$u(5,1) = 0.00$	$w(5,1) = 1.00$
Total $U = 4.25$	$W = 8.75$

Li shows that U/W, the ratio of the totals, is then an estimate of φ_1. This is essentially because by definition

$$\frac{u(c,a)}{w(c,a)} = \frac{\alpha(c,a)}{\beta(c,a)} = \frac{n(c,a+1) + n(c,a+2) + \ldots}{n(c,a) \qquad + n(c,a+1) + \ldots}. \tag{6.5}$$

Because the expected values of the frequencies $n(c,a)$, $n(c,a+1)$, $n(c,a+2)$, ... form a geometric progression with ratio φ_1, each term in the numerator of the fraction on the right is in expected value φ_1, times the corresponding term in the denominator. Hence, in a large sample, this fraction is approximately φ_1, i.e., $u(c,a)$ approximately φ_1 times $w(c,a)$. When we sum over-all values of c and a, the total U of the $u(c,a)$ will be approximately φ_1 times the total W of the $w(c,a)$. The object of bringing in the γ's and δ's is to give an efficient weighting system, so that each part of the data contributes to the correct extent. Here we find

$$U/W = 4.25/8.75 = .49. \tag{6.6}$$

Its standard error is

$$\sqrt{(\varphi_1\varphi_0/W)} = \sqrt{(.486 \times .514/8.75)} = .17. \tag{6.7}$$

Thus, the estimate is again consistent with $\varphi_1 = .5$, i.e., a 1:1 segregation. We can also combine this with our previous estimate, based on the children following the first g. Let W' denote the total number of such children, and U' the number of type G. Let $W'' = W + W'$, and $U'' = U + U'$. Then U''/W'' is the estimate of φ_1 obtained from the whole sample, with standard error $\sqrt{(\varphi_1\varphi_0/W'')}$. Thus, in our case we have

U	$-$	4.25	W	$-$	8.75
U'	$=$	16.00	W'	$=$	42.00
U''	$=$	20.25	W''	$=$	50.75

Estimate of $\varphi_1 = 20.25/50.75 = .40$

with S.E. $\sqrt{(.40 \times .60/50.75)} = .070$.

It is also quite easy to find the maximum likelihood estimate of φ_1. We may do this either for the data of Table X-5 or for the complete data as originally given in Table X-3. The easiest method is the counting method of Ceppellini, Siniscalco, and Smith. A paper by Smith (1957) explained how to apply this to the complete data; we, therefore, just indicate here how it can be applied to Table X-5. In order to see how the analysis works, we can imagine that the data were arrived at as follows (this is not quite identical with the real situation but has the same observed consequences). An investigator finds (or constructs) a number of families which arise from a random process in which each child has a probability φ_1 of being G, $\varphi_0 = 1 - \varphi_1$ of being g. Having collected this information, he deletes from it (1) all information about families with only G children and (2) all information about children following the first g child in a family, except that he retains the total number of children. He passes on the remaining information to the statistician, in the form of Table X-5, and asks him to estimate φ_1. Now the statistician can hope to estimate φ_1 if he can put back at least an estimate of the numbers of children which have been deleted and then take the proportion of G children among all children. He need not worry about the children following the first g child, however, since they will occur in expected proportions $\varphi_1 G + \varphi_0 g$, and, hence, all he needs to do is to add the children deleted in families with all G children, to the children already known from Table X-5, i.e., those up to and including the first g child, and then find the proportion of G in the total.

To see in more detail how this is done, consider families of three children. The probability that such a family from a $Gg \times gg$ mating will have all G children, and, hence, be excluded from our sample, is $\varphi_1{}^3$; the probability that it will be included is, accordingly, $(1 - \varphi_1{}^3)$. There are $n(3) = 11$ families included; hence, we can estimate that there are $n(3)\varphi_1{}^3/(1 - \varphi_1{}^3)$ families excluded. Since in each of these families there are three G children, this means that we estimate that there are $3n(3)\varphi_1{}^3/(1 - \varphi_1{}^3)$ G children excluded. Now we can count the children in families of three in Table X-5, up to and including the first g child, and add to them the estimated excluded G children. Since there are altogether $n(3) = 11$ families of three children, each having only one g recorded, there are 11 g children. The number of G children, including the rejected ones, is estimated to be

$$0 \times 3 + 1 \times 5 + 2 \times 3 + 3 \times n(3)\varphi_1{}^3/(1 - \varphi_1{}^3)$$
$$= 11 + 3n(3)\varphi_1{}^3/(1 - \varphi_1{}^3).$$

Similarly, for families of two children we count 24 g's and $15 \times 0 + 9 \times 1 + 2 \times 24\varphi_1{}^2/(1 - \varphi_1{}^2)$ G's. The procedure then follows the iteration

125

method explained in more detail by Smith (1957). We take some provisional value of φ_1, say $\varphi_1 = .58$. We estimate the numbers of G and g children (up to the first g child plus all rejected families) as shown in Table X-6.

TABLE X-6
COUNT OF G AND g CHILDREN FROM TABLE X-5

FAMILY SIZE	g	G (ESTIMATED)	TOTAL
2	24	39.0	63.0
3	11	21.3	32.3
4	5	5.5	10.5
5	1	1.5	2.5
Total	41	67.3	108.3

We now find an improved estimate of φ_1 as $67.3/108.3 = .629$, and repeat the process. By iteration, this leads eventually to the final estimate $.63 \pm .14$, which is the maximum likelihood estimate. It again agrees with a possible 1:1 ratio, and it does not differ significantly from the estimate .38 based on the children following the first recessive. We can equally well apply the same counting method to the whole sample, including children up to and after the first recessive; it is only necessary to count all the observed children plus the estimated excluded ones (Smith, 1957). This leads to the estimate $.44 \pm .065$.

The same method of analysis can be applied to G × G matings. Whenever there is at least one g child, the mating can be inferred to be $Gg \times Gg$, with expected Mendelian proportion $\varphi_1 = \frac{3}{4}$ of dominants. The actual proportion φ_1 can be estimated from the families containing at least one g child as above. The simplicity of the method (particularly in Li's form) is at the price of losing some information by ignoring families containing all dominants. There is a method by Fisher which will take this information also into account fairly simply (Smith, 1956).

APPLICATION TO OTHER SYSTEMS

The methods of analysis described above can be applied at once to the ABO blood group system. Some matings will reveal at once the genotypes of the parents and, hence, the segregations expected on the basis of Mendelian theory. For example, $A_1B \times O$ is genotypically $A_1B \times OO$ and, hence, should give $\frac{1}{2}A_1O + \frac{1}{2}OO - \frac{1}{2}A_1 + \frac{1}{2}O$ children, similarly $A_1B \times A_2B$ should give
$$\frac{1}{4}A_1A_2 + \frac{1}{4}A_1B + \frac{1}{4}BA_2 + \frac{1}{4}BB = \frac{1}{4}A_1 + \frac{1}{4}A_1B + \frac{1}{4}A_2B + \frac{1}{4}B.$$

A mating B × O will be of the same type as G × g with g recessive, already discussed in Section 6. We can select families with at least one O child. The mating is then known to be $BO \times OO$ for certain. Similarly a mating B $\times$ B will be known to be $BO \times BO$ if it has an O child. It will then be expected to give a 3:1 ratio, as would a G $\times$ G mating. Consider now a more complicated case, such as A_1 (mother) $\times A_2$ (father). We can at once see that if the mother is homozygous A_1A_1, all children necessarily must be A_1, whatever the genotype of the father. If any child, however, has a blood group different from A_1, the mother must be heterozygous, i.e., A_1A_2 or A_1O, and the segregation in the mother's genes is shown by the segregation between children who are A_1 and those who are not A_1. This, again, is analogous to the G $\times$ g case, with "A_1" instead of G and "not A_1" instead of g, and can be analyzed in a similar way.

Thus, suppose we had the following families from $A_1 \times A_2$ matings:

(1) Children A_1, A_1, A_1
(2) Children A_1, A_2, A_2
(3) Children A_2, A_1, O, A_2, O, A_1.

Family (1) would show no segregation in the mother's genes and would be ignored. Family (2) would be similar to a G $\times$ g mating with children G, g, g, and family (3), similar to such a mating with children g, G, g, g, g, G. We sometimes also can get information about segregation in the father's genes. For this purpose, children which are A_1 are quite uninformative and would be left out of consideration. Thus, family (1) above would be ignored and families (2) and (3) would be simplified to:

(2) Children A_2, A_2
(3) Children A_2, O, A_2, O.

We now observe that if any child in the family is not A_2 (i.e., is O) the father is certainly heterozygous (i.e., A_2O), and the segregation in the father is shown by the division into A_2 and not A_2 children. That is, as regards segregation of the father's genes, family (3) would behave as would a G $\times$ g mating with children G, g, G, g. Family (2) would be like a G $\times$ g mating with children G, G and would be ingored in the method of analysis suggested above.

A mating A_1B (mother) $\times A_2$ (father) combines the features of $A_1B \times O$ and $A_1 \times A_2$ matings. It shows the segregation in the mother's genes for certain; the children are divided into those of group A_1, who get the mother's A_1 gene, and those carrying a B gene (and being, therefore, A_2B or B) who get the mother's B gene. In considering the possible segregation in the father's genes, we must first reject all A_1 children as uninformative, i.e., we retain only those children who carry a B gene. If any of these have a blood group different from A_2B, the father must be

127

heterozygous, and the segregation of the father's genes is shown in those children carrying a B gene by being either A_2B or not A_2B. Again, we have an analogy to the G $\times$ g mating.

A mating $A_2B \times A_1$ will show segregation in the mother's genes (according to whether a child does or does not carry a B gene). If there is any child not carrying an A_1 gene, the family also will show segregation in the father's genes, each child being scored according to whether it carried A_1 or not. Note that in this case all the children are scored for the segregation in the father's genes, not merely some of them as in the $A_1B \times A_2$ mating.

A mating B (mother) $\times A_1$ (father) will show segregation in the mother's genes if there is any child not carrying a B. It, therefore, behaves as would a G $\times$ g mating as far as the mother is concerned. The same applies, quite independently, to segregation in the father's genes, which will be shown if there is any child not carrying an A_1.

We can imagine a generalization of the ABO system to one in which we have series of alleles $A_1, A_2, A_3, \ldots, A_a, B_1, B_2, \ldots, B_b, C_1, C_2, \ldots, C_c$, etc., and O, where O is recessive to all the others, A_r is recessive to A_s if $r > s$, B_r is recessive to B_s if $r > s$, and so on, but there are no other recessivity relations. The analysis of segregations for this system is exactly analogous to that for the usual ABO blood groups. If the two parents have different phenotypes, it is possible to consider the segregations separately in the mother's genes and the father's genes, with effectively the same patterns of segregation as we have already considered. If the mother and father have the same phenotype, only three patterns of segregation can arise; no segregation (as with O $\times$ O); 1:2:1 (as with $A_1B \times A_1B$); a possible 3:1 segregation, shown by the appearance of a recessive offspring (as with B $\times$ B).

Unfortunately, there does not seem to be any simple or obvious way to extend this type of analysis to more complicated systems of alleles, such as those of rhesus. Let us suppose that we have a pair of antisera, which, by analogy with rhesus we might call anti-R_1 and anti-R_2. We may suppose that there are four alleles, which we may call R_1, R_2, R_{12}, and r; here the presence of allele R_1 is sufficient to ensure a positive reaction with anti-R_1; similarly, the presence of R_2 ensures a positive reaction with anti-R_2; R_{12} reacts with both; and r, with neither. Any individual can be classified into one of four phenotypes, such as (R_1 | $R_2$0) which means positive reaction with anti R_1, no reaction with anti R_2. An individual of phenotype ($R_1 + R_2 +$) could be genotypically $R_{12}r$, $R_{12}R_1$, $R_{12}R_2$, $R_{12}R_{12}$, or $R_{12} r$; and a mating ($R_1 + R_2 +$) $\times$ ($R_1 + R_2 +$) can, therefore, be any one of fifteen different types, even when reciprocal matings are not distinguished. If it should happen that one of the children is ($R_1$0$R_2$0) $= rr$, we can infer that the mating must be $R_{12}r \times R_{12}r$. Otherwise, we cannot infer either the mating type or the segregation ratio for certain. Suppose, for example, that we have observed at least one child of each of the phenotypes ($R_1 + R_2 +$), ($R_10R_2 +$), ($R_1 + R_20$). Then the different matings and segregation ratios in Table X-7 are possible.

TABLE X-7

MATING	OFFSPRING			
	($R_1 + R_2 +$)	($R_10R_2 +$)	($R_1 + R_20$)	(R_10R_20)
$R_1R_2 \times R_1R_2$	½	¼	¼	0
$R_1R_2 \times R_{12}r$	½	¼	¼	0
$R_1R_2 \times R_1r$	¼	½	¼	0
$R_1R_2 \times R_2r$	¼	¼	½	0
$R_1r \times R_2r$	¼	¼	¼	¼

Thus, for a complete analysis of these more complicated systems with multiple alleles a more sophisticated approach seems necessary. We can retain the simplicity, however, in the following way: Consider, firstly, only one of the antisera, say anti-R_1, on its own. We can then classify individuals as dominants, ($R_1 +$) or (G) and recessives, (R_10) or (g), and analyze as with a single pair of alleles $R_1 = G$ and *not* $R_1 = g$, verifying that the segregations agree with expectation. We can now repeat with anti-R_2 on its own. Naturally, these two tests are not independent of one another, and they will not show any interaction which may occur between different alleles, but the analysis may be sufficient to establish the mode of inheritance with reasonable certainty.

REFERENCES

GOOD, I. J. 1950. *Probability and the Weighting of Evidence*. Griffin, London.
GOODMAN, L. A. 1964. Some possible effects of birth control on the incidence of disorders and on the influence of birth order. *Ann. Human Genet.*, 27:41–52.
HALDANE, J. B. S. 1932. A method for investigating recessive characters in man. *J. Genet.*, 25:251–55.
———. 1938. The estimation of the frequency of recessive characters in man. *Ann. Eugen.*, 8:255–62.
———. 1947. The mutation rate of the gene for haemophilia, and its segregation ratios in males and females. *Ann. Eugen.*, 13:262–71.
———. 1956. Mutation in the sex-linked recessive type of muscular dystrophy. A possible sex-difference. *An. Human Genet.*, 20:344–47.
LI, C. C. 1964. Estimation of recessive proportion by first appearance time. *Ann. Human Genet.*, 28:177–80.
———. 1966. A new method of studying Mendelian segregation in man. *In Mutation in Population*, R. Hončarir (ed.), pp. 155–66. Czechoslovak Academy of Sciences, Prague.

CEDRIC A. B. SMITH

MORTON, N. E. 1959. Genetic tests under multiple ascertainment. *Amer. J. Human Genet.*, 11:1–16.

SAVAGE, L. J. 1954. *The Foundations of Statistics.* Wiley, New York.

SMITH, C. A. B. 1956. A test for segregation ratios in family data. *Ann. Human Genet.*, 20:257–65.

————. 1957. Counting methods in genetical statistics. *Ann. Human Genet.*, 21:254–76.

————. 1959. A note on the effects of ascertainment on segration ratios. *Ann. Human Genet.*, 23:311–23.

————. 1965. Personal probability and statistical analysis. *J. Roy. Statist. Soc.*, A., 128:469–99.

WOOLF, B. 1957. The log likelihood ratio test (G-test). *Ann. Human Genet.*, 21:397–409.

EVOLUTIONARY BIOLOGY AND BIOMETRICS

MOTOO KIMURA
National Institute of Genetics,
Mishima, Japan

XI. HALDANE'S CONTRIBUTIONS TO THE MATHE-MATICAL THEORIES OF EVOLUTION AND POPULATION GENETICS[1]

Among Haldane's multitudinous contributions to biology, those to the mathematical theories of evolution and population genetics should occupy a central position. It is now well known that he laid the foundation, together with R. A. Fisher and S. Wright, to the mathematical theory of population genetics. He published many important papers on this subject until his death, and it appears that this was his favorite field, one where he felt at home and was proud of his contributions.

Starting in 1924, he published a series of papers entitled "A Mathematical Theory of Natural and Artificial Selection." The first paper of this series (Part I) was also his first paper on the subject. With this paper, he opened up a new field of study in which the process of change in gene frequencies by natural selection is treated mathematically. The work is based on his belief that "a satisfactory theory of natural selection must be quantitative" and that only through quantitative investigation can the adequacy be tested of the genetic theory of natural selection. He considered various kinds of selection such as zygotic, gametic, familial selection, or selection involving sex-linked loci. A typical example is as follows: In a very large random-mating population, the dominants (AA, Aa) are favored, and, as compared with them, $1 - k$ of the recessive (aa) individuals survive to breed, where k is termed "coefficient of selection." Writing $u_n A : 1a$ for the proportion of two types of gametes produced by the $(n - 1)$th generation, he derived the recurrence equation,

$$u_{n+1} = u_n(1 + u_n)/(1 + u_n - k).$$

This is a nonlinear equation and he could not obtain the exact solution, but he did work out approximate solutions. He then constructed a table from which one can readily find out the relation between temporal change of genotypic frequencies and selection intensity. He applied this theory to a

[1] Contribution number 639 from the National Institute of Genetics, Mishima, Shizuoka-ken, Japan.

case of industrial melanism that occurred in Manchester and found that the value of k is at least 0.332 and probably as large as 0.5. Now, it is well known, thanks mainly to the work of Kettlewell, that selection intensities of this magnitude commonly are involved in industrial melanisms, but less known is the remarkable fact that the prediction was made by Haldane some forty years ago. It is often remarked, especially by those who are not well acquainted with the mathematical theory of population genetics, that the classical works of Fisher, Haldane, and Wright are all based on the assumption of small selection intensities and, therefore, are inadequate for the handling of actual situations. This single example shows how wrong such a statement is. Admittedly, the solutions of the recurrence equation which he obtained were approximations, but this does not prevent his solutions from being satisfactory for most practical purposes. Nevertheless, he appears to have kept a strong interest in the mathematical investigations of this type of equation throughout his life, judging from the numerous papers in which the subject is treated. In his last paper on the subject (Haldane and Jayakar, 1963a), he finally showed how to solve such equations in terms of automorphic functions.

Such treatment, as initiated by Haldane, of the change of gene frequencies can be called deterministic, since no random elements, e.g., random sampling of gametes, are taken into account. Even if more sophisticated stochastic treatments have been developed since (cf. Kimura, 1964), the deterministic treatment is still widely used and usually is found satisfactory when the population is large. Indeed, because of its simplicity, it still remains the most useful, and sometimes the only manageable, approach to many problems. As a deterministic theory, and as far as a single locus with a pair of alleles is concerned, his treatment is unlikely to be surpassed for many years to come.

In Parts II, III, IV, and VI (1924b, 1926, 1927a, 1930a) of the series on mathematical theory, he investigated the effects of various factors on the change of gene frequencies, such as partial inbreeding, partial assortative mating, incomplete dominance (including over-dominance) for autosomal as well as sex-linked loci, multifactorial inheritance, linkage (but without selection), polyploidy, generation overlap, and isolation. (Some of these topics were elaborated more extensively in other papers, as in "Theoretical Genetics of Autopolyploids" (1930b).) These papers contain results which are still useful but often overlooked. In Part V (1927b) he took up a stochastic problem and investigated the probability of fixation of mutant genes, using the method of generating function suggested by Fisher (1922). He showed for the first time that a dominant mutant gene having a small selective advantage k (>0) in a large random-mating population has a probability of about 2k of ultimately becoming established in the population. The probability of fixation is much more difficult to evaluate if the advantageous mutation is completely recessive, but, with remarkable insight, he estimated it as of the order of $\sqrt{k/N}$, where k is the selective advantage of the recessives and N is the population number. Later investigations have fully confirmed the validity of his results. In the same paper, he also considered the equilibrium between recurrent mutation and selective elimination and the rate by which such an equilibrium is reached in case of complete dominance.

Another outstanding paper in the series is Part VIII. "Metastable Populations" (1931), in which he investigated the situation where mutant genes are disadvantageous singly but become advantageous in combination. For example, in the case of two dominant genes A and B, he expressed the relative fitnesses of the four phenotypes as follows: AB 1, aaB 1 $-$ k_1, Abb 1 $-$ k_2, $aabb$ 1 $+$ K. Assuming no linkage complications, he treated the two-loci case with extreme elegance, determining trajectories of points representing the genetic composition of a population in a two-dimensional co-ordinate system. He then argued that, for m genes, a population can be represented by a point in m-dimensional space. He also suggested that in many cases related species represent stable types such as he had described and that "the process of species formation may be a rupture of the metastable equilibrium." According to him "such rupture will be specially likely when small communities are isolated." It is interesting to note the similarity of this work to the well-known theory of S. Wright, which was propounded independently and which describes evolution as a trial and error process in terms of multidimensional adaptive surfaces.

Haldane's works up to this stage are summarized in his book *The Causes of Evolution*, published in 1932, and, together with contributions made by R. A. Fisher (1930) and S. Wright (1931) in this period, may truly be called classical. Despite the simplifying assumptions they contain, they should be the basis for any future development in the theory of population and evolutionary genetics. No serious student in the field can work successfully without studying them. It is regrettable therefore, that in recent years a tendency has developed, especially in the United States, among the naturalistic workers on evolution to deprecate these classical works as "beanbag genetics," without supplying adequate models for quantitative treatments. As mathematical education becomes widespread among biology students, it is hoped that these classical works will receive greater appreciation.

135

Haldane took many opportunities to write on the use of mathematics in biology, especially in relation to the genetic theory of evolution. He wrote in "Forty Years of Genetics" as follows: "At present one may say that the mathematical theory of evolution is in a somewhat unfortunate position, too mathematical to interest most biologists, and not sufficiently mathematical to interest most mathematicians. Nevertheless, it is reasonable to suppose that in the next half century it will be developed into a respectable branch of Applied Mathematics" (Haldane, 1938).

The recent development of theories which treat the change of gene frequencies as stochastic processes certainly bears out his prediction made a quarter of a century ago.

Based on the mathematical tools that he had developed, he continued to work on various problems of mutation and selection. I would like to mention two outstanding papers published in 1935 and 1937. One yielded the first estimation of the mutation rate in man (Haldane, 1935), based on his calculation of the equilibrium between mutation and selection. Thus, he established what is now called the indirect method of estimating mutation rates. The other (Haldane, 1937*a*) is entitled "The Effect of Variation on Fitness." Here he derived the principle that the loss of population fitness as a result of recurrent harmful mutations depends entirely on the mutation rate and not on the degree of harmfulness of the mutant genes to an individual, provided that the harmful effect is large enough to keep the gene rare. We estimate that the loss of fitness due to such mutations amounts to about 3 or 4 per cent in *Drosophila* and roughly 10 per cent in man. This remarkable principle was later discovered independently by Muller (1950) who expressed it in terms of "genetic death." Since then the principle has played a fundamental role in assessing the genetic damage of ionizing radiation to human populations. In the same paper, Haldane also investigated a case where the heterozygote is fitter than either homozygote (a situation now known as over-dominance) and showed that such a gene pair lowers the fitness of the species far more than do recurrent harmful mutations. Herein we can see the first attempt at calculating the amount of genetic elimination which results from natural selection acting on genotypic differences. Thus, Haldane created the basis from which the concept of genetic load was developed later by Crow and his associates (cf. Crow and Kimura, 1965), a concept which recently is proving to be increasingly useful in spite of several criticisms, some of which are based on misconceptions.

"The measurement of natural selection" seems to be one of Haldane's favorite topics, and his contributions to it are fundamental. In a paper bearing this title (Haldane, 1954), he proposed to measure the intensity of selection by $I = \log_e s_0 - \log_e S$, where s_0 is the fitness of the optimum phenotype and S is that of the whole population. Applying this relation to the data obtained by Karn and Penrose (1951) on birth weight and mortality, he found that the selection intensity involved is about 2.4 per cent. He pointed out also that natural selection tends to reduce variance by weeding out extreme forms.

In his attempts to create a quantitative evolutionary theory, he suggested (Haldane, 1949a) the term *darwin* as a unit of evolutionary rate, one darwin standing for the rate of change of 10^{-6} per year. He showed that the average rate for horse teeth was around 40 millidarwins. The rate of one darwin appears to be exceptional in nature, whereas the rate of change under artificial selection may reach kilodarwins, or more. With the slow rate of evolution in nature, he conjectured that the majority of genes responsible for the variation were replaced by allelomorphs in a few million generations. His calculations revealed the important point that the selective force responsible for evolution is usually extremely small.

In order to obtain quantitative information regarding the intensity of natural selection, he explored many aspects of variation in nature. Thus, he showed that in certain cases a cline may supply such an information. His mathematical theory of cline (Haldane, 1948) appears to have stimulated Fisher's work on the same subject published a couple of years later.

In discussing Haldane's contributions to the genetic theory of natural selection, one can scarcely go without mentioning "The Cost of Natural Selection" (1957a). In this paper he showed mathematically that in the process of substituting one allele for another by natural selection, the total number of genetic deaths is almost independent of the selection coefficient, but rather depends on the initial frequency, say p_0, and the degree of dominance of the allele used for substitution. For example, if the allele is completely dominant, the sum of the fractions of selective deaths is approximately $D = -\ln p_0$, while if it is semidominant, $D = -2\ln p_0$. Then he suggested that the typical value for the number of deaths involved in one gene substitution is about 30 times the population number in one generation and that, in horotelic (standard rate) evolution, the mean time taken for each gene substitution is about 300 generations. This seems to explain the slowness of evolution. This paper follows the same line of thought as "The Effect of Variation on Fitness" (1937a.) At the moment, opinion seems to be divided on the importance of his concept of the "cost." For myself, I share with him the belief that "quantitative arguments of the kind here put forward should play a part in all future discussions of evolution." It must have been this belief that made him later work out "More Precise Expressions for the Cost of Natural Selection" (1960), in which, however, he warned the reader against extending the theory to cover biological situations to which it does not, in fact, apply. The most important of these situations appears to be the case where a genotype which is originally unfavorable gradually becomes neutral and then favorable. Thus he concluded: "This fact may lead to some modifications in the application of the theory of 'cost' or 'substitutional load' to evolution, but a full consideration is reserved until the theory of evolution under a slowly changing selective intensity in diploids has been worked out."

Besides his work on selection, his contributions to the theory of inbreeding are important, even if some of his results since have been superseded. In 1931 in collaboration with C. H. Waddington, he investigated the amount of crossing-over found in a final population produced by continued inbreeding, such as self-fertilization, brother-sister mating, and so on. The treatment was quite laborious, and a better treatment and more general results were supplied soon by Wright (1933). In 1934, in collaboration with M. S. Bartlett, he investigated the rate of decrease of heterozygosis under brother-sister mating in tetraploids. They also investigated in 1935 an interesting situation in which inbreeding is continued while a particular gene locus is kept heterozygous. In 1937 Haldane studied the effect of continued brother-sister mating for autosomal and sex-linked loci in a diploid, assuming multiple alleles. The method employed in these papers is equivalent to the matrix method later used by Fisher (1949). His study with P. Moshinsky on human inbreeding, especially on marriages of cousins (Haldane and Moshinsky, 1939), must be a classic in the field of consanguinity study in man. If most of it now appears rather elementary, I suppose that this paper contributed a great deal to bring about such an advance in the knowledge of human genetics! The elegant treatment of the inbreeding coefficient in this paper anticipates the later work of Malécot (1948) who completed the probabilistic interpretation of the inbreeding coefficient. Also, Haldane extended the concept of inbreeding to cover linked loci in order to treat the problem of "The Association of Characters as a Result of Inbreeding and Linkage" (1949*b*).

In the field of human genetics in general, Haldane supplied many valuable methods for estimating gene frequencies, detecting linkage, testing randomness of mating, and so on. He also wrote a large number of papers on mathematical statistics, treating such problems as inverse probability and parameter estimation. Though I am not competent

138

enough to judge the real significance of these works in the field of theoretical statistics, it appears to me that he was carrying on the tradition of Pearsonian biometry, trying to extend the application of statistics to biology, as Haldane's Centenary Lecture "Karl Pearson, 1857–1957" testifies (Haldane, 1957b).

With his versatility, he treated many subjects and produced many new ideas throughout his life. One may even say that almost no fundamental subject exists in evolutionary biology which he did not touch. His ideas are often overlooked.

His prodigious brain was kept active until his old age, and after he moved to India he still kept publishing original works despite "a huge burden of research supervision, teaching, editing, and administration" as he wrote in one of his letters. His elegantly written short paper with his colleague Jayakar entitled "Polymorphism Due to Selection of Varying Direction" bears witness to his continued productivity.

Haldane's courageous and immensely stimulating paper entitled "A Defense of Beanbag Genetics" (1964) appears to be his last serious writing on the genetic theory of natural selection. At the end of this paper he wrote: "Meanwhile, I have retired to a one-storied 'ivory tower' provided for me by the Government of Orissa in this earthly paradise of Bhubaneswar and hope to devote my remaining years largely to beanbag genetics."

It is a real pity that the remaining years were too short.

REFERENCES

BARTLETT, M. S., AND J. B. S. HALDANE. 1934. The theory of inbreeding in autotetraploids. *J. Genet.*, 29:175–80.

———. 1935. The theory of inbreeding with forced heterozygosis. *J. Genet.*, 31: 327–40.

CROW, J. F., AND M. KIMURA. 1965. The Theory of Genetic Loads. *Proc. XI Int. Congr. Genet.* Vol. 3. pp. 495–505.

FISHER, R. A. 1922. On the dominance ratio. *Proc. Roy. Soc. Edinburgh*, 42:321–41.

———. 1930. *The Genetical Theory of Natural Selection.* Clarendon Press, Oxford.

———. 1949. *The Theory of Inbreeding.* Oliver and Boyd, Edinburgh.

HALDANE, J. B. S. 1924. A mathematical theory of natural and artificial selection. Part I. *Trans. Camb. Phil. Soc.*, 23:19–41.

———. 1925. A mathematical theory of natural and artificial selection. Part II. *Proc. Camb. Phil. Soc.*, 1:158–63.

———. 1926. A mathematical theory of natural and artificial selection. Part III. *Proc. Camb. Phil. Soc.*, 23:363–72.

———. 1927a. A mathematical theory of natural and artificial selection. Part IV. *Proc. Camb. Phil. Soc.*, 23:607–15.

———. 1927b. A mathematical theory of natural and artificial selection. Part V. *Proc. Camb. Phil. Soc.*, 23:838–44.

————. 1930*a*. A mathematical theory of natural and artificial selection. Part VI. *Proc. Camb. Phil. Soc.*, 26:220–30.

————. 1930*b*. Theoretical genetics of autopolyploids. *J. Genet.*, 22:359–72.

————. 1931. A mathematical theory of natural selection. Part VIII. *Proc. Camb. Phil. Soc.*, 27:137–42.

————. 1932. *The Causes of Evolution*. Harper, New York and London.

————. 1935. The rate of spontaneous mutation of a human gene. *J. Genet.*, 31: 317–26.

————. 1937*a*. The effect of variation on fitness. *Amer. Natur.*, 71:337–49.

————. 1937*b*. Some theoretical results of continued brother-sister mating. *J. Genet.*, 34:265–74.

————. 1938. Forty years of genetics. *In Background to Modern Science*, J. Needham & W. Pagel (eds.), pp. 225–43, Cambridge Univ. Press, Cambridge.

————. 1948. The theory of a cline. *J. Genet.*, 48:277–84.

————. 1949*a*. Suggestions as to quantitative measurement of rates of evolution. *Evolution*, 3:51–56.

————. 1949*b*. The association of characters as a result of inbreeding and linkage. *Ann. Eugen.*, 15:15–23.

————. 1954. The measurement of natural selection. *Caryologia*, 6 (Suppl.):480–87.

————. 1957*a*. The cost of natural selection. *J. Genet.*, 55:511–24.

————. 1957*b*. Centenary lecture: Karl Pearson, 1857–1957. *Biometrika*, 44:303–13.

————. 1960. More precise expressions for the cost of natural selection. *J. Genet.*, 57:351–60.

————. 1964. A defense of beanbag genetics. *Perspect. Biol. Med.*, 7:343–59.

HALDANE, J. B. S., AND S. D. JAYAKAR. 1963*a*. The solution of some equations occurring in population genetics. *J. Genet.*, 58:291–317.

————. 1963*b*. Polymorphism due to selection of varying direction. *J. Genet.*, 58:237–42.

HALDANE, J. B. S., AND P. MOSHINSKY. 1939. Inbreeding in Mendelian populations with special reference to human cousin marriage. *Ann. Eugen.*, 9:321–40.

HALDANE, J. B. S., AND C. H. WADDINGTON. 1931. Inbreeding and linkage. *Genetics*, 16:357–74.

KARN, M. N., AND L. S. PENROSE. 1951. Birth weight and gestation time in relation to maternal age, parity, and infant survival. *Ann. Eugen.*, 16:147–64.

KIMURA, M., 1964. Diffusion models in population genetics. *J. Appl. Probabil.*, 1:177–232.

MALÉCOT, G., 1948. *Le mathématiques de l'hérédité*. Masson, Paris.

MULLER, H. J. 1950. Our load of mutations. *Amer. J. Human Genet.*, 2:111–76.

WRIGHT, S. 1931. Evolution in Mendelian populations. *Genetics*, 16:97–159.

————. 1932. The roles of mutation, inbreeding, crossbreeding, and selection in evolution *Proc. 6th Int. Congr. Genet.*, 1:356–66.

————. 1933. Inbreeding and recombination. *Proc. Nat. Acad. Sci.*, Wash., 19:420–33.

YU. M. SVIREZHEV and N. W. TIMOFÉEFF-RESSOVSKY
Institute of Medical Radiology,
Obninsk, Kaluga Region, U.S.S.R.

XII. SOME TYPES OF POLYMORPHISM IN POPULATIONS

INTRODUCTION

In some natural populations of various animal and plant species, a rather long state of polymorphism of this or that character is observed (Ford, 1940). This state is supposed to be due to the maintenance by certain mechanisms of two or more forms in the state of dynamic equilibrium.

In experiments on the relative viability of various mutations and their combinations in *Drosophila funebris* at various temperatures and degrees of overpopulation of cultures (Timoféeff-Ressovsky, 1934), it was found that some mutations which sharply decreased the viability in the homozygous state increased the relative viability of heterozygotes (in comparison with a normal parent homozygote). Based on this, one could suppose that in some cases a state of dynamic equilibrium between normal and mutant forms can be established in the population because of the increased viability of heterozygotes, which constantly segregate a less viable mutant form. These experiments led to a number of special investigations on the relative viability of some mutations in *Drosophila melanogaster* in homo- and heterozygous states and their compatibility with the normal form in stable model populations of this species. The first publications of the results of such experiments were made by Ph. l'Héritier and G. Teissier, who described competitive relations of various mutations of *Drosophila melanogaster* with a normal form, as well as of two *Drosophila* species: *D. melanogaster* and *D. funebris* (l'Héritier, 1936, 1937; l'Héritier and Teissier, 1933, 1934, 1935).

On the other hand, more than ten years of observations of and collections in the same population of the ladybug *Adalia bipunctata* have shown that a more or less permanent ratio of black to red forms of this bug in the population is due to various selection pressures on these forms. This difference is caused by their relative viability in different seasons. Black forms have the advantage (connected apparently with more intensive reproduction) during the vegetative period, and red forms survive winter

141

better. As a result, the last (fall) population contains more black forms and the first one after winter, the spring population, more red forms. Permanent polymorphism in the population is, thus, maintained by oppositely directed selection pressure on these forms in winter and in summer (Timoféeff-Ressovsky, 1940).

In the cases described above we distinguish two types of polymorphism. We shall refer to the first type as heterozygotic, and the second as adaptational polymorphism. The meaning of these terms will become clear below.

We shall show how the quantitative mathematical model of these two phenomena not only will confirm already known experimental data (which is undoubtedly useful since it, in turn, confirms experimentally the adequacy of the constructed model), but also will allow us to consider the problem of polymorphism in populations from another point of view.

The probabilistic interpretation of the Mendelian rules of heredity, strictly made for the first time by Hardy (1908), helped to construct quantitative models of the influence of selection pressure on genotypic composition of population (Jennings, 1916; Chetverikov, 1926; Wright, 1939). One of the pioneers in this trend in population genetics, the trend based on probabilistic-statistical methods and using an accurate language of numbers, devoid of ambiguous interpretation, was J. B. S. Haldane. At the same time, the works of Haldane usually are based on experimental facts and are never just speculative figures (Haldane, 1932, 1935, 1938, 1957; Haldane and Jayakar, 1963).

QUANTITATIVE MODEL OF GENOTYPIC EQUILIBRIUM IN POPULATIONS

In this section a model will be constructed describing the time change of the genotypic composition of population under various selection pressures.

Let there be a sufficiently large, numerically stable, panmictic population of organisms containing only three genotypes: AA, Aa, and aa. This means that heredity in the population is determined only by two allelic genes A and a. Let us assume that all organisms in the population at any moment of time are the same according to all characteristics with the exception of genotypic difference in alleles A and a. Let us take average longevity of one generation for a time unit. Let us assume that at a certain moment of time t, organisms, having appeared at the moment $t - 1$, produce a progeny, after which they leave the population, so that in the time interval from t to $t + 1$ only organisms of the next generation exist. By index $(-)$ we shall denote such values, meanings of which are taken to the left of point t, by index $(+)$, those to the right of point t.

Let us introduce the following symbols:

$$u(t) = \text{frequency of genotype } AA;$$
$$2v(t) = \text{frequency of genotype } Aa;$$
$$w(t) = \text{frequency of genotype } aa;$$
$$p(t) = \text{frequency of allele } A;$$
$$q(t) = \text{frequency of allele } a.$$

Normalization conditions are:

$$u(t) + 2v(t) + w(t) = 1;$$
$$p(t) + q(t) = 1.$$

Let frequencies of corresponding genotypes in the population, equal, by the moment t (moment of reproduction), $u_-(t)$; $2v_-(t)$; $w_-(t)$. Then frequencies of alleles A and a correspondingly equal:

$$p_-(t) = u_-(t) + v_-(t)$$
$$q_-(t) = v_-(t) + w_-(t). \tag{1.1}$$

Owing to the assumption of panmixia, frequencies of zygotes in the progeny produced at the moment t will be written as:

$$u_+(t) = p_-^2(t);$$
$$2v_+(t) = 2p_-(t)q_-(t);$$
$$w_+(t) = q_-^2(t). \tag{1.2}$$

It is easy to see that at the moment t, frequencies of zygotes, considered as time functions, undergo a break. Gene frequency however, remains continuous.

Indeed:

$$p_+(t) = u_+(t) + v_+(t);$$

but from (1.2) it follows that:

$$p_+ = u_+ + v_+ = p_-^2 + p_-q_- = p_-^2 + p_-(1 - p_-) = p_-$$

which confirms the above statement.

Since differing selection pressure affects various genotypes, the frequency relation of genotypes must change by the end of the generation.

143

Let genotype frequencies become as follows as a result of selection effect by the moment $t + 1$ (moment of reproduction of the next generation):

$$u_-(t + 1) = \frac{\alpha u_+(t)}{w};$$

$$2v_-(t + 1) = \frac{2\beta v_+(t)}{w};$$

$$w_-(t + 1) = \frac{\gamma w_+(t)}{w} \qquad (1.3)$$

where $1/w = 1/(\alpha u_+(t) + 2\beta v_+(t) + \gamma w_+(t))$ is normalization factor.

Here α, β, γ are certain coefficients, which, in general, may depend on time and the introduction of which allows us to take into account the influence of selection pressure. Indeed, α, β, γ are certain not normalized probabilities of attainability of reproduction age by an individual of corresponding genotype. Values of these probabilities depend on conditions under which the population lives (degree of overpopulation, influence of temperature, humidity, and so on). It is conceivable that these values are determined by the viability of each genotype under given environmental conditions.

Now we shall try to determine these coefficients. Let genotype frequencies be known to us (for instance, from the experiment) at the beginning and the end of life of a certain generation. From (1.3) we shall have

$$\alpha u(u^* - 1) + 2\beta u^* v + \gamma u^* w = 0;$$
$$\alpha uv^* + \beta(2v^* - 1)v + \gamma v^* w = 0;$$
$$\alpha uw^* + 2\beta vw^* + \gamma w(w^* - 1) = 0.$$

Here $u = u_+(t)$; $u^* = u_-(t + 1)$. Similar symbols are introduced for other values.

We obtained a homogeneous set of three linear algebraic equations for the determination of values α, β, γ. A matrix rank of coefficients of this set is less than three. Hence, the set has a non-trivial solution. One of the unknown quantities must be given beforehand. Not interfering with the general pattern, let us assume that the coefficient, corresponding to genotype, viability of which is the highest, is equal to 1. Then other coefficients will be less than 1. In this way we have done the normalization and determined the coefficients α, β, γ as probabilities of corresponding genotypes to attain the reproduction age, on condition that one of the genotypes always reaches this age (probability unit). The following cases are possible:

1) The homozygote AA is the most viable. Then

$$\alpha = 1; \qquad \beta = \frac{uv^*}{u^*v}; \qquad \gamma = \frac{uw^*}{u^*w}.$$

2) The heterozygote Aa is the most viable. Then

$$\beta = 1; \qquad \alpha = \frac{u^*v}{uv^*}; \qquad \gamma = \frac{vw^*}{v^*w}.$$

3) The homozygote aa is the most viable. Then

$$\gamma = 1; \qquad \alpha = \frac{u^*w}{uw^*}; \qquad \beta = \frac{v^*w}{wv^*}.$$

Let us term factors α, β, γ the relative viability coefficients of genotypes AA, Aa, and aa, correspondingly. In general, α, β, γ can be time functions.

We have determined genotype frequencies in the population by the moment $t + 1$. Correspondingly, for frequency of allele A, we shall have:

$$p_-(t + 1) = u_-(t + 1) + v_-(t + 1).$$

The increase of frequency p during the lifetime of a generation equals:

$$\delta p = p_-(t + 1) - p_+(t) = u_-(t + 1) - u_+(t) + v_-(t + 1) - v_+(t).$$

With a sufficient degree of precision, one can assume that during the lifetime of one generation the increase of gene frequency is linear in time. Thus, the increase of gene frequency for the time $\delta t (\delta t \leq 1)$ equals:

$$p_-(t + \delta t) - p_+(t) = [u_-(t + 1) - u_+(t) + v_-(t + 1) - v_+(t)] \cdot \delta t. \quad (1.4)$$

Substituting in (1.4) the values $u_-(t + 1)$, $v_-(t + 1)$ from (1.3) and keeping in mind that

$$u_+(t) + v_+(t) = p_+(t);$$
$$u_+(t) = p_-^2(t);$$
$$v_+(t) = p_-(t)[1 - p_-(t)];$$
$$p_+(t) = p_-(t)$$

we have

$$p_-(t + \delta t) - p_-(t) = \frac{(2\beta - \gamma - \alpha)p_-^3 - (3\beta - 2\gamma - \alpha)p_-^2 + (\beta - \gamma)p_-}{\gamma + 2(\beta - \gamma)p_- - (2\beta - \gamma - \alpha)p_-^2} \cdot \delta t.$$

$$(1.5)$$

145

Since, as shown above, $p(t)$ is a continuous function of t, it is possible to show that $dp_-/dt = \dot{p}_-$ exists and is determined at point t. Passing in (1.5) to the limit at $\delta t \to 0$ we have:

$$\frac{dp}{dt} = \frac{(2\beta - \gamma - \alpha)p^3 - (3\beta - 2\gamma - \alpha)p^2 + (\beta - \gamma)p}{\gamma + 2(\beta - \gamma)p - (2p - \gamma - \alpha)p^2} \qquad (1.6)$$

From here on, we shall omit symbol $(-)$ in p_-. In the initial condition: $p(t_0) = p_0$ with α, β, γ being constant, the equation (1.6) is integrable and its integral equals:

$$\left\{\frac{p}{p_0}\right\}^{\gamma/\beta-\gamma} \left\{\frac{1-p}{1-p_0}\right\}^{\alpha/\beta-\alpha} \left\{\frac{\epsilon-p}{\epsilon-p_0}\right\}^{\alpha\gamma-\beta^2/(\beta-\gamma)(\beta-\alpha)} = e^t; \qquad (1.7)$$

where

$$\epsilon = \frac{\beta - \gamma}{2\beta - \gamma - \alpha}.$$

From (1.7), it is clear that depending on relations between α, β, γ at $t \to \infty$ three states may be reached:

$$p_\infty = 0; \qquad p_\infty = 1; \qquad p_\infty = \epsilon.$$

Let us consider this problem in detail. Equation (1.6) can be rewritten in the form:

$$\dot{p} = \frac{p(1-p)(\epsilon-p)}{\delta + 2\epsilon p - p^2}; \qquad (1.8)$$

where

$$\delta = \frac{\gamma}{2\beta - \gamma - \alpha}.$$

We shall investigate phase trajectories of the set described by this equation on the phase plane $(\dot{p}, p; p\epsilon[0,1])$. The following cases are possible:

1) The homozygote AA is the most viable. Then $\alpha = 1$; $\beta < 1$; $\gamma < 1$. Let $\beta \geq \gamma$. In this case either $\epsilon > 1$, or $\epsilon \leq 0$. Function $f(p) = \delta + 2\epsilon p - p^2$ is positive at $\epsilon > 1$ and negative at $\epsilon \leq 0$ for any $p\epsilon[0.1]$. Then $\dot{p}$ is always positive. Hence, only one steady state $p^* = 1$ is realized. In Fig. XII 1(a) a phase trajectory at $\beta = 0.9$, $\gamma = 0.5$ is shown.
Let $\beta < \gamma$. Then $0 < \epsilon < 1$ function $f(p)$ is always negative. Therefore, $\dot{p} < 0$ at $p_0 < \epsilon$, $\dot{p} > 0$ at $p_0 > \epsilon$. Hence, there are two steady states $p^* = 0$ and $p^* = 1$. The first one is reached if $p_0 < \epsilon$, the second, if $p_0 > \epsilon$. In Fig. XII-1(b), phase trajectory at $\beta = 0.5$, $\gamma = 0.9$ is shown.

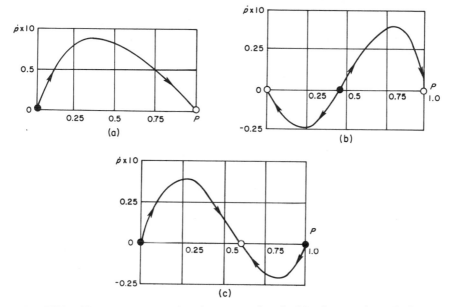

Fig. XII-1. The phase trajectories of a system, described by the equation 1.6. $\bigcirc =$ the stable state, $\bullet$ = the unstable state. (a) $\alpha = 1$; $\beta = 0.9$; $\gamma = 0.5$. (b) $\alpha = 1$; $\beta = 0.5$; $\gamma = 0.9$. (c) $\beta = 1$; $\alpha = 0.8$; $\gamma = 0.7$.

2) The heterozygote Aa is the most viable. Then $\beta = 1$; $\alpha < 1$; $\gamma < 1$. At any α and γ less than 1, $0 < \epsilon < 1$, $f(p) > 0$ for $p\epsilon[0.1]$. Therefore $\dot p > 0$ at $p_0 < \epsilon$, $\dot p < 0$ at $p_0 > \epsilon$. Hence, there is one steady state $p^* = \epsilon$, the so-called polymorphism state. In Fig. XII-1(c) a phase trajectory at $\alpha = 0.8$, $\gamma = 0.7$ is shown.

3) The homozygote aa is the most viable. In this case, by substituting A for a, we have again the first case, and it, therefore, will not be considered in detail.

Let us consider the case when $\dot p = 0$ for all p. It is clear that for this condition it is necessary and sufficient that the right part in (1.6) equals 0 at any p. This requirement is met if

$$2\beta - \gamma - \alpha = 0;$$
$$3\beta - 2\gamma - \alpha = 0;$$
$$\beta - \gamma = 0.$$

This set has a non-trivial solution: $\alpha = \beta = \gamma$. If we assume that one of the relative viability coefficients equals 1, the rest will also equal 1, which means that selection pressure is absent. Thus, we have proved in a different way Hardy's theorem (Hardy, 1908) which states that in the absence of selection pressure in a panmictic population there is no time change of the frequency ratio of genotypes.

Experimental Heterozygotic Polymorphism in Model Populations; Comparison of Theoretical and Experimental Results

The mutation ebony in *Drosophila melanogaster* (allele e^b) was used for the experiments below. In this allele heterozygotes differ from the parent normal form by a darker color, a clearly pronounced dark strip on the prothorax and a darker ventral side of the abdomen. Because of these indications of partial dominance, it is possible, practically without failure, to distinguish the flies which are heterozygous for ebony from normal ones. As a control, parallel to experiments on ebony mutation, esperiments on plexus mutation were performed, the latter being practically the same in relative viability as normal flies.

Studies on Relative Viability of Ebony Mutation in Homo- and Heterozygous States

Ebony and plexus cultures were crossed repeatedly with the same inbred normal culture for two years. As a result, homozygous ebony, plexus, and normal cultures with little genotypic difference were obtained.

In the first series the ebony flies were crossed with normal ones; then in F_2 the number of homozygous ebony flies was calculated, as well as the heterozygous and homozygous normal ones. In standard tubes with food, about 50, 150, or 300 eggs were placed per tube, laid by heterozygous flies of the first generation. The tubes with 50 eggs were not overpopulated, with 150 eggs, slightly, and with 300 eggs, severely overpopulated. All these F_1- crosses were repeated some hundredfold to obtain enough F_2- flies. The results of these experiments are shown in Table XII-1. It is clear from this table that in tubes not overpopulated the percentage of homozygous normal, heterozygous, and homozygous ebony flies corresponded well with the expected ratio 1:2:1. Accordingly, viabilities of heterozygous and homozygous ebony flies, expressed as percentages of homozygous normal in the table, were practically indistinguishable from 100 per cent.

At slight overpopulation, a positive deviation in the percentage of heterozygous flies and a vegetative deviation in that of the homozygous ebony flies was observed (about 105 and 80 per cent, respectively). At

TABLE XII-1

DETERMINATION OF RELATIVE VIABILITY OF HETEROZYGOUS AND HOMOZYGOUS EBONIES BASED ON DEPARTURES FROM EXPECTED F_2-SEGREGATION (1 : 2 : 1) IN CULTURES OVERPOPULATED TO DIFFERENT DEGREES

EGGS PER VIAL	NUMBER AND %	NUMBER AND PERCENTAGE OF FLIES				PERCENTAGE VIABLE	
		$+/+$	$+/e$	e/e	Total		
50	No.	3,201	6,407	3,183	12,791	$+/e$	100.1
	%	25.03	50.10	24.87	100	e/e	99.5
150	No.	5,341	11,183	4,262	20,786	$+/e$	104.7
	%	25.7	53.8	20.5	100	e/e	79.8
300	No.	3,887	8,423	2,791	15,101	$+/e$	108.3
	%	25.7	56.4	17.9	100	e/e	71.8

severe overpopulation, these deviations in relative viability were more pronounced: heterozygous flies gave 108 per cent and homozygous ebony, 72 per cent.

Since an error is possible in the classification of heterozygous ebony flies, a second experimental series was performed. In standard tubes with food, the following kinds and numbers of eggs were placed per tube: 100 eggs from the aforementioned plexus culture or 100 eggs of homozygous normal flies, or 100 eggs of heterozygous ebony or 100 eggs of homozygous ebony flies. The results of this experimental series are shown in Table XII-2.

In these experiments the results of the previous series were confirmed: relative viability of heterozygous ebony flies was 108.5 per cent, and homozygous ebony, 77.6 per cent of plexus, while normal and plexus had the same relative viabilities.

TABLE XII-2

RELATIVE VIABILITY OF NORMAL HOMOZYGOTES, HETEROZYGOTES, AND EBONY HOMOZYGOTES CALCULATED AS PERCENTAGE OF VIABILITY OF PLEXUS MUTATION IN OVERPOPULATED CULTURES (200 EGGS PER VIAL)

EGGS PER VIAL	NUMBER AND %	NUMBER AND PERCENTAGE OF FLIES			PERCENTAGE VIABLE (OF PLEXUS)
		px	(e)	Total	
100 px +100 $+/+$	No.	3,817	3,841	7,658	
	%	49.8	50.2	100	100.7
100 px +100 $+/e$	No.	4,281	4,537	8,719	
	%	47.3	52.7	100	108.5
100 px +100 e/e	No.	3,453	2,681	6,134	
	%	56.3	43.7	100	77.6

Thus, both experimental series showed that mutation e^b in the heterozygous state had a higher relative viability as compared to its parent normal form, while homozygous e^b flies had a rather decreased relative viability as compared to their parent form.

Experiments with Ebony in Stable Model Populations

Based on the results of the experiments described above, experiments on supplanting of ebony flies by normal ones in stable model populations were carried out.

Model populations of *Drosophila* were obtained in the following way: Twenty pairs of flies were released in boxes with thirty holes made in the bottom to place the standard feeding cups with usual food. Every day a new feeding cup with food was placed in a subsequent hole until all thirty holes were filled. Then, in the same order, an old feeding cup was replaced by a new one with fresh food and so on. This rotation of trophic medium was maintained for several years.

After about six months the number of flies in the box reached the stable level of 14,000–17,000. Later, only insignificant fluctuations from this level were observed. Two of the boxes with quantitatively stabilized populations were "infected" with 50 pairs of normal flies. Every 50 days the number of flies in these boxes was thoroughly calculated, distinguishing normal (including heterozygous ebony) and homozygous ebony flies.

In Tables XII-3 and XII-4, the results of these experiments are shown. In both boxes the supplanting of ebony by normal flies occurred rather

TABLE XII-3

DISPLACEMENT OF EBONY FLIES FROM STABLE MODEL POPULATION WITH 30-DAY FOOD CYCLE (FIRST BOX)

	NUMBERS OF FLIES			PERCENTAGE	
DAYS	e	+	Total	e	+
0	14,380	0	14,380	100	0
50	10,107	6,104	16,211	62.5	37.5
100	7,402	7,925	15,327	48.4	51.6
150	5,883	11,680	17,563	33.4	66.6
200	3,140	12,131	15,271	20.6	79.4
250	1,388	12,354	13,742	10.1	89.9
300	1,118	14,512	15,630	7.2	92.8
350	1,237	13,644	14,881	8.3	91.7
400	1,511	14,641	16,152	9.4	90.6
450	1,126	16,086	17,212	6.5	93.5
500	1,131	14,215	15,346	7.4	92.6
550	1,374	14,496	15,870	8.6	91.4
600	1,113	14,403	14,516	7.6	92.4
650	1,320	14,852	16,172	8.2	91.8

TABLE XII-4

DISPLACEMENTS OF EBONY FLIES FROM STABLE MODEL POPULATION WITH 30-DAY FOOD
CYCLE (SECOND BOX)

DAYS	NUMBER OF FLIES			PERCENTAGE	
	e	+	Total	e	+
0	15,281	0	15,281	100	0
50	9,972	6,377	16,349	58.5	41.5
100	7,336	8,374	15,710	48.9	53.1
150	5,329	9,564	14,893	35.8	64.2
200	3,161	12,689	15,850	19.9	80.1
250	1,301	14,331	15,632	8.3	91.7
300	1,601	14,523	16,124	9.9	90.1
350	1,201	13,075	14,276	8.0	92.0
400	1,347	14,067	15,414	8.7	91.3
450	1,591	15,134	16,725	9.5	90.5
500	1,548	13,789	15,337	10.1	89.9
550	1,427	14,753	16,180	8.8	91.2

quickly. After about 250 days the number of ebony flies had fallen to less than 10 per cent of the total number of flies in the box; then it became stabilized, fluctuating insignificantly about a certain mean value (8–9 per cent). In the first box calculations were performed for 650 days, in the second, for 550 days, counting from the moment of release of normal flies into the ebony population. Both populations gave very similar results as far as total number of flies in the boxes was concerned, as well as time changes and changes of stabilization level of percentage of normal and ebony flies. Fig. XII-2 shows the average percentage curve of time change

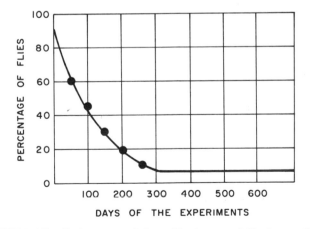

Fig. XII-2. The displacement of ebony flies by normal flies in a stable model population experiment.

of ebony flies for both boxes. Thus, both of the investigated, quantitatively stable fly populations showed that, despite a rather quick supplanting of ebony flies by normal flies at the beginning, ebony flies did not disappear from the population and were stabilized at a certain level, about which only insignificant fluctuations were observed later. It is conceivable to assume that this was due to the interaction of negative selection of homozygous ebony flies (in connection with their lowered relative viability) and positive selection of heterozygotes, which, as was shown above, are of higher relative viability.

Comparison of Theoretical and Experimental Results

In the experiments described above, a steady polymorphism state, connected with the highest viability of heterozygous flies, was observed. In the model constructed by us the following condition corresponds to this case:

$$\beta = 1; \quad \alpha < 1; \quad \gamma < 1.$$

Note that all results are preserved if we take that $\alpha = 1$, and, correspondingly, $\beta > 1$. Since in our experiments relative viability was determined in relation to normal form, we shall use the last symbols. Because the dynamics of the substitution of ebony flies was observed in quantitatively stabilized populations, it is only natural to assume the values of relative viability coefficients obtained under the conditions of highly overpopulated cultures. The following values of these coefficients were received:

$$\alpha = 1 \text{ for genotype } +/+$$
$$\beta = 1.083 \text{ for genotype } +/e$$
$$\gamma = 0.718 \text{ for genotype } e/e.$$

In control experiments with plexus mutation:

$$\beta = 1.085 \text{ for genotype } +/e$$
$$\gamma = 0.776 \text{ for genotype } e/e.$$

Let us assume the mean values of these two as relative viability coefficients for the comparison of theoretical and experimental results:

$$\beta = 1.084; \quad \gamma = 0.747.$$

The value of the polymorphous level of the wild allele (+) frequency for these values of β and γ equals:

$$p^* = \epsilon = \frac{\beta - \gamma}{2\beta - \gamma - 1} = 0.8.$$

Correspondingly, polymorphous levels for genotype frequencies will be as follows:

frequency of genotype $+/+$ $= (p^*)^2$ $= 64\%$
frequency of genotype $+/e$ $= p^*(1 - p^*) = 32\%$
frequency of genotype e/e $= (1 - p^*)^2 = 4\%$.

In our experiment the polymorphous level of genotype e/e was about 8 per cent. Correspondingly, the polymorphous level of allele $(+)$ was about 72 per cent in contrast to the theoretical level of 80 per cent. In Fig. XII-3 are shown the theoretical and experimental time-dependences of the percentage of allele $(+)$ in population. Mean longevity of one *Drosophila* generation was assumed to be 15 days (720 hours). Experimental frequency p of allele $(+)$ was calculated by formula:

$$p = 1 - \sqrt{w}$$

where w = percentage of ebony flies in population. Theoretical frequency p was calculated by formula (1.7). Since it was rather difficult at the beginning of the experiment to determine the initial frequency p_0, the frequency of allele $(+)$ 50 days (~ 3.3 generations) after the beginning of the experiment equal to 22.5 per cent was assumed for p_0.

It is seen that at the point where the experimental curve reaches the plateau (20 generations and 300 days after the beginning of the experiment), the theoretical and experimental values of p coincide. Then the theoretical value of p increases, very slowly reaching its asymptotic 80 per cent value. Apparently, the very slow substitution of allele (e) could not be determined experimentally, since it would have demanded about 100 generations to obtain a marked difference between values $p(20)$ and $p(100)$. Besides, at small values of polymorphous level of ebony homozygote ($\sim 4\%$), even rather small absolute errors in the determination

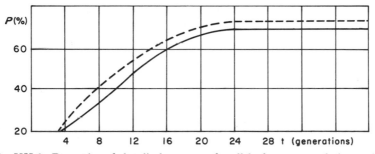

Fig. XII-3. Dynamics of the displacement of e allele from a population and the establishment of polymorphism (- - - - theoretical; —— experimental).

of percentage of homozygous ebony flies lead to greater relative errors. All these factors may somehow explain the discrepancy between theoretical and experimental results.

It is conceivable however, that a quite good correlation was obtained between theoretical and experimental data describing the dynamics of the establishment of polymorphism in population (taking into account difficulties in obtaining similar experimental data and the high probability of error). It indicates that a considerably accurate quantitative description of the real biological system was performed with the help of a mathematical model constructed by us.

ADAPTATIONAL POLYMORPHISM IN NATURAL POPULATIONS OF *Adalia bipunctata*; THEORETICAL ANALYSIS OF ADAPTATIONAL POLYMORPHISM

A population of *Adalia bipunctata* on the Institute territory in the vicinity of Berlin was chosen as material for this investigation. There was a stone building of an old church with deep crevices between stones in the southern wall. These crevices were chosen by *Adalia* and (in less quantities) other ladybug species for mass wintering places. During first two or three sunny warm days (usually in the first days of April) a mass emergence of overwintering ladybugs occurred. In the fall after the last warm period (usually at the end of October), a mass accumulation of ladybugs on the southern wall occurred. Then they crept into crevices for wintering. During these periods it was easy to collect large quantities of *Adalia* on the southern stony wall. The bugs were collected indiscriminately (all specimens) from a certain area of the wall, then divided into two main forms (red and black), scored separately, and released in the same place of wintering. In this simple way for ten years the composition of population which overwintered at a certain place was accurately estimated before and after wintering.

It is known that in many *Adalia bipunctata* populations, eight varying forms are found. Of these, three forms have black spots against brick-red background, the rest, red spots against black background. Under middle European conditions *Adalia*, as a rule, produce three generations during the vegetative period. In especially favorable years (an early spring and a late autumn), a fourth generation may appear in the fall, though such cases must be rare, according to laboratory data. In general, the last generation is most likely to overwinter, creeping into wintering places.

Adalia genetics was studied by Lus (1928, 1932, 1961) who found a simple monohybrid segregation in inheritance of red and black forms. The majority of variations of these forms described by systematists comprise a series of multiple alleles, black forms being dominant. In the population investigated by us, more than 97 per cent of all bugs belonged to forms *typica*, 4-*maculata*, 6-*pustulata*; the quantities of the remaining forms were negligible. As stated above, in our work we divided all bugs into two forms: red (*f. typica* and an insignificant number of two variants of *f. annulata*) and black (*f. 6-pustulata*, *f.* 4-*maculata* and an insignificant number of forms 2-*maculata*, *lunigera*, and *sublunata*).

After the emergence of all overwintering bugs, a rather large number of individuals which had died during winter remained in crevices, serving as wintering places. One of the large crevices was emptied thoroughly for three years before spring emergence of bugs. All *Adaliae* found were placed in glass containers. Forty-eight hours later all bugs that survived winter revived. The next day the number of live and dead bugs was estimated according to two main forms, which gave direct data on the overwintering of both forms.

Results of Quantitative Estimation of Two Main Forms in Population

The counts of bugs were performed from 1930 to 1940, excluding 1932. Altogether, in spring collections more than 55,000 individuals were registered, in autumn collections, more than 105,000. Yearly results of collections of two forms, red and black, are shown in Table XII-5.

It is clear from this table that in all cases red bugs prevailed in spring collections and black bugs in autumn ones. In spring collections the percentage of red bugs varied, during the ten years, from 57 to 71 per cent and in autumn ones, from 30 to 49 per cent.

The results obtained show that the relative viability of the red form in the winter period is higher than is that of the black one. The picture reverses in the summer period apparently because of increased rates of development and fecundity (in comparison with red form), as well as a higher rate of survival of the black form under summer conditions.

It is possible to assume that constant dimorphism in *Adalia* populations is due to differently directed selection pressure on each of the forms in different seasons. During wintering, the red form is subject to positive selection, whereas the black form is in the breeding period, the warm time of the year.

To confirm this assumption, for three years the live and dead bugs of both forms were counted at a certain wintering place, just before spring emergence. The results are shown in Table XII-6. Data in this table confirm conclusions drawn from the data of Table XII-5. For all three years, among the total number of live and dead bugs in the wintering place, the black form prevailed. Among surviving bugs, however, the red

TABLE XII-5

Number of Black and Red Forms of *Adalia* in Spring (April) and Autumn (October) Collections at the Wintering Place During Ten Years

Year	Spring					Autumn				
	Total	Black No.	Black %	Red No.	Red %	Total	Black No.	Black %	Red No.	Red %
1930	604	176	29.1	428	70.9	1,244	783	70.2	461	29.8
1931	777	334	43.0	443	57.0	1,116	622	55.7	494	44.3
1933	570	213	38.1	357	61.9	1,009	675	66.9	334	33.1
1934	432	149	34.5	283	65.5	1,237	708	66.1	529	33.9
1935	553	199	36.2	354	63.8	981	500	51.0	481	49.0
1936	492	171	34.7	321	65.3	818	435	53.2	383	46.8
1937	397	162	40.8	235	59.2	921	513	55.7	408	44.3
1938	471	192	40.7	279	59.3	880	448	51.0	432	49.0
1939	687	234	34.1	453	65.9	1,223	686	56.1	537	43.9
1940	571	239	41.8	332	58.2	1,142	755	66.1	387	33.9
Total	5,554	2,069	37.3	3,485	62.7	10,571	6,125	58.0	4,446	42.0

form predominated, exceeding the percentage of the black form by two to three times. It is quite clear that the red form has an essential advantage in winter season. In Fig. XII-4 are presented diagrams showing changes in the relative percentages of black and red forms and frequencies of corresponding alleles by years.

TABLE XII-6

<small>WINTER SURVIVAL OF *Adalia*. DATA ON THREE WINTER SEASONS FOR ONE OF THE WINTERING PLACES</small>

		TOTAL		SURVIVORS		
YEAR	FORM	No.	%	No.	%	% of Total Beetles
	Black	1,845	63.9	78	40.2	4.2
1930	Red	1,044	36.1	116	59.8	11.1
	Total	2,889	100.0	194	100.0	6.7
	Black	2,018	58.7	121	41.8	6.0
1931	Red	1,416	41.3	168	58.2	11.9
	Total	3,434	100.0	289	100.0	8.4
	Black	1,983	66.1	63	40.1	3.1
1933	Red	1,018	33.9	94	59.9	9.2
	Total	3,001	100.0	157	100.0	5.2

Theoretical Analysis of Adaptational Polymorphism

Since in the panmictic, rather large *Adalia* population, a simple monohybrid segregation takes place, one can assume that allele *A* determines black form, and allele *a*, the red one, *A* being dominant. Then heterozygotes *Aa* do not differ phenotypically from homozygotes *AA*. Hence, it is possible to assume that the relative viability of homozygote *AA* equals that of heterozygote *Aa*. As was shown above, *Adalia* usually produces three generations during the vegetative period, the third generation generally overwintering. Let us assume that two summer generations are subject to one selection pressure and the wintering generation, to another, each of these pressures being quantitatively constant during the lifetime of two summer and one wintering generations, and, correspondingly, changing abruptly from summer to wintering generations, and vice versa. The same can be said about values quantitatively characterizing these selection pressures—relative viability coefficients.

Let us consider wintering generations. Experimental data in Tables XII-5 and XII-6 allow one to determine the relative frequencies of genotypes at the beginning of the life of the wintering generation (autumn collections) and at the end of it (spring collections). Indeed, if u, $2v$, w are

157

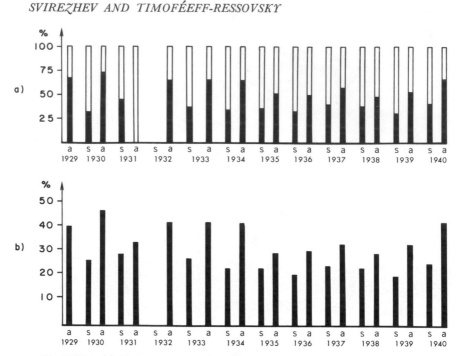

Fig. XII-4. (a) The percentage of the black and red forms of *Adalia* in spring (*s*) and autumn (*a*) populations. The dark sections of the columns indicate the black form. (*b*) The frequency of the dominant gene *A* (the black) in the population in spring (*s*) and autumn (*a*) yearly collections.

frequencies of genotypes *AA*, *Aa* (black form), and *aa* (red form) at the beginning of the life of population, and u^*, $2v^*$, w^*— at the end, then values $u + 2v$, w; $u^* + 2v^*$, w^* are the relative percentages of the black and red forms in the population in the autumn collection of the previous year and spring collection of the next year, respectively. It was shown above that the red form has maximum viability in the winter period. It is natural to assume, therefore, that the relative viability coefficient of homozygote *aa* equals 1. As above, let us denote relative viability coefficients of genotypes *AA*, *Aa*, and *aa* by α, β, γ, respectively. Then $\gamma = 1$; $\alpha = \beta$. If

$$\gamma = 1, \text{ then } \alpha - \beta = \frac{u^*v}{uv^*} - \frac{v^*w}{w^*v}.$$

From this, it is easy to calculate

$$\alpha = \beta = \frac{u^* + 2v^*}{u + 2v} \cdot \frac{w}{w^*}. \tag{3.1}$$

158

Using the results of Tables XII-5 and XII-6 and employing (3.1), it is possible to calculate the relative viability coefficients $\alpha = \beta$ for the wintering population for almost all winters from 1928 to 1940 (excluding the winter of 1931–32). Values of these coefficients are presented in Table XII-7.

Let us note that for the winter of 1930–31, we obtained two different values $\alpha = \beta$. One value $\alpha = \beta = 0.32$ was calculated according to data of Table XIII-5, when autumn and spring collections were made on the wall before the bugs crept in for wintering and immediately after emergence from wintering places. The second value $\alpha = \beta = 0.506$ was calculated according to data of Table XII-6, when before emergence from one of the crevices a relative percentage of live and dead red and black forms was calculated. However, quantitative discrepancy in the relative viability coefficients, calculated according to two different series of experimental results, is not of major importance. It can be explained by the influence of a large number of non-controlled random factors leading to considerable variations in these values.

Let us consider now the summer generations. In this case, however, we cannot calculate the relative viability coefficients directly on the ground of experimental data, because frequencies of corresponding genotypes at the beginning and end of life of the summer generations are unknown. We shall, therefore, proceed as follows. (Let us first note that since in the summer period black form has the highest relative viability, then $\alpha = \beta = 1; \gamma < 1.$)

Let us consider three generations in turn. In the wintering generation we know the frequencies of corresponding genotypes at the beginning of life of the generation. Then p_0 frequency of gene A at the moment equals

$$p_0 = 1 - \sqrt{w_0}\,; \tag{3.2}$$

where w_0 = frequency of zygote aa at the beginning of life of the wintering generation. Since we know the relative viability coefficient $\alpha = \beta$ of genotypes AA and Aa in the winter period, then from formula (1.5) we shall have (at $\alpha = \beta; \gamma = 1$)

$$p_1 = \frac{\alpha p_0}{p_0^2(1 - \alpha) - 2p_0(1 - \alpha) + 1}; \tag{3.3}$$

where p_1 = frequency of gene A at the end of the life of the wintering generation. Quite similarly (at $\alpha = \beta = 1$) for the frequency of gene A at the end of the first generation, we shall have:

$$p_2 = \frac{p_1}{p_1^2(\gamma - 1) - 2p_1(\gamma - 1) + \gamma}; \tag{3.4}$$

159

and for the frequency of gene A at the end of the life of the second summer generation:

$$p_3 = \frac{p_2}{p_2{}^2(\gamma - 1) - 2p_2(\gamma - 1) + \gamma}. \tag{3.5}$$

Here we assume that during the lifetime of two summer generations the relative viability coefficients do not change, and, finally, for the frequency of gene A at the beginning of the life of the next wintering generation we shall have:

$$p_3 = 1 - \sqrt{w_1}. \tag{3.6}$$

Here w_1 = the frequency of genotype aa at the beginning of life of the next wintering generation. Since α is known, values p_1 and p_3 may be estimated easily by formulas (3.2), (3.3), and (3.6) from experimental data in Tables XII-5 and XII-6. Excluding value p_2 from (3.4) and (3.5), we shall have an equation for estimation of

$$(1 - p_1)^4\gamma^3 + 2p_1(1 - p_1)^3\gamma^2 + p_1(1 - p_1)^2(p_1 - \delta)\gamma$$

$$= p_1{}^2[1 + \delta(2 - p_1)]; \qquad \delta = \frac{1 - 2p_3}{p_3}. \tag{3.7}$$

With the help of data in Tables XII-5, XII-6, and XII-7, let us determine from equation (3.7) the values of the relative viability coefficients γ of genotype aa for all summer periods from 1930 to 1940, excluding the summer of 1932. These values are presented in Table XII-8. For the summer of 1931, for the same reasons as for the winter of 1931–32, two values of γ are presented. In addition, calculated according to formulas (3.2), (3.3), and (3.6), the frequencies of gene A in spring and autumn of

TABLE XII-7

COEFFICIENTS OF RELATIVE VIABILITY
OF *AA* AND *Aa* ZYGOTES IN WINTER
SEASON

YEAR	$\alpha = \beta$
1929–30	0.380
1930–31	0.320 (0.506)
1932–33	0.343
1933–34	0.261
1934–35	0.291
1935–36	0.510
1936–37	0.605
1937–38	0.545
1938–39	0.498
1939–40	0.560

TABLE XII-8

COEFFICIENTS OF RELATIVE VIABILITY
OF *aa* ZYGOTES IN SUMMER SEASON

YEAR	γ
1930	0.415
1931	0.780 (0.820)
1933	0.473
1934	0.400
1935	0.775
1936	0.656
1937	0.736
1938	0.850
1939	0.612
1940	0.550

every year (beginning with the autumn of 1929 and ending with the autumn of 1940, excluding the spring of 1932) are presented in Table XII-9.

TABLE XII-9

FREQUENCIES OF GENE A (DOMINANT ALLELE) IN STUDIED POPULATION OF *Adalia* IN SPRING (s) AND AUTUMN (a)

YEAR	SEASON	FREQUENCY OF A(p)
1929	a	0.400
1930	s	0.254
1930	a	0.454 (0.400)
1931	s	0.282 (0.300)
1931	a	0.335 (0.357)
1932	s	—
1932	a	0.418
1933	s	0.254
1933	a	0.425
1934	s	0.221
1934	a	0.418
1935	s	0.228
1935	a	0.300
1936	s	0.202
1936	a	0.315
1937	s	0.241
1937	a	0.334
1938	s	0.236
1938	a	0.300
1939	s	0.202
1939	a	0.338
1940	s	0.252
1940	a	0.417

Dynamics of Adaptational Polymorphism in Adalia bipunctata Population

To receive a clearer picture of intra-population polymorphism in *Adalia bipunctata*, let us construct a phase trajectory of the dynamic system describing the change of frequency of gene A in the population under the influence of selection pressure.

Since in the summer $\alpha = \beta = 1$; $\gamma < 1$, and in the winter $- \alpha = \beta < 1$; $\gamma = 1$, equation (1.8) for summer will be written as follows:

$$\frac{dp}{dt} = \frac{p(1 - p)^2}{[\gamma/(1 - \gamma)] + 2p - p^2}; \tag{3.8}$$

and for winter as:

$$\frac{dp}{dt} = \frac{p(1 - p)^2}{[1/(\alpha - 1)] + 2p - p^2}. \tag{3.9}$$

161

SVIREZHEV AND TIMOFÉEFF-RESSOVSKY

With the help of viability coefficients taken from Tables XII-8 and
XII-9, let us construct phase trajectories of the system described by
equations (3.8), (3.9), as shown in Fig. XII-5.

It is seen from the considered phase picture that the system fluctuates
within a yearly period about a certain slowly drifting center, the deviation
of which occurs apparently as a result of changes from year to year in
climatic conditions. Since climatic conditions have a certain periodicity,
one can assume that the drift of the center also occurs about some
equilibrium and that, consequently, such state of polymorphism can be
regarded stable.

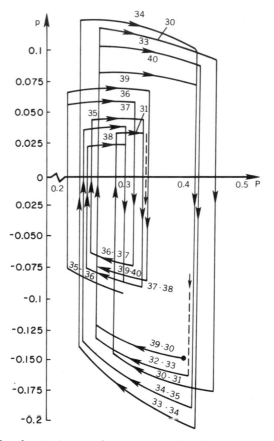

Fig. XII-5. The phase trajectory of a system describing the changes in the frequency
of gene A in the population under the action of the oppositely directed selection pressures during the different seasons of the year. The phase cycles of the winter season of
1931–32 and the summer season of 1932, for which we have no experimental data, are
dotted.

Unlike the previous case of heterozygote polymorphism, where a steady polymorphous state was secured by a higher relative viability of heterozygote and was described by a point on axis p, in this case we deal with a whole area of polymorphism, in which the describing point can not be in the state ($\hat{p} = 0; 0 < p < 1$). If environmental conditions were constant, the system would be polymorphically unstable (stable states: $p \equiv 0; p \equiv 1$), but seasonal changes of environmental conditions ensure the steady polymorphous state. It is conceivable that intra-population polymorphism in the case of *Adalia bipunctata* is ensured by different adaptation of various genotypes to environmental conditions in the winter and summer seasons, and therefore it can be termed the "adaptational polymorphism."

Conclusion

Two essentially different types of polymorphism—heterozygotic and adaptational—were studied. It was shown, both theoretically and experimentally, that in the case of heterozygotic polymorphism the stabilization of mutant homozygotes in a population is due to high relative viability of heterozygotes. Naturally, similar polymorphic conditions may be attained at some other quantitative relations between the relative viabilities under question: a necessary and sufficient requirement for such stable state of polymorphism to exist is higher relative viability of the heterozygote as compared to both the homozygotes.

Unlike the heterozygotic polymorphism, which was attained at constant values of coefficients of relative viability, the adaptational polymorphism in a population of *Adalia bipunctata* was established on the basis of periodic changes in the coefficients, connected with the various degrees of adaptation of the red and the black forms in winter and summer seasons.

References

CHETVERIKOV, S. S. 1926. On certain aspects of the evolutionary process from the standpoint of modern genetics. *Z. Exp. Biol.* (Russian), 2:3–54.

FORD, E. B. 1940. Polymorphism and taxonomy. *The New Systematics*. Oxford.

HALDANE, J. B. S. 1932. *The Causes of Evolution*. London.

————. 1935. The rate of spontaneous mutation of a human gene. *J. Genet.*, 31: 317.

————. 1938. Indirect evidence for the mating system in natural populations. *J. Genet.*, 36:213.

————. 1957. The conditions for coadaptation in polymorphism for inversion. *J. Genet.*, 55:218.

HALDANE, J. B. S., AND S. D. JAYAKAR. 1963. The solution of some equations occurring in population genetics. *J. Genet.*, 58:291.

HARDY, J. H. 1908. Mendelian proportions in a mixed population. *Science*, 5:49.

L'Héritier, Ph. 1936. Contribution a l'étude de la concurrence lavrair chez les D-S. *C. R. Soc. Biol.*, 122:264.

———. 1937. Elimination des formes mutantes dans les populations de D. *C. R. Soc. Biol.*, 124:881.

L'Héritier, Ph., and G. Teissier. 1933. Etude d'une population de D. en équilibre. *C. R. Acad. Sci.*, *Paris*, 197:1765.

———. 1934. Une éxperience de selection naturelle Courbe d'élimination du gêne "Bar" dans une population de D. équilibre. *C. R. Soc. Biol.*, 117:1049.

———. 1935. Recherches sur la concurrence vitale. Etude de populations mixtes de D. melanogaster et D. funebris. *C. R. Soc. Biol.*, 118:1396.

Jennings, H. S. 1916. The numerical results of diverse systems of breeding. *Genetics*, 1:53.

Ludwig, W. 1939. Der Begriff Selektionsvorteil und die Schnelligkeit der Selektion. *Zool. Anz.*, 126:209.

Lus, Ya. Ya. 1928. On the heredity of colour and pattern in lady-bugs, Adalia bipunctata and Adalia decempunctata. [In Russian.] *Izvestiya Buro genet.*, 6:89.

———. 1932. Analysis of dominance in heredity of elytrae and foreback pattern in Adalia bipunctata. [In Russian.] *Trudy lab. genet.*, 6:135.

———. 1961. On the biological significance of colour polymorphism in two-punctated lady-bug, Adalia bipunctata. *Latvijas entomol.*, 4:3.

Svirezhev, Yu. M., and N. W. Timoféeff-Ressovsky. 1966. On the genotypes equilibrium in model populations D. melanogaster. *Problemy kibernetiki*, vyp. 16.

Teissier, G. 1942. Persistance d'une gêne lethal dans une population de D-s. *C. R. Acad. Sci.*, Paris, 214:327.

Timoféeff-Ressovsky, N. W. 1934. Über die Vitalität einiger Genmutationen und ihrer Kombinationen bei D. funebris und ihre Abhängigkeit vom genotypischen und vom äusseren Milieu. *Z. Ind. Abst. Vererbl.*, 66:319.

———. 1940. Zur Analyse des Polymorphismus bei Adalia bipunctata. I. *Biol. Zentralbl.*, 60:130.

Timoféeff-Ressovsky, N. W., and Yu. M. Svirezhev. 1966. On the adaptational polymorphism in populations Adalia bipuncata. *Problemy kibernetiki*, vyp. 16.

Wright, S. 1939. *Statistical Genetics in Relation to Evolution.* Hermann, Paris.

JAMES F. CROW
Genetics Laboratory,
University of Wisconsin,
Madison, Wisconsin

XIII. THE COST OF EVOLUTION AND GENETIC LOADS[1]

A satisfactory theory of natural selection must be quantitative. In order to establish the view that natural selection is capable of accounting for the known facts of evolution we must show not only that it can cause a species to change, but that it can cause it to change at a rate which will account for present and past transmutations (*A Mathematical Theory of Natural and Artificial Selection* [Haldane, 1924]).

Every species observed with sufficient care has been found to include members less fit than the average and whose lack of fitness is heritable. Their number in a sufficiently large population is approximately constant, and in spite of selection does not diminish, either because the genes or chromosomal abnormalities responsible for them are continually being replenished as the result of mutation, or because they are advantageous in a different combination. We shall discuss the effect of such deleterious genes on the fitness of the species (*The Effect of Variation on Fitness* [Haldane, 1937]).

In this paper I shall try to make quantitative the fairly obvious statement that natural selection cannot occur with great intensity for a number of characters at once unless they happen to be controlled by the same genes (*The Cost of Natural Selection* [Haldane, 1957]).

Haldane's earliest work in population genetics, from which the first quotation is taken, was concerned with the dynamics of evolution. He found equations relating the rate of change in the composition of a population to the intensity of selection. Starting with the simplest cases—a single pair of alleles, random mating, discrete generations—he successively treated more and more complex problems. These included non-Mendelian inheritance, different intensities of selection in the two sexes, family selection, sex linkage, inbreeding and assortative mating, multiple factors, linkage, polyploidy, and overlapping generations. These early studies are summarized in his 1932 book, *The Causes of Evolution*, which has become a classic and was recently reissued in paperback form. One of his last articles was a witty and spirited justification of this work, entitled "A Defense of Beanbag Genetics" (1964).

[1] Paper #1135 from the Genetics Laboratory.

In his early papers he derived a number of nonlinear recurrence equations for which the mathematical solutions were not known. He could get simple solutions only for very weak and very strong selection. He was able to obtain numerical answers for intermediate selection intensities, however, that were entirely satisfactory for any datum available then (or now). He retained an interest in such equations throughout his life and 40 years later published a solution to some of them (Haldane and Jayakar, 1963).

Haldane's main object in these early investigations was to see if selection of a reasonable intensity is sufficient to account for known rates of evolution. In his very first paper he showed that the selective advantage of the melanotic form of the peppered moth would have to be at least 50 per cent to account for the observed increase in dark forms between 1848 and 1900 in the industrial areas around Manchester. In general, however, only exceedingly slight selective advantages are needed to account for most evolutionary rates.

Molecular biology has at last made possible the study of evolution in terms of actual gene substitutions rather than externally visible characters. I shall return to this subject later in considering Haldane's work on the cost of natural selection.

Haldane was concerned with the *statics* of evolution as well as the dynamics. He once remarked that biology differed from classical mechanics in that the study of dynamics came before that of statics. His early papers considered the now familiar equilibria where mutation is balanced by selective disadvantage of the mutant and where the heterozygote enjoys a competitive advantage over either homozygote. He also considered the metastable equilibrium that arises when non-allelic genes are disadvantageous individually but enter into adaptively superior combinations (Haldane, 1930). This interest, too, continued throughout his life; one of his last papers gave in a very elegant form the conditions for stability of an intermediate gene frequency at a sex-linked locus (Haldane and Jayakar, 1964).

Thus, Haldane was the first person to consider in a quantitative way the adequacy of the theory of natural selection as the underlying mechanism for evolution and the origins of species. He, along with R. A. Fisher and Sewall Wright, founded population genetics theory, and Haldane continued to contribute to this throughout his long productive life

I should like to discuss in more detail two of Haldane's papers, two that to me have been of the greatest interest and significance. In both instances he was able to see a quantitative relation of a totally new sort. Both papers have had a large impact on the thinking of population geneticists, and both (along with natural extensions by other authors) have aroused considerable controversy.

The Cost of Natural Selection

I shall consider the more recent paper (Haldane, 1957) first, since it deals more with the dynamics of evolution than with equilibria. It is therefore closely related to, and a natural extension of, his earliest work. Its purpose is set forth in the third quotation above.

In this article Haldane investigated mathematically the following situation: A population is assumed to be at equilibrium between mutation and selection. An environmental change, such as an alteration in climate, a new predator, a new source of food, or migration to a new habitat, renders the species somewhat less well adapted. The adaptation improves through natural selection, but this necessitates a certain amount of differential mortality or fertility. Concentrating on a particular locus, Haldane showed that the total number of selective deaths (or the equivalent in lowered fertility) required for this process depends mainly on p_0, the initial frequency of the gene that subsequently is favored by natural selection. If the cost, for example, were ten this would mean that during the process of gene substitution the number of selective deaths is ten times the population number in a single generation.

For a haploid organism the cost is $- \ln p_0$, which for $p_0 = 10^{-4}$ is 9.2. The value is nearly independent of the selective advantage, if this is small. With diploidy and varying degrees of dominance, Haldane estimated the cost of a gene substitution to be between 10 and 100, with 30 as a representative value. He also considered sex-linked loci and inbreeding.

To summarize, in Haldane's words: "The unit process of evolution, the substitution of one allele by another, if carried out by natural selection based on juvenile deaths, usually involves a number of deaths equal to about ten or twenty times the number in a generation, always exceeding this number, and perhaps rarely being 100 times this number. To allow for occasional high values I take thirty as a mean. If natural selection acts by diminished fertility the effect is equivalent."

I shall formulate the problem in a way that differs slightly from Haldane's original method. It turns out that this formulation makes Haldane's equations more nearly exact and, to me at least, offers a more transparent interpretation. Since Haldane's paper has raised doubts in some minds (see, for example, Brues, 1964; Van Valen, 1963), this way of presentation may help resolve some of the doubts.

167

Consider first a single locus in a haploid organism with discrete generations. The parameters are as follows:

Genotype	A	A'
Frequency	p	$q = 1 - p$
Relative fitness	1	$1 - s$

Assume that A is initially rare but is now favored by selection, perhaps because of a change in environment.

In the first generation (generation 0) the frequency of A is p_0. Relative to the A genotype, a fraction s of the A' genotype will fail to survive or reproduction will be lower by an equivalent amount. In the whole population the ratio of individuals (or genes) eliminated (i.e., not represented in the next generation because of preadult death or differential fertility) to those not eliminated will be $sq_0/(1 - sq_0)$. Next generation the proportion of A' genes will be $q_1 = q_0(1 - s)/(1 - sq_0)$ and so on in successive generations.

To be concrete, I am thinking of a population with a reproductive excess but which, because of mortality, has an adult population that is roughly constant from generation to generation. The size of the adult population will probably be regulated mainly by density-dependent factors. In this population, if $sq_0 = .2$ and therefore $1 - sq_0 = .8$, the ratio of eliminated to non-eliminated is .2/.8 or .25. In other words, to have this much selection there must be a reproductive capacity of 25 per cent in excess of the adult number if the population size is to be maintained.

I shall call the quantity $sq/(1 - sq)$, summed over all the generations involved in a gene substitution, the *cost of a gene substitution*. Designating this by C, we have

$$C = \sum \frac{sq_t}{1 - sq_t} \qquad (1)$$

If the population number at birth is N_b and at the adult stage is N_a, then $N_a = (1 - sq)N_b$ (assuming for the moment that there are no other causes of differential mortality or fertility). If, as is probably the case in most organisms, the number is regulated by other factors than this gene, N_a will be roughly constant throughout the gene substitution, although it may increase slightly as the population increases in fitness. (Haldane simply summed sq_t, which therefore measures the ratio of eliminations to the number of zygotes rather than to the number of adults.)

Notice that, if we multiply both numerator and denominator by N_b and recall that $N_a = (1 - sq)N_b$, equation (1) becomes $C = E/N_a$, where $E = \Sigma N_b sq$ is the total number of eliminations. Thus, if N_a and N_b are roughly constant, C measures the ratio of the total number of eliminations throughout the process to the number of adults in a single generation.

Here are values of C corresponding to several values of s, assuming that the initial frequency, p_0, is 0.01.

s	1.00	.99	.50	.10	.01	limit
C	99	52	6.2	4.8	4.63	4.61

Three features of these numbers are evident. The first is that the values are large. For example, if $s = .1$, the total cost is 4.8; that is to say, that the total number of "genetic deaths" during the gene substitution is about five times the number of adults in a single generation. The second feature is that the total cost is less if s is small, that is, if selection takes place slowly. Thirdly, the cost does not change much after s becomes as small as .10 and hardly at all when s is less than .01.

It is quite likely, of course, that s changes as it is placed in combination with other genes, as the population density changes, and as environmental fluctuations occur. It is not necessary for s to be constant during this process as long as it remains small and positive. On the other hand, if the sign of s varies during the process or differs in different gene combinations the total cost may be increased correspondingly.

Most evolutionists have placed major emphasis on genes of small effect. The third feature, as Haldane noted, means that the cost for such genes is nearly independent of s and depends solely on p_0, as will now be shown.

I shall assume that the change in gene frequency is slow enough that the addition in equation (1) can be replaced by integration. Thus, to a satisfactory approximation for most instances,

$$C = \int_0^\infty \frac{sq}{1 - sq}\, dt. \qquad (2)$$

From Haldane's first paper on this subject (1924), however, the increment in gene frequency for one generation is

$$\Delta p = \frac{spq}{1 - sq} \qquad (3a)$$

or, approximately,

$$dt = \frac{1 - sq}{spq}\, dp. \qquad (3b)$$

169

Substituting (3*b*) into (2) gives

$$C = \int_{p_0}^{1} \frac{dp}{p} = - \ln p_0 \tag{4}$$

as was to be shown. (As I mentioned before, Haldane's original formulation did not include the denominator in equation (2). Since he neglected the denominator in (3*a*) as being sufficiently close to unity, he also arrived at equation (4). Thus his equation (4) is a more accurate answer to the question I asked than it is to his original question. Of course, as *s* approaches 0, the distinction disappears.)

The upper limit should not be exactly 1 because the gene frequency is kept from reaching this value by reverse mutation, but that makes only a trivial difference in the cost. Furthermore, since the cost depends on the logarithm of the initial frequency, it changes rather slowly with changes in the initial frequency, as the following examples show:

p_0	$C = - \ln p_0$
10^{-6}	14
10^{-4}	9
10^{-2}	4.6
10^{-1}	2.3

The cost, therefore, is determined more easily than might have been thought.

Most of the cost is during the early generations of the gene substitution while the favorable gene is rare and the ratio of eliminations to non-eliminations is high. This means that genes that are initially common, either because of a high mutation rate or because they were only mildly disadvantageous previously, are the least costly to substitute. Moreover, it is probably just such genes with very slight effects that are most important in evolution, not only because they are initially less rare, but because a gene that is only mildly deleterious in the old environment has the best chance of being beneficial in the new. The lower cost of a gene replacement is one more argument for a micromutational view of evolution.

In a diploid species the cost is greater. The procedure for calculating it is much the same as before. I again assume discrete generations with random mating, and let *h* be a measure of dominance. The parameters are as follows:

Genotype	AA	AA'	$A'A'$
Frequency	p^2	$2pq$	q^2
Fitness	w	$w(1 - hs)$	$w(1 - s)$.

The change in frequency of gene A in one generation (Wright, 1949) is

$$\Delta p = \frac{p(w_A - \bar{w})}{\bar{w}} \approx \frac{dp}{dt} \tag{5}$$

where w_A is the average fitness of individuals carrying gene A, weighted by the number of A genes carried, and $\bar{w}$ is the average fitness of the population.

$$\bar{w} = w[1 - s(1 - p)(1 - p + 2hp)] \tag{6}$$

$$w_A = w[1 - hs(1 - p)] \tag{7}$$

By analogy with (2) the cost is

$$C = \int_0^\infty \frac{w - \bar{w}}{\bar{w}} \, dt. \tag{8}$$

Substituting from (5), (6), and (7) into (8), changing the integration limits as in (4) and integrating, we arrive at

$$C = \frac{-1}{1 - h}\left[ln\, p_0 + h\, ln\, \frac{h}{1 - h - (1 - 2h)\, p_0} \right] \tag{9}$$

when $h \neq 1$, and

$$C = - ln\, p_0 + \frac{1 - p_0}{p_0} \tag{10}$$

when $h = 1$. Note that again the equations are wonderfully free of any dependence on s.

Here are some approximate representative values.

h	p_0	Approx. C	
0	10^{-4}	9	A dominant
0.5	10^{-4}	18	
.9	10^{-3}	50	partial dominance
.99	10^{-2}	70	
1.00	10^{-2}	100	A recessive

A quantity analogous to the cost of a gene substitution is

$$C' = \sum \frac{w_A - \bar{w}}{\bar{w}} \approx \int_0^\infty \frac{w_A - \bar{w}}{\bar{w}} \, dt \tag{11}$$

which is easily calculated. Substituting from equation (5), we obtain

$$C' = \int_{p_0}^1 \frac{dp}{p} = - ln\, p_0 \tag{12}$$

which is the same as for a haploid organism.

C' will be less than C, because $w_A < w$; thus, this is a lower limit. Furthermore, C' is completely general as regards dominance, epistasis, linkage, and mating system. It is useful, therefore, in setting a lower limit on the cost of a gene substitution. Notice that in equation (9) when $h = 0$, $C = -\ln p_0$, so the least cost is with a fully dominant mutant.

Thus, in a diploid system, the cost of substituting a moderately rare mutant (e.g., one previously maintained by a mutation rate of 10^{-5} to 10^{-4}) is from 10 to 100. That is to say, the total number of eliminated individuals is 10 to 100 times the number of adults in any single generation. Haldane suggested 30 as a representative number.

With this cost value, a species that effected one gene substitution every 300 generations would have to have an average of 10 per cent reproductive excess during the process. If a pair of species differ by 1,000 loci, and 10 per cent reproductive excess were devoted (with perfect efficiency) to this process, it would have required about 300,000 generations for this divergence to take place.

These considerations show that the observed rates of amino acid changes in proteins such as hemoglobin, cytochrome C, and ribonuclease, which average very roughly one amino acid change per 10 million years in recent mammalian history, are consistent with a reasonable amount of natural selection during this period; 10,000 gene loci, each with a nucleotide substitution every two million generations, would require (if we again take 30 as the cost per substitution) a reproductive excess of $10^4 \times .5 \times 10^{-6} \times 30$, or 15 per cent.

The remarkable property that C is not dependent on s when s is small means that for a given initial frequency and dominance all substitutions have the same cost. This would make it appear that twice as much selection (on this metric) would be required to increase human height 2 mm by substituting two independent genes, each contributing 1 mm, as by one gene with twice as much effect. This is mitigated, however, by the fact that genes with small effects are likely to have higher initial frequencies.

Somewhat similar considerations apply to gene combinations. For example, if two or more linked genes are required to produce an effect, it might be possible to substitute all for the price of one, but, again, the multiple mutant genotype is likely to be initially very rare, and the cost is thereby enhanced.

Sewall Wright has suggested several times that much of evolution may depend not on substitution of initially rare mutants but on minor shifts in frequency of a number of genes with intermediate frequencies. To change one gene from a frequency of .001 to .999 is far more costly than to shift ten independent genes from .45 to .55. If these accomplished the same phenotypic effect, as might well be the case, Wright's model would require less reproductive excess.

I have assumed that the environment changed suddenly so that a previously deleterious gene immediately became favorable, as might be the case if a species migrated to a new locale. On the other hand, the change might be gradual, so that s slowly changes from negative to positive values. Fortunately, this makes only a small change in the calculations, as Kimura (1967) has shown, and the general conclusions remain essentially unchanged. For example, if s changes from $-.01$ to 0 in 10,000 generations rather than immediately, the total cost is reduced by about one-third.

An interesting application and extension of Haldane's principle has been made by Kimura (1960, 1967), who calculated the evolutionary adjustment of dominance and of mutation rates on the assumption that selection tends to minimize the sum of the cost and the mutation load.

Most organisms have a reproductive rate far in excess of that required to maintain the population size in the absence of preadult mortality. Haldane was concerned with only that part of mortality and sterility that was selective, that is to say, different for different genotypes. A million-fold reproductive excess, such as is found in some plants and invertebrates, is not necessarily more effective in selection than is an excess of a few percentages in which the differences are mainly genetic. Observations on the total reproductive rate only set an upper limit on the amount of gene substitution that could take place. We have no way, from this measurement alone, to determine whether or not Haldane's 10 per cent is a reasonable value for the amount of reproductive excess that is genetically selective.

We can go one step further by considering the *differential* contribution of various individuals. In this way fertility differences can also be taken into account. One way of looking at this is given in the next section.

A VARIANCE APPROACH TO THE COST OF NATURAL SELECTION

Another of the great generalizations in evolutionary theory is Fisher's "fundamental theorem of natural selection" (1930). This states that the rate of increase in fitness at a particular time is equal to the genetic variance in fitness at that time. I should like to attempt an application of this principle to Haldane's problem.

Letting $\overline{m}$ be the average fitness of the population, measured in Malthusian parameters (Fisher, 1930), and V_g the genic variance in fitness, the theorem states that

$$d\overline{m} = V_g dt. \qquad (13)$$

173

The genic variance (Fisher's genetic variance, Wright's additive genetic variance) is the variance associated with the least squares regression of phenotype on genotype, where each gene is assigned the same value in any genotypic combination (i.e., as if there were no dominance or epistasis). The conditions under which the theorem is exactly correct are somewhat restricted, but it is a satisfactory approximation in a great many circumstances.

Integrating both sides of (13)

$$\Delta m = m_1 - m_0 = \int_{t_0}^{t_1} V_g \, dt \tag{14}$$

where Δm is the increase in fitness during the time interval. If V_g is approximately constant

$$\Delta m = V_g(t_1 - t_0) = nV_g \tag{15}$$

where n is the number of generations involved.

This gives a way of relating the change in fitness associated with a gene substitution to the genic variance and the rate of evolution. For example, if a gene substitution produces a fitness change of Δm (or s in the earlier notation) the average number of generations required for a fitness change equivalent to a gene substitution is

$$n = \frac{\Delta m}{V_g} . \tag{16}$$

A relation quite similar to (16) has been obtained by Sved (1968) through consideration of selection based on a threshold model of gene action.

It is difficult to measure V_g from census data. One can get an upper limit by measuring the total variance in the number of progeny per individual (counted as zygotes or at birth). The appropriate measure is the variance in progeny number divided by the square of the mean—what I have called the Index of Opportunity for Selection (Crow, 1958, and later; in the 1958 paper, it was called the Index of Total Selection).

Even in those human populations with very low death rates and fairly uniform birth rates, however, the index is rather large—large enough that if all the variances were efficiently utilized for gene frequency change there would be enormous rates of evolution (Crow, 1966). The difficult question is to assess the genic component of the variance, that portion that *is* efficiently utilized. Until this can be done, I am not at all sure that a variance approach is any improvement over Haldane's principle.

The two approaches might better be regarded as complementary. The variance approach differs from Haldane's method in not being independent of s and in measuring not the number of gene substitutions but the change in fitness (or a trait correlated with fitness).

It is too soon to assess the true value of Haldane's paper. As more data from amino-acid analyses of proteins from related species are accumulated, it will be possible to see if the observed rates of evolution are consistent with a simple model of substitution of previously deleterious genes and a moderate level of selection. As stated above, this is what the earliest data seem to show. In any case I should like to quote Haldane's concluding sentence from the 1957 paper: "To conclude, I am quite aware that my conclusions will probably need drastic revision. But I am convinced that quantitative arguments of the kind here put forward should play a part in all future discussions of evolution."

Genetic Loads

Haldane's 1937 paper, from which the second quotation at the beginning of this article is taken, is much better known. One of Haldane's major points was independently discovered by Muller (1950).

In this paper Haldane showed that the effect of mutation on the fitness of a population is independent of how deleterious the mutant phenotype is but is instead determined almost entirely by the mutation rate. The reduction in fitness is equal to the total mutation rate per gamete multiplied by a factor that is between 1 and 2, depending on the dominance of the mutant genes. In this same paper Haldane demonstrated that, for a given s, the effect on fitness is much larger for a locus maintained by superior fitness of the heterozygote than for one maintained by recurrent mutation.

Haldane's paper gave the first basis for assessing the impact of mutation on the population. It also showed that any increase in mutation rate would have an effect on fitness ultimately equal to this increase. This principle, widely used by Muller and others, provided a basis for various assessments of the genetic effect of radiation at a time when the question first became one of social and political importance.

The proportion by which mutation lowers the fitness (or other trait of interest) in an equilibrium population compared to a hypothetical population without mutation I have called the mutation load. The effect of Mendelian segregation in comparison with a nonsegregating equilibrium population (i.e., one that is asexual) I have called the segregation load. This seemed to me preferable to Dobzhansky's designation as the balanced load, since the mutation load is also determined by the balance of mutation with selection.

175

The relative magnitude of the expressed mutation and segregation load in natural populations has been a subject for much discussion, and the answer is not yet clear in any diploid population that I know of.

Since I have already written a great deal on the subject of genetic loads (Crow, 1958, 1961, 1963; Morton *et al.*, 1956; Crow and Kimura, 1965), I shall not repeat it here.

The mutation load has been treated more generally with various epistatic models by Kimura (1961) and by Kimura and Maruyama (1966). The striking increase of the load in finite populations has been discussed by Kimura *et al.* (1963). A very fruitful application of the principle has been made by Morton and his colleagues in the analysis of human consanguinity effects.

I should like here to discuss only one aspect of the subject.

As Haldane first pointed out, the segregation load is much greater than the mutation load for a comparable value of *s*. Although it is difficult to place an exact limit—this is likely to differ in different organisms—it is clear that the segregation load cannot be indefinitely large; there is some sort of limit on the number of strongly selected polymorphisms.

It is important to realize, however, that segregation load considerations do not limit the number of polymorphisms per se but the total selection expended. There is no limit, according to this principle, on the number of neutral or nearly neutral polymorphisms.

Recent studies in human genetics have revealed a large number of polymorphisms. More quantitative have been the studies of Hubby and Lewontin (1966; Lewontin and Hubby, 1966), who showed that the average *Drosophila pseudoobscura* is heterozygous for at least one-eighth of its loci, if the protein sampled can be taken as representative. The authors raise the question whether this would create an inordinately large segregation load.

An alternative hypothesis based on a threshold effect has been presented in three very similar papers that appeared simultaneously (King, 1967; Sved *et al.*, 1967; Milkman, 1967). All three suggested that individuals with more than a certain number of heterozygous loci are alike, or at least not very different. In order to keep from having excessively drastic inbreeding effects—contrary to observations in many species—it is necessary to postulate also a threshold below which additional homozygotes have little or no effect.

To me, the necessity to postulate a threshold at both ends of the heterozygosity scale reduces the attractiveness of these models. In our present ignorance we cannot rule out the possibility of an upper threshold, but experimental observations suggest that whatever departures from independent gene action occur with inbreeding are in the direction of rein-forcing rather than diminishing harmful effects.

On the other hand, I agree with these authors in preferring not to postulate multiple-heterozygous genotypes that are many times as fit as the average individual in the population, but are prevented from occurring with more than an infinitesimal probability by the Mendelian mechanism. Under these circumstances I would be surprised by the ubiquity of the Mendelian form of inheritance and would expect it to be largely replaced by asexual and Oenothera-like mechanisms.

I suggest that the explanation may be a simpler, and perhaps less interesting, one. The loci that Lewontin and Hubby are studying, I suggest, are in the main not strongly selected. They may be maintained at intermediate frequencies by mutation pressure or by slight heterozygote advantage. The problem, then, becomes one of how great is the fixation tendency of random drift. An effective population number of 10^4 would maintain the majority of loci heterozygous if the total mutation rate from one to another of many neutral mutant states were 10^{-4} (Kimura and Crow, 1964). If there were slight heterosis, the number would increase, of course. This doesn't seem an excessively large effective population number for a species of *Drosophila* where migration is a real possibility.

FINAL REMARK

I hope I have written enough to make convincing the assertion that Haldane's work has stimulated a great deal of thought and research. He has more than contributed greatly to the quantification of the theories of natural selection: he has opened the ways for others to continue. The theory is on a much firmer basis, and we can now accept as the grossest of understatements Haldane's opening sentence in his famous 1937 paper: "There is good reason to believe, with Darwin, that natural selection has played a very important part in evolution."

REFERENCES

BRUES, ALICE M. 1964. The cost of evolution vs. the cost of not evolving. *Evolution*, 18:379–83.

CROW, J. F. 1958. Some possibilities for measuring selection intensities in man. *Human Biol.*, 30:1–13.

———. 1961. Population genetics. *Amer. J. Human. Genet.*, 13:137–50.

———. 1963. The concept of genetic load: a reply. *Amer. J. Human Genet.*, 15:310–15.

———. 1966. The quality of people: human evolutionary changes. *BioScience*, 16:863–67.

CROW, J. F., AND M. KIMURA. 1965. The theory of genetic loads. *Proc. XI Int. Congr. Genet.*, 3:495–505.

FISHER, R. A. 1930. *The Genetical Theory of Natural Selection*. Clarendon Press, Oxford. (Rev. ed., 1958. Dover Press, New York.)

HALDANE, J. B. S. 1924. A mathematical theory of natural and artificial selection. Part I. *Trans. Camb. Phil. Soc.*, 23:19–41.

———. 1930. A mathematical theory of natural and artificial selection. Part VIII. Metastable populations. *Proc. Camb. Phil. Soc.*, 27:137–42.

———. 1932. *The Causes of Evolution.* Harper, New York and London.

———. 1937. The effect of variation on fitness. *Amer. Natur.*, 71:337–49.

———. 1957. The cost of natural selection. *J. Genet.*, 55:511–24.

———. 1964. A defense of beanbag genetics. *Perspect. Biol. Med.*, 7:343–59.

HALDANE, J. B. S., AND S. D. JAYAKAR. 1963. The solution of some equations occurring in population genetics. *J. Genet.*, 58:291–317.

———. 1964. Equilibria under natural selection at a sex-linked locus. *J. Genet.*, 59:29–36.

HUBBY, J. L., AND R. C. LEWONTIN. 1966. A molecular approach to the study of genic heterozygosity in natural populations. I. The number of alleles at different loci in *Drosophila pseudoobscura. Genetics*, 54:577–94.

KIMURA, M. 1960. Optimum mutation rate and degree of dominance as determined by the principle of minimum genetic load. *J. Genet.*, 57:21–34.

———. 1961. Some calculations on the mutational load. *Jap. J. Genet.*, 36 (Suppl): 179–90.

———. 1967. On the evolutionary adjustment of spontaneous mutation rates. *Genet. Res.*, 9:23–34.

KIMURA, M., AND J. F. CROW. 1964. The number of alleles that can be maintained in a finite population. *Genetics*, 49:725–38.

KIMURA, M., AND T. MARUYAMA. 1966. The mutational load with epistatic gene interactions in fitness. *Genetics*, 54:1337–51.

KIMURA, M., T. MARUYAMA, AND J. F. CROW. 1963. The mutation load in small populations. *Genetics*, 48:1303–12.

KING, J. L. 1967. Continuously distributed factors affecting fitness. *Genetics*, 55: 483–92.

LEWONTIN, R. C., AND J. L. HUBBY. 1966. A molecular approach to the study of genic heterozygosity in natural populations. II. Amount of variation and degree of heterozygosity in natural populations of *Drosophila pseudoobscura. Genetics*, 54:595–609.

MILKMAN, R. D. 1967. Heterosis as a major cause of heterozygosity in nature. *Genetics*, 55:493–95.

MORTON, N. E., J. F. CROW, AND H. J. MULLER. 1956. An estimate of the mutational damage in man from data on consanguineous marriages. *Proc. Nat. Acad. Sci.*, Wash., 42:855–63.

MULLER, H. J. 1950. Our load of mutations. *Amer. J. Human Genet.*, 2:111–76.

SVED, J. A. 1968. Possible rates of gene substitution in evolution. *Amer. Natur.* (in press).

SVED, J. A., T. E. REED, AND W. F. BODMER. 1967. The number of balanced polymorphisms that can be maintained in a natural population. *Genetics*, 55:469–81.

VAN VALEN, L. 1963. Haldane's dilemma, evolutionary rates and heterosis. *Amer. Natur.*, 97:185–90.

WRIGHT, S. 1949. Adaptation and selection, pp. 365–89. *In* G. L. Jepson, G. G. Simpson, and E. Mayr (eds.), *Genetics, Paleontology, and Evolution.* Princeton Univ. Press, Princeton.

A. C. ALLISON
Clinical Research Centre Laboratories,
Mill Hill, London, England

XIV. GENETICS AND INFECTIOUS DISEASE

In his now celebrated paper on "Disease and Evolution" published in 1949, Haldane suggested that the struggle against disease, particularly infectious disease, has been a very important evolutionary agent, and that some of its results have been rather unlike those of the struggle against natural forces, hunger, and predators, or with members of the same species.

> The first question which we should ask is this. How important is disease as a killing agent in nature? On the one hand, what fraction of members of a species die of disease before reaching maturity? On the other, how far does disease reduce the fertility of those members which reach maturity?

> There is however a general fact which shows how important infectious disease must be. In every species at least one of the factors which kills it or lowers its fertility must increase in efficiency as the species becomes denser. Otherwise the species, if it increased at all, would increase without limit. A predator cannot in general be such a factor, since predators are larger than their prey, and breed more slowly. . . . Of course the density-dependent check may be lack of food or space. . . . I believe however that the density-dependent limiting factor is more often a parasite whose incidence is disproportionately raised by overcrowding.

The paper contains many other fertile ideas:

> It is an advantage for a species to be biochemically diverse, and even to be mutable as regards genes concerned in disease resistance. For the biochemically diverse species will contain at least some members capable of resisting any particular pestilence. . . . Now every species of mammal or bird so far investigated has shown a quite surprising diversity revealed by serological tests. . . . I wish to suggest that they may play a part in disease resistance, a particular race of bacteria or virus being adapted to individuals of a certain range of biochemical constitution, while those of other constitutions are relatively resistant.

In the discussion following this paper, the possibility that resistance of thalassemic heterozygotes against malaria contributed to the high frequency of that condition was mentioned. Another possibility was that "(by analogy with the advantage possessed by vermilion *Drosophila* on media deficient in tryptophan) microcythemic heterozygotes may be at

179

an advantage on diets deficient in iron or other substances, thus leading to anemia." Haldane concluded his paper "In this brief communication I have no more than attempted to suggest some lines of thought. . . . Few of them can be followed profitably except on the basis of much field work." In this respect also his insight was prophetic.

MALARIA AND THE ABNORMAL HEMOGLOBINS

While these suggestions were being presented at a Symposium on Ecological and Genetic Factors in Animal Speciation in Italy in 1949, I was working as anthropologist to the Oxford University Mount Kenya Expedition. In between periods of helping my colleagues with their collections of plants and insects, I was accumulating blood specimens from East Africans for studies of blood groups, sickling, and other genetic characters (Allison *et al.*, 1952). I noticed that the sickle-cell trait was common in tribes of different ethnic composition living near the coast of Kenya or Lake Victoria but rare in the tribes living in the high or dry country between. About this time it was also being recognized that sickle-cell anemia is relatively frequent among East African children and usually lethal. It seemed obvious that something must be counterbalancing the loss of sickle-cell genes, and, in view of the distribution of sickling and the likelihood that some blood factor was responsible, I speculated that resistance against malaria might be involved.

There was no opportunity to test the hypothesis until I had finished my medical studies and returned to East Africa in 1953. As a medical student at Oxford, I had been stimulated by the ideas of E. B. Ford on polymorphism and had helped Sir William MacArthur with his lectures and demonstrations on tropical medicine. In this way I had learned something about genetics and malaria. Two-thirds of the 1953 work in East Africa was well designed, the remaining third—as it turned out—ill designed. The first point which I recognized was the necessity of analyzing the effects of the sickle-cell trait in young children. In regions where malaria is hyperendemic the most severe effects of the disease are upon children in the age group six months to about four years. Older children and adults have considerable acquired immunity to the disease. Hence, if the sickle-cell trait exerted any protective effect against natural infections, it would have to be sought in children of the appropriate age group. This would greatly increase the difficulty of obtaining enough subjects, because it is a lot easier to carry out tests on school children and adults than on young children, but there was no alternative. Moreover, the rates and counts of *Plasmodium falciparum* in peripheral blood constituted the only index of susceptibility or resistance that one could hope to use in a short time. This was obviously less satisfactory than direct evidence of mortality, but again no alternative existed. So, collecting and staining specimens by day, and counting them by night, I steadily accumulated data on young children from Bugunda which—to my joy—showed significantly lower parasite rates and counts in those with the sickle-cell trait than in others (Allison, 1954a).

The second approach was the ecological one. I travelled extensively throughout East Africa and tested nearly 5000 subjects for sickling. High rates—up to 40 per cent—were found in tribes living in malarious areas and low rates in non-malarious areas in several different parts of Kenya, Uganda, and Tanganyika (Allison, 1954b). This distribution cut across accepted tribal affinities based on language and other anthropological characters and was, of course, the result expected if one environmental factor, namely, incidence of malaria, were particularly important in maintaining high frequencies of sickling in populations.

The third investigation was of the effects of inoculation of *P. falciparum* on subjects belonging to the same tribe with and without the sickle-cell trait (Allison, 1954a). A large difference between the two groups was found. Again, I had to use the only subjects available, and these were adults of the Luo tribe who had had prior exposure to malaria, although they had lived in a non-malarious environment for some time. Neither I nor the various experts consulted appreciated at that time how powerful and long-lasting the effects of acquired immunity to malaria can be, and, in retrospect, it seems clear that this part of the investigation was seriously biased because of greater residual immunity in the sickling than in the non-sickling group.

On return to England, my results were presented at a seminar at the Galton laboratory. Afterwards, Haldane invited me up to his room and we had a long and interesting discussion, in which I remember trying to keep him from following too many tangential arguments—on thrushes and worms and palmtrees, on everything but cabbages and kings and what I wanted to discuss! He was kind enough not to disappoint me by mentioning that he had already published the essential idea in connection with thalassemia, but others were pleased soon afterwards to draw attention to my lack of originality, concluding also that I must be wrong: the whole thing was far too simple to be true. As a result of the Galton meeting, Sheila Maynard Smith and I got together and worked out the thematic implications of the sickling problem (Allison, 1954c; Smith, 1954). The analysis still stands.

As everyone knows, the malaria hypothesis was attacked vigorously. Workers in Africa failed to find any difference in malaria parasite rates and counts between sickling and non-sickling adults and schoolchildren, who were highly immune. Later Raper (1955, 1956), Foy *et al.* (1955)—Foy had started as my most severe critic—and others looked at young children of the appropriate age groups and had no difficulty in confirming the difference between sickling and non-sickling children. In Table XIV-1, all the published observations are summarized and analyzed by the method of Woolf (1955), which allows comparisons to be made between populations with different gene frequencies and attack rates. The relative incidence of *P. falciparum* infections in non-sickling and sickling children is always above unity, the weighted mean being 1.46. The differences are significant at the 5 per cent level in eight of the ten groups. The probability is much less than 1 in 1000 that the total difference from unity would occur by chance; and the heterogeneity between groups, despite the differences in conditions under which the observations were made, is no more than would be expected by chance.

In Table XIV-2, the incidence of heavy *P. falciparum* infections is compared in sickling and non-sickling subjects. The differences are even more striking: the weighted mean relative incidence is 2.17, and the difference from unity is very significant ($\chi^2 = 51.379$ for 1 d.f.) with only slight heterogeneity between groups.

As these observations accumulated, the attack on the malaria hypothesis shifted to other ground. It was argued, chiefly by Wilson (1961), that malaria parasite counts were unrelated to potential mortality and therefore useless as an indication of the selective effects operating. In a classical study in Malaya, Field (1949), however, had shown unambiguously that the risk of fatality in falciparum malaria was closely related to the parasite count in the peripheral blood, and Vandepitte and Delaisse (1957) produced similar data from the Congo. Hence, the results in Table XIV-2 provide strong, though indirect, evidence that sickle-cell trait carriers are more likely to survive in malarious environments than non-sickling children. Direct evidence that this is so has been provided by Raper and others who have examined the hemoglobins of children dying of complicated malaria. The data are summarized in Table XIV-3. The probabilities of obtaining the observed results by chance are calculated from the binomial distribution and combined by the method of Fisher (1949), giving $\chi^2 - 46.4$ (p < 0.001). The recent data of Gilles *et al.* (1967) from Nigeria support this association still further.

Critics of the malaria hypothesis derived encouragement from the conclusion of Beutler *et al.* (1955) that there was no difference in the course of induced malaria in United States Negroes with and without the sickle-cell

TABLE XIV-1

P. falciparum Parasite Rates in African Children

Authors[a]	Subjects and Age in Years	Sickle-Cell Trait		Non-Sickle-Cell Trait		Relative Incidence[b]	Weight	Woolf χ^2	Probability
		Falciparum	Total	*Falciparum*	Total				
(1) Allison (1954a)	Uganda, <6	12	43	113	247	2.18	7.58	4.60	0.05 > p > 0.02
(2) Foy *et al.* (1955)	Kenya, <6	131	241	154	241	1.49	28.81	4.53	0.05 > p > 0.02
(3) Raper (1955)	Uganda, <10	73	191	494	1,009	1.55	38.26	7.36	0.01 > p > 0.001
(4) Colbourne and Edington (1956)	S. Ghana	42	173	270	842	1.47	27.10	4.05	0.05 > p > 0.02
(5) Colbourne and Edington (1956)	N. Ghana, <5	11	15	165	177	5.00	2.32	6.01	0.02 > p > 0.01
(6) Walters and Chwatt (1956)	Nigeria, <5	162	213	680	890	1.02	31.24	0.01	p > 0.99
(7) Edington and Laing (1957)	N. Ghana, <4	13	19	109	127	2.79	3.24	3.24	0.10 > p > 0.50
(8) Garlick (1960)	Nigeria, <6	51	91	245	342	1.98	16.95	7.93	0.01 > p > 0.001
(9) Allison and Clyde (1961)	Tanganyika, <5	77	136	272	407	1.54	24.38	4.60	0.05 > p > 0.02
(10) Thompson (1962, 1953)	S. Ghana	34	123	176	593	1.10	20.52	0.20	p > 0.50

Notes: Weighted mean relative incidence = 1.46.

Difference from unity, $\chi^2 = 29.2$ for 1 d.f., $p < 0.001$.

Heterogeneity between groups $\chi^2 = 13.5$ for 9 d.f., $0.20 > p > 0.10$.

[a] Further references in Allison (1964a).

[b] Incidence of *P. falciparum* infections in non-sickle-cell trait groups relative to unity in corresponding sickle-cell trait groups.

TABLE XIV-2

INCIDENCE OF HEAVY *P. falciparum* INFECTIONS IN AFRICAN CHILDREN

AUTHORS	CLASSIFICATION OF INFECTION	SICKLE-CELL TRAIT		NON-SICKLE-CELL TRAIT		RELATIVE INCIDENCE[a]	WEIGHT	WOOLF χ^2	PROBABILITY
		Heavy Infections	Total	Heavy Infections	Total				
(1) Allison (1954a)	Group 2 or 3	4	43	70	247	3.86	3.38	6.16	$0.02 > p > 0.01$
(2) Foy et al. (1955)	Heavy	21	241	38	241	1.96	11.99	5.43	$0.02 > p > 0.01$
(3) Raper (1955)	$> 1000/\mu l$	35	191	374	1,009	2.63	25.49	23.74	$p < 0.001$
(4) Colbourne and Edington (1956)	$> 1000/\mu l$	3	173	57	842	4.11	2.79	5.59	$0.02 > p > 0.01$
(5) Colbourne and Edington (1956)	$> 1000/\mu l$	5	15	75	177	1.47	3.07	0.46	$p > 0.50$
(8) Garlick (1960)	$> 1000/\mu l$	25	91	147	342	1.99	14.91	7.06	$0.01 > p > 0.001$
(9) Allison and Clyde (1961)	$> 1000/\mu l$	36	136	152	407	1.66	20.71	5.27	$0.05 > p > 0.02$
(10) Thompson (1962, 1963)	$> 5630/\mu l$	3	123	42	593	3.05	2.72	3.38	$0.10 > p > 0.05$

Notes: Weighted mean relative incidence = 2.17.

Heterogeneity between groups $\chi^2 = 5.719$ for 7 d.f., $0.7 > p > 0.5$.

[a] Incidence of heavy *P. falciparum* infections in non-sickle-cell trait groups relative to unity in corresponding sickle-cell trait groups.

TABLE XIV-3

DEATHS FROM MALARIA IN RELATION TO THE SICKLE-CELL TRAIT IN AFRICAN CHILDREN

AUTHOR	SUBJECTS	NO. OF DEATHS	NO. WITH SICKLE-CELL TRAIT	INCIDENCE OF SICKLE-CELL TRAIT IN POPULATION	PROBABILITY
Raper (1956)	Uganda (Kampala)	16	0	0.20	0.028148
J. and C. Lambotte-Legrand (1958)	Congo (Leopoldville)	23	0	0.235	0.0021095
Vandepitte (1959)	Congo (Luluaborg)	23	1	0.25	0.115938
Edington and Watson-Williams (1964)	Ghana (Accra)	13	0	0.08	0.33826
Edington and Watson-Williams (1964)	Nigeria (Ibadan)	29	0	0.24	0.00034953

Note: $\chi^2 = 46.4$ (10 d.f.), $p < 0.001$.

trait. These subjects were highly susceptible, having lived in a non-malarious environment. For those who read more than the summary of the paper, however, there were indications of differences between the two groups. The logarithms of parasite counts in sickling subjects were significantly lower than in subjects without the trait. It was necessary to interrupt the course of the infection in five out of eight subjects without the sickle-cell trait earlier than this was done in any of the trait carriers. What emerges is the unsuitability of the test system. The disease is induced in highly susceptible subjects by inoculation of trophozoites and cannot be allowed to run its course. It is now known that complicating factors, such as acquired immunity, greatly affect the outcome of such infections. The situation is very different from infection of infants in the field, and it is doubtful whether any useful information can be gleaned from induced infections in adult subjects.

DISTRIBUTION OF THE ABNORMAL HEMOGLOBINS

Some hundreds of thousands of individuals have now been examined for abnormal hemoglobins in different parts of the world, and the association of high frequencies with the distribution of falciparum malaria is no longer in dispute. In Africa sickling is common only in malarious areas, and the pattern is repeated in the Mediterranean countries, Arabia, India, and the West Indies (Allison, 1964a). Ceppellini (1955) drew attention to the fact that in Sardinia the thalassemia gene frequency is much higher in the formerly malarious low country than it is in the mountains, although similar blood group frequencies are found in both. In general, the pattern is repeated in New Guinea (Kidson and Gorman, 1962), in Greece (Barnicot et al., 1963; Stamatoyannopoulos and Fessas, 1964), and in Cyprus (Plato, 1964). There are, however, some malarious areas of New Guinea where low thalassemia frequencies exist (but not the reverse), and there are three non-malarious parts of Greece and Cyprus where frequencies of thalassemia carriers are of the order of 12 per cent; in malarious areas frequencies approach 30 per cent. It also has been established that most β-thalassemia homozygotes die before reaching reproductive age. Hence, there must have been some counterbalancing advantage, and even in the absence of direct evidence the distribution makes it likely that resistance of heterozygotes against malaria is the most likely main factor.

When two or more abnormal hemoglobins co-exist in the same area, an interesting problem in population genetics arises. Often individuals heterozygous for two abnormal hemoglobin genes are at a disadvantage compared with those heterozygous for one or with normal homozygotes, e.g., those with S and β-thalassemia, S and C, or E and β-thalassemia. Many years ago I predicted (Allison, 1955) that as a result of selection abnormal hemoglobin genes ought to be mutually exclusive in populations. It is now widely accepted that this is the case. In West Africa, as the frequency of Hb-C rises, toward Northern Ghana and High Volta, the frequency of Hb-S falls. In Liberia both genes are uncommon, but the frequency of β-thalassemia is reported to be higher than it is elsewhere in Africa (Allison, 1964b). In Greece frequencies of β-thalassemia are lower in areas of high sickling than in other malarious areas (Barnicot et al., 1963; Stamatoyannopoulos and Fessas, 1964). In Southeast Asia, as frequencies of β-thalassemia rise, those of Hb-E fall (Flatz et al., 1965). Considering all the factors that intervene, the distribution of abnormal hemoglobins in different parts of the world is remarkably like the predictable distribution of relatively rare mutations that have become polymorphic as a result of selection by an important infectious disease, malaria, and by diseases due to the abnormal hemoglobins themselves.

MALARIA AND GLUCOSE-6-PHOSPHATE DEHYDROGENASE DEFICIENCY

When it was becoming apparent that glucose-6-phosphate dehydrogenase (G-6-PD) deficiency of red blood cells had a distribution similar to that of abnormal hemoglobins in tropical countries, Motulsky (1960) and Allison (1960) suggested that it might also confer protection against falciparum malaria. Allison and Clyde (1961) and Harris and Gilles (1961) found lower malarial parasite counts in young East and West African children than in children with normal enzymes, which has been confirmed recently in extensive data from Nigeria (Gilles et al., 1967). On the other hand, in a small series from Nigeria (Porter et al., 1964) and a Thailand study (Kruatrachne et al., 1962) no significant differences were found in parasite counts among children with and without G-6-PD deficiency. Powell and Brewer (1965) noted no significant difference in the course of induced falciparum malaria in American Negro adults with and without enzyme deficiency; but the remarks above on similar work on sickling subjects apply also to this finding.

Some of these studies were inadequately controlled for possible complications (e.g., malaria may temporarily raise G-6-PD levels, and post-mortem specimens give very unreliable results). Control was carefully exercised in the study of Gilles et al. (1967) which provides strong evidence of protection, although it seems to be less powerfully and consistently manifested than is that provided by sickling.

The distribution of G-6-PD deficiency among different parts of the world and the clear positive correlation with the incidence of abnormal hemoglobins strongly support the interpretation that malaria has been an important selective factor (Motulsky, 1964; Allison, 1964*a*, *b*).

BLOOD GROUPS, DISEASE, AND SELECTION

Studies of blood groups, and similar antigens or leucocytes and tissue cells eliciting homograft reactions, have revealed an astonishing range of genetically controlled diversity. Arguing from a conviction that all polymorphisms are stabilized by selection, Ford (1940) suggested that blood-group polymorphisms in man might be maintained by selective forces arising because of inequalities in the susceptibility of persons possessing different blood groups to specific diseases. In the same year a striking example was discovered: hemolytic disease of the newborn was shown to be caused by Rh incompatibility. This phenomenon produces a direct selective effect on blood-group genes, the implications of which were discussed by Wiener (1942) and more fully by Haldane (1942). Inevitably, selection due to fetal-maternal blood-group incompatibility acts against heterozygotes, and such selection leads to an unstable equilibrium or a situation in which the less common (Rh-negative) gene will be eliminated from populations. Regarding the persistence of polymorphism at the Rh locus, in 1955 I drew attention to two possible explanations. The first is that the heterozygote might have a net advantage, which would be difficult to recognize in practice because of inability to distinguish serologically between heterozygotes and homozygotes. The second rests upon the known effect of ABO status upon Rh immunization. It can be shown theoretically (Kimura, 1956) that if genes at two loci interact in such a way that the selective effects upon the one set of genes are dependent upon the constitution of the other set and if selection maintains polymorphism at one locus, stability also can be achieved at the second locus. Hence, if the ABO polymorphism is maintained by selection, stability at the Rh locus might follow. Although either of these explanations is theoretically sound, we do not know what actually happens in populations. We can, however, be confident that other suggested explanations, such as that selection against the Rh-negative gene operates indirectly through malaria (Gorman, 1964), are incorrect (*see* Allison, 1964*a*).

The general point that people with different ABO blood groups show unequal susceptibility to particular diseases has been firmly established for some time (Roberts, 1959). The main examples are well known and need no recapitulation. Unfortunately, the biochemical factors underlying the susceptibility differences are unknown, and the associations between blood group and disease tell us very little about the action of selection on the blood-group genes. This is so because most of the diseases involved take their toll after reproductive age (*see* Reed, 1960) and because it is not known whether the associations are different for homozygous and heterozygous A or B subjects, which is important for theoretical analysis.

An interesting general field of study has been opened by the finding that certain bacteria, protozoa, and helminths have antigens related to blood-group substances. The observations are old and well authenticated. Now that the chemical constitutions of carbohydrates determining antigenic specificity are becoming known (Morgan, 1964; Lüderitz *et al.*, 1966), reasons for sharing of antigens are apparent. Only a finite number of combinations of constituent disaccharides, trisaccharides, and so forth exist, so that some overlap between hosts and parasites is inevitable.

Several investigators have suggested that particular organisms might be resisted unequally by subjects possessing different blood groups, either because of "naturally occurring antibodies" or because of immunological tolerance which inhibits the ability to produce antibodies against antigens resembling those possessed by the host. The whole approach has been discredited somewhat by the controversy following the claim of Vogel *et al.* (1960) that the present-day distribution of blood groups might be explained largely in terms of host selection through smallpox, plague, and syphilis. These suggestions have met with severe criticism, but the recent report by Chakravarti *et al.* (1966) claims such a strong relation between the incidence and course of virulent smallpox and ABO blood groups that an independent re-examination of the problem is called for.

There is little doubt that sharing of antigens between host and parasite sometimes can be important in the etiology of disease. Well-known examples include the demonstration of antigenic similarity between cardiac tissue and certain streptococci (Kaplan, 1964). The current hypothesis is that streptococcal infection induces autoimmunity, rheumatic fever, and glomerulonephritis. There is also an antigenic similarity between group A streptococci which give rise to glomerulonephritis in the rat and the renal glomeruli of that animal (Markowitz *et al.*, 1960). Some individuals showing good immunological responses to most stimuli show specific failures to respond. Thus, patients with vaccinia gangrenosa do not have circulating antibody against vaccinia virus, although their γ-globulin levels are normal (Kempe *et al.*, 1956). Children, apparently normal immunologically, suffering from recurrent staphylococcal infections, lack antibodies which inhibit the Müller reaction (Quic and Wanamaker, 1960). One explanation is that such individuals share antigenic determinants with the parasites in question that are lacking in normal individuals; hence they are less immunologically responsive, or more readily paralyzed by abundant antigen, than are normal subjects. Rowley and Jenkin

(1962) concluded that sharing of antigens between mouse tissues and *Salmonella typhimurium* CS contributes to the pathogenicity of this organism for mice. Other evidence that sharing of antigens between parasites and hosts may affect susceptibility to disease is reviewed by Jenkin (1963) and Boyden (1963).

Considering the problem from the wider evolutionary viewpoint, the only plausible explanation so far advanced for the existence of blood groups and similar antigens giving rise to homograft reactions seems to be the maintenance of variability in host populations in respect of resistance against disease. Cell-mediated immune responses themselves presumably arose in the first place as part of the defense against parasites, and they are clearly important in resistance against some infectious agents, such as mycobacteria. Later, as Burnet (1964) and others have suggested, cell-mediated immune responses may have been mobilized as a policing system to dispose of malignant cells with antigens different from those of the host.

But why should heterogeneity of antigenic make-up have arisen in the first place? Its presence poses biological problems, including maternal-fetal incompatibility. A reasonable answer seems to be that it is advantageous for a population to maintain variability in respect of genetic constitution, including blood-group constitution, and capacity to resist a wide variety of diseases. Any homogeneous population might be exterminated by a particular epidemic infection.

In discussions of the mechanisms by which such polymorphisms are maintained, one point appears to have been overlooked. This is that if sharing of antigens between hosts and parasites is disadvantageous, then heterozygotes (having a wider range of antigens) will be at a greater disadvantage than homozygotes. Hence, selection will tend to operate against heterozygotes, which cannot lead to stable polymorphism. It therefore seems likely that other factors—of which we know very little—may be operating so as to relate blood-group constitution in a more positive way to susceptibility to disease.

That such relations do, in fact, exist is established in man and experimental animals. Thus, McDonald and Zuckerman (1962) found that among Air Force recruits exposed to a new strain of influenza A2 virus, those infected showed a highly significant excess of group O, and a corresponding deficiency of A, compared with controls in all three regions tested. Lilly *et al.* (1964) found a relation between susceptibility to leukemogenesis by Gross virus and H-2 genotype. The H-2 antigens are present on erythrocytes and many other cells and are determined by a series of closely linked genes. Mice homozygous for H-2K were much more susceptible to virus oncogenesis than were mice heterozygous for or lacking H-2k.

The whole question has been taken a step further by Bailey (1966). In a series of five large experiments he analyzed gene mutation histocompatibility by tail skin-graft tests in isogenic mice. The observed mutation rate per zygote was more than 1 per cent; most mutational changes were gains in an antigen; the number of mutants was not increased by paternal X-ray treatment; and the environment in which the parents were born and raised affected the incidence of "mutations." To explain the results Bailey suggests that the observed changes in histocompatibility were the result of the incorporation of viral genomes into germinal cells of parents in a manner paralleling the phenomenon of lysogeny and lysogenic conversion in bacteria. The hypothesis was then extended to explain the origin and function of the histocompatibility and blood-group genes. There is no space here for full discussion of these generalizations, which are stimulating but not without their difficulties. Some points are mentioned below.

The data already accumulated are sufficient to bear out Haldane's suggestions regarding the relation between antigenic variability and susceptibility to infectious disease. In general, from the Rh case and other examples we can be certain that selection is operating on human blood-group genes, and observations in animals indicate that the effects can be quite strong. Thus, several small inbred lines of chickens have remained polymorphic for one or more blood-group systems. All of the highly inbred white leghorn lines studied by Gilmour (1962) still show segregation of at least one to four blood-group loci. The levels of inbreeding reached are the result of from 21 to 26 generations of full sibmatings, corresponding to computed coefficients of 98.9 to 99.6 per cent. Briles (1960) sampled 73 different closed populations (inbred up to coefficients of 86 per cent) and found segregation at the B locus in all but two of them; most were polymorphic for other blood-group systems as well. This type of evidence argues powerfully for heterozygous advantage, because in the absence of selection many of the populations should have become homozygous for the blood-group alleles. Morton et al. (1966) found that blood-group and transferrin genotypes were related to the mortality of chick embryos, thus providing direct evidence of selection. Though the general effect was of over-dominance, the observed genotypic mortality differences by themselves could not explain the persistence of polymorphisms at the loci in question.

Genetic Basis of Resistance Against Bacteria or Viruses

Considering resistance against infections from the genetic standpoint, two aspects have to be borne in mind: genetically controlled variation in the invading organism giving rise to differences in pathogenicity and genetically controlled variation in the resistance of host organisms. The outcome of an infection depends mainly on the interaction of these two factors, though nutrition and other environmental factors may also be contributory. Analyzing the host response, a distinction also must be made between cases of resistance which are under control of single, major genetic factors and those which are determined by many genes. Where single genetic factors are important, plots of susceptibility to a given organism show a bimodal or trimodal distribution, some hosts being much more resistant than others, and the resistance segregates among the progeny of resistant and susceptible hosts. On the other hand, when many genes are involved, plots of susceptibility show a continuous distribution and there is no clear-cut segregation among progeny.

Single-gene mechanisms of resistance against parasites or noxious chemicals are widespread among living organisms. As a rule, resistance against drugs or insecticides is inherited in this way. Turning to viruses, single-gene mutations often allow bacteria to resist infection by bacteriophages that can multiply in the parental host strains; single-gene mutations in the phages can sometimes overcome this resistance (*see* Adams, 1959; Stent, 1964). Special interest attaches to the so-called conditional lethal mutations which impair complete development under certain conditions, for these have provided useful information about the genetic control of synthesis of virus components (Epstein *et al.*, 1963).

Numerous examples of single-gene resistance against infection come from plant genetics (*see* Walker, 1951; Holmes, 1965). This type of resistance is fortunately common and allows ready fixation of resistance genes in desirable stocks by suitable breeding programs. It is no exaggeration to state that present-day civilization is dependent on efficient agricultural production, and the latter has been possible only because cereals and other plants resistant to pandemics have been developed.

In mammals resistance against pathogens is complicated by a variety of immune responses, which are themselves more or less directly under genetic control. The interplay between other forms of innate resistance and immune responses is a delicate one. There is, nevertheless, good evidence that single genes can make a major contribution to resistance or susceptibility. I have reviewed the situation with regard to viruses (Allison, 1965). Several examples of single-gene resistance, sometimes dominant, sometimes recessive, are found in mice. Bang and Warwick (1960) showed, moreover, that cultures of macrophages from susceptible mice were destroyed by mouse hepatitis virus, whereas cultures of cells from resistant strains of mice were not. This finding also has been demonstrated in the case of arboviruses of the B group. Thus, the susceptibility of an individual cell to infection parallels that of the whole animal, and resistance is not due to an orthodox immune response.

A relatively common situation, however, seems to be graded and continuous distribution of host resistance factors, which are inherited in a manner suggesting segregation of several gene pairs. Gowen (1961) has summarized much information of this kind. Thus the outcome of infections of chickens with *Salmonella pullorum* or mice with *Salmonella typhimurium* depends upon the virulence of the strain of infecting organism used and the inherited resistance of the host.

The well-known work of Fenner and his colleagues (*see* Fenner and Ratcliffe, 1965) on myxomatosis illustrates the potency of infectious disease as a selective agent under natural conditions. When the virus was first introduced into the Australian rabbit population, it was highly virulent and killed more than 95 per cent of the infected animals. The small proportion of survivors multiplied, and some of their progeny were still susceptible, so there was a series of epidemics. When rabbits were trapped year by year and tested under conditions which precluded effects of antibody, however, the wild populations were found to have markedly increased resistance to a standard challenge dose of virus. The virus itself changed, isolates from wild animals becoming less virulent than the parent virus but virulent enough to attain high concentrations in skins of infected animals, thereby ensuring continued transmission under natural conditions. It is also interesting that the virus has remained more virulent in England, where flea transmission would be facilitated by killing the host, than it has in Australia. This is a nice example of evolution of host and parasite so as to ensure survival of both. Other examples of interactions between genetic factors and infectious agents are not yet fully understood. Different breeds of sheep show wide variation in susceptibility to scrapie, a degenerative disease of the nervous system, and Parry (1962) concluded that the disease is inherited as a simple Mendelian recessive character. Since a virus with unusual properties can reproduce scrapie in mice (*see* Chandler, 1963), a reasonable conclusion is that genetic factors of the sort analyzed by Parry were influencing susceptibility to infection by the agent. Kuru, a degenerative disease of the human nervous system, shows a familial concentration in certain New Guinea highlanders, and Gajdusek (1963) has suggested that it may be analogous to scrapie. Intracerebral inocula of brain extracts from subjects with kuru reproduced a

193

similar disease in chimpanzees, which now has been passed to other chimpanzees (Gajdusek *et al.*, 1967). Hence, it seems that an infectious agent probably is involved, to which the New Guineans are unusually susceptible.

For reasons which are sufficiently obvious, analysis of genetic components in resistance against infectious disease is much more difficult in man than in experimental animals. Exceptions are the undue susceptibility to infection of subjects with certain rare inherited conditions, such as hypogammaglobulinemia and the Chediak-Higashi syndrome. There can be little doubt, however, that genetically controlled resistance is powerful and differs among the several races of mankind. Thus, United States Negroes show considerable resistance against the malaria parasites *Plasmodium vivax* (Boyd and Stratman-Thomas, 1933) and *P. knowlesi* (Milam and Coggeshall, 1938). This is not due to acquired immunity, abnormal hemoglobins, or glucose-6-phosphate dehydrogenase deficiency. On the other hand, Africans and some other populations are more susceptible to measles than western Europeans. Thus, African children exposed to a standard vaccine strain of measles virus showed more severe effects than were produced by the same virus in European children (Morley *et al.*, 1963). It is unlikely that diet and other environmental factors alone can account for these differences.

GENETIC CHANGES AS A RESULT OF INFECTION

So far, genetic factors in hosts influencing the course of infectious disease have been considered. Equally interesting is the fact that infection actually can produce genetic changes in host cells. The most obvious example is the malignant growth following virus infection in experimental animals or tissue cultures. The malignant potentialities are perpetuated in the progeny cells, so this must be regarded as a genetic change. Furthermore, virus-specific antigens are demonstrable in the tumor cells by transplantation resistance, complement fixation, and other tests (see Hellström and Möller, 1965). This again fits the formal definition of a genetic change.

Recently, we have been looking at quite another situation, in which we suspect that infectious disease also may be producing a genetic change (Allison and Paton, 1966). This is in the trisomy of human chromosome 21 producing Down's syndrome (mongolism), the incidence of which rises markedly with increasing maternal age (Fig. XIV-1). Earlier suggestions that Down's syndrome might follow parental tuberculosis or infective hepatitis seem unlikely, but antibodies to *Mycoplasma hominis* type 1 are commoner and attain higher levels in women toward the end of repro-

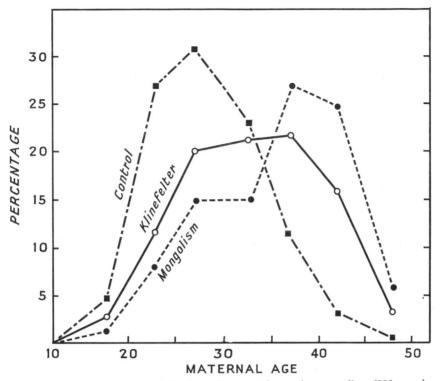

Fig. XIV-1. Percentage distribution of maternal ages in mongolism (883 cases), XXY Klinefelter's syndrome (175 cases), and a control population. (By courtesy of Prof. L. S. Penrose and Dr. M. A. Ferguson-Smith [from Allison and Paton, 1966].)

ductive life than in younger or older women (Fig. XIV-2). Mycoplasmas have been isolated from the female reproductive tract, including the fallopian tube and ovary, and we suggest that mycoplasma infection might result in abnormal meiotic division and trisomy. The relation of Klinefelter's syndrome to maternal age (Fig. XIV-1) suggests that the maternal age effect is common to several trisomies, and is not specific for Down's syndrome. There is a simple biochemical mechanism by which mycoplasmas might produce a disorder in spindle functioning, namely, production of hydrogen peroxide. This substance is the hemolysin of mycoplasmas and is produced in large amounts by $M.$ $pneumoniae$ and in smaller amounts by other mycoplasmas. Exposure of cells to hydrogen peroxide is known to produce chromosomal abnormalities, some apparently owing to malfunctioning of mitotic spindles (see Biesele, 1958). When human diploid cells were cultured in the presence of $M.$ $hominis$ type 1, significantly increased numbers of endoreduplications and chromosome

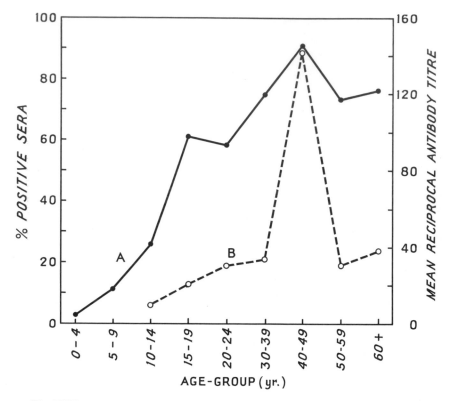

Fig. XIV-2. Antibody to *M. hominis* type 1 (strain DC 63) measured by indirect hemagglutination (from Taylor-Robinson *et al.*): (*A*) percentage of sera with antibody titre of 1:10 or greater; (*B*) geometric mean titre of antibody expressed as a reciprocal (from Allison and Paton, 1966).

aberrations were observed (Allison and Paton, 1966). Any extrapolation from these results *in vitro* to what happens *in vivo* in the reproductive tract must be tentative, but a comparison of the antibody status of mothers of mongols and carefully matched controls is in progress at present. If the association with *M. hominis* type 1 infection holds up, the results will be important because they may provide a way of preventing the occurrence of such trisomies, which represent a high proportion of all congenital defectives.

PROSPECTS

There has been considerable progress during the past fifteen years. When Haldane wrote his paper on disease and evolution in 1949, the concept was hypothetical. Now we can be quite confident that natural selection *does* operate in human populations, and that disease *is* a potent cause of selection. A great deal of information about the genetic basis of disease resistance in plants and experimental animals has accumulated, and the chemistry underlying the resistance is coming to light here and there. The structure of abnormal hemoglobins is known, as is that of many blood-group specific substances and antigens in bacteria. The main focus of attention at present seems to be on defining more precisely genetic factors underlying resistance against certain viruses, such as the leukosis viruses in chickens, and genetic factors influencing the capacity of hosts to respond immunologically against defined antigens. The nature of new antigens induced by viruses in hosts also attracts a great deal of interest. The possibility that these processes resemble lysogenic conversion in bacteriophages deserves careful analysis. Now that such conversion is explicable in precise chemical terms, the extension of such work to mammalian cells should take place before too long. The borderlines between genetics, immunology, infectious disease, and molecular biology are becoming blurred. Haldane, who was himself no respecter of boundaries and was a pioneer in biochemical genetics, surely would have viewed these trends with satisfaction.

REFERENCES

ADAMS, M. H. (ed.). 1959. *Bacteriophages.* Interscience, New York.

ALLISON, A. C. 1954a. Protection afforded by the sickle-cell trait against subtertian malarial infection. *Brit. Med. J.*, 1:290.

———. 1954b. The distribution of the sickle-cell trait in East Africa and elsewhere, and its apparent relationship to the incidence of subtertian malaria. *Trans. Roy. Soc. Trop. Med. Hyg.*, 48:312.

———. 1954c. Notes on sickle-cell polymorphism. *Ann. Human Genet.*, 19:39.

———. 1955. Aspects of polymorphism in man. *Cold Spr. Harb. Symp. Quant. Biol.*, 20:239.

———. 1960. Glucose-6-phosphate dehydrogenase deficiency in red blood cells of East Africans. *Nature*, 186:431.

———. 1964a. Polymorphism and natural selection in human populations. *Cold Spr. Harb. Symp. Quant. Biol.*, 29:137.

———. 1964b. Population genetics of abnormal haemoglobins and glucose-6-phosphate dehydrogenase deficiency, p. 365. *In* J. H. P. Jonxis (ed.), *Abnormal haemoglobins in Africa.* Blackwell, Oxford.

———. 1965. Genetic factors in resistance against virus infections. *Archiv. Ges. Virusforsch.*, 17:280.

ALLISON, A. C., AND D. F. CLYDE. 1961. Malaria in African children with deficient glucose-6-phosphate dehydrogenase. *Brit. Med. J.*, 1:1346.

ALLISON, A. C., E. W. IKIN, AND A. E. MOURANT. 1952. Blood groups in some East African tribes. *J. Roy. Anthropol. Inst.*, 82:55.

ALLISON, A. C., AND G. R. PATON. 1966. Chromosomal abnormalities in human diploid cells infected with mycoplasma and their possible relevance to the aetiology of Down's syndrome (Mongolism). *Lancet*, 2:1229.

BAILEY, D. W. 1966. Heritable histocompatibility changes: lysogeny in mice? *Transplantation*, 4:482.

BANG, F. B., AND A. WARWICK. 1960. Mouse macrophages as host cells for the mouse hepatitis virus and the genetic basis of susceptibility. *Proc. Nat. Acad. Sci., Wash.*, 46:1065.

BARNICOT, N. A., A. C. ALLISON, B. S. BLUMBERG, G. DELIYANNIS, C. KRIMBAS, AND A. BALLAS. 1963. Haemoglobin types in Greek populations. *Ann. Human Genet.*, 26:229.

BEUTLER, E., R. J. DERN, AND C. L. FLANAGAN. 1955. Effect of sickle-cell trait on resistance to malaria. *Brit. Med. J.*, 1:1189.

BIESELE, J. J. 1958. *Mitotic Poisons and the Cancer Problem.* Elsevier, London.

BOYD, M. F., AND W. K. STRATMAN-THOMAS. 1933. Studies on benign tertian malaria; on the refractoriness of negroes to infection *P. vivax. Amer. J. Hyg.*, 14:485.

BOYDEN, S. V. 1963. Cellular recognition of foreign matter. *Int. Rev. Exp. Pathol.*, 2:311.

BRILES, W. E. 1960. Blood groups in chickens, their nature and utilization. *World's Poultry Sci.*, 16:223.

BURNET, F. M. 1964. Immunological factors in the process of carcinogenesis. *Brit. Med. Bull.* 20:154.

CEPPELLINI, R. 1955. Discussion of polymorphism in man. *Cold Spr. Harb. Symp. Quant. Biol.*, 20:252.

CHAKRAVARTI, M. R., B. K. VERMA, T. V. HANUROV, AND F. VOGEL. 1966. Relation between smallpox and the ABO blood groups in a rural population in West Bengal. *Humangenetik*, 2:78.

CHANDLER, R. L. 1963. Experimental scrapie in the mouse. *Res. Vet. Sci.*, 4:276.

COLBOURNE, M. J., AND G. M. EDINGTON. 1956. Sickling and malaria in the Gold Coast. *Brit. Med. J.*, 1:784.

EDINGTON, G. M., AND W. N. LAING. 1957. Relationship between haemoglobins S. and C. and malaria in the Gold Coast. *Brit. Med. J.*, 11:143.

EDINGTON, G. M., AND G. J. WATSON-WILLIAMS. 1964. Sickling, haemoglobin C, glucose-6-phosphate dehydrogenase deficiency and malaria in Western Nigeria. *In*, J. H. P. Jonxis, ed., *Abnormal Haemoglobins in Africa.* Blackwell, Oxford.

EPSTEIN, R. H., A. BALLE, C. M. STEINBERG, E. KELLENBERGER, R. S. EDGAR, M. SUSMAN, H. G. DENHARDT, AND A. LIELAUSIS. 1963. Physiological studies on conditional lethal mutants of bacteriophage T_4D. *Cold Spr. Harb. Symp. Quant. Biol.*, 28:375.

FENNER, F., AND F. N. RATCLIFFE. 1965. *Myxomatosis.* Univ. Press, Cambridge.

FIELD, J. W. 1949. Blood examination and prognosis in acute falciparum malaria. *Trans. Roy. Soc. Trop. Med. Hyg.*, 43:33.

FISHER, R. A. 1959. *Statistical Methods for Research Workers.* Oliver and Boyd, Edinburgh, p. 99.

FLATZ, G., C. PIK, AND S. SRINGAM. 1965. Haemoglobin E and β-thalassaemia: their distribution in Thailand. *Ann. Human Genet.*, 29:151.

FORD, E. B. 1940. *Genetics for Medical Students.* Methuen, London.

Foy, H., W. Brass, R. A. Moore, G. Timms, A. Kondi, and T. Oluoch. 1955. Two surveys to investigate the relation of the sickle-cell trait and malaria. *Brit. Med. J.*, 1:289.

Gajdusek, D. C. 1963. Kuru. *Trans. Roy. Soc. Trop. Med. Hyg.*, 57:151.

Gajdusek, D. C., C. J. Gibbs, and M. Alpers. 1967. Transmission and passage of experimental "kuru" to chimpanzees. *Science*, 155:212.

Garlick, J. P. 1960. Sickling and malaria in South West Nigeria. *Trans. Roy. Soc. Trop. Med. Hyg.*, 54:146.

Gilles, H. M., K. A. Fletcher, R. G. Hendrickse, R. Lindner, S. Reddy, and N. Allan. 1967. Glucose-6-phosphate dehydrogenase deficiency, sickling and malaria in African children in South-Western Nigeria. *Lancet*, 1:138.

Gilmour, D. G. 1962. Blood groups in chickens. *Ann. N.Y. Acad. Sci.*, 97:166.

Gorman, J. G. 1964. Selection against the Rh-negative gene by malaria. *Nature*, 202:676.

Gowen, J. W. 1961. Experimental analysis of genetic determinants in resistance to infectious disease. *Ann. N.Y. Acad. Sci.*, 91:689.

Haldane, J. B. S. 1942. Selection against heterozygosis in man. *Ann. Eugen.*, 11:333.

———. 1949. Disease and evolution. *La Ricerca Sci.*, 19 (Suppl.):68.

Harris, R., and H. M. Gilles. 1961. Glucose-6-phosphate dehydrogenase deficiency in the peoples of the Niger delta. *Ann. Human Genet.*, 25:199.

Hellström, K. E., and G. Möller. 1965. Immunological and immunogenic aspects of tumour transplantation. *Progr. Allergy*, 9:158.

Holmes, F. O. 1965. *Advances in Virus Res.*, 11:139.

Jenkin, C. R. 1963. Heterophile antigens and their significance in host-parasite relationship. *Advance Immunol.*, 3:351.

Kaplan, M. H. 1964. Immunological cross-reaction between group A streptococcal cells and mammalian tissues; a possible relationship to induction of autoimmunity in rheumatic fever. *In* J. W. Uhr (ed.), *The Streptococcus, Rheumatic Fever and Glomerulonephritis*. Williams and Wilkins Co., Baltimore.

Kempe, C. H., T. O. Berge, and B. England. 1956. Hyperimmune vaccinal gamma globulin; source, evaluation and use in prophylaxis and therapy. *Pediatrics*, 18:177.

Kidson, C., and J. G. Gorman. 1962. A challenge to the concept of selection by malaria in glucose-6-phosphate dehydrogenase deficiency. *Nature*, 196:49.

Kimura, M. 1956. A model of a genetic system which leads to closer linkage by natural selection. *Evolution*, 10:278.

Kruatrachne, M., P. Charoenlarp, T. Chongsuphajaisiddhi, and C. Harinasuta. 1962. Erythrocyte glucose-6-phosphate dehydrogenase and malaria in Thailand. *Lancet*, 2:1183.

Lambotte-Legrand, J., and C. Lambotte-Legrand. 1958. Notes complémentaires sur la drépanocytose. II. Sicklémi et malaria. *Ann. Soc. Belge Med. Trop.*, 38:45.

Lilly, F., E. A. Boyse, and L. J. Old. 1964. Genetic basis of susceptibility to viral leukemogenesis. *Lancet*, 2:1207.

Lüderitz, O., A. M. Staub, and O. Westphal. 1966. Immunochemistry of the O and R antigens of *Salmonella* and related *Enterobacteriaceae*. *Bacteriol Rev.*, 30:192.

McDonald, J. C., and A. J. Zuckerman. 1962. ABO blood groups and acute respiratory virus disease. *Brit. Med. J.*, 2:89.

MARKOWITZ, A. S., S. H. ARMSTRONG, AND D. S. KUSHNER. 1960. Immunological relationships between the rat glomerulus and nephritogenic streptococci. *Nature*, 187:1095.

MILAM, F., AND L. T. COGGESHALL. 1938. Duration of *Plasmodium knowlesi* infections in man. *Amer. J. Trop. Med. Hyg.*, 18:331.

MORGAN, W. T. J. 1964. Some aspects of immunological specificity in terms of carbohydrate structure. *Bull. Soc. Chim. Biol.*, 46:1627.

MORLEY, D., N. WOODLAND, AND W. J. MARTIN. 1963. Measles in Nigerian children; a study of the disease in West Africa, and its manifestations in England and other countries, during different epochs. *J. Hyg., Camb.*, 61:115.

MORTON, J. R., D. G. GILMOUR, E. M. McDERMID, AND A. L. OGDEN. 1965. Association of blood group and protein polymorphisms with embryonic mortality in the chicken. *Genetics*, 51:97.

MOTULSKY, A. G. 1960. Metabolic polymorphisms and the role of infectious diseases in human evolution. *Human Biol.*, 32:28.

————. 1964. Theoretical and clinical problems of glucose-6-phosphate dehydrogenase deficiency, p. 143. *In* J. H. P. Jonxis (ed.). *Abnormal Haemoglobins in Africa*. Blackwell, Oxford.

PARRY, H. B. 1962. Scrapie: a transmissible and hereditary disease of sheep. *Heredity*, 17:75.

PLATO, C. C., D. L. RUCKNAGEL, AND H. GERSHOWITZ. 1964. Studies on the distribution of glucose-6-phosphate dehydrogenase deficiency, thalassemia and other genetic traits in the coastal and mountain villages of Cyprus. *Ann. Human Genet.*, 16:267.

PORTER, I. H., S. H. BOYER, E. J. WATSON-WILLIAMS, A. ADAM, A. SZEINBERG, AND M. SINISCALCO. 1964. Variation of glucose-6-phosphate dehydrogenase in different populations. *Lancet*, 1:895.

POWELL, R. D., AND G. J. BREWER. 1965. Glucose-6-phosphate dehydrogenase deficiency and falciparum malaria. *Amer. J. Trop. Med.*, 14:358.

QUIE, P. G., AND L. W. WANNAMAKER. 1960. An unusual staphylococcal product and its host interactions. *Univ. Minn. Med. Bull.*, 32:125.

RAPER, A. B. 1955. Malaria and the sickling trait. *Brit. Med. J.*, 1:1186.

————. 1956. Sickling in relation to morbidity from malaria and other diseases. *Brit. Med. J.*, 1:965.

REED, T. E. 1960. Polymorphism and natural selection in blood groups. In *Genetic Polymorphisms and Geographic Variations in Disease*. U.S. Public Health Service, Washington.

ROBERTS, J. A. F. 1959. Some associations between blood groups and disease. *Brit. Med. Bull.*, 15:129.

ROWLEY, D., AND C. R. JENKIN. 1962. Antigenic cross-reaction between host and parasite. *Nature*, 193:151.

SMITH, S. M. 1954. Appendix to notes on sickle-cell polymorphism. *Ann. Human. Genet.*, 19:39.

STAMATOYANNOPOULOS, G., AND R. FESSAS. 1964. Thalassemia and glucose-6-phosphate dehydrogenase, sickling and malarial endemicity in Greece; a study of five areas. *Brit. Med. J.*, 1:875.

STENT, G. S. 1964. *Molecular Biology of the Bacterial Viruses*. W. H. Freeman and Co., San Francisco.

THOMPSON, G. R. 1962. Significance of haemoglobins S and C in Ghana. *Brit. Med. J.*, 1:682.

————. 1963. Malaria and stress in relation to haemoglobins S and C. *Brit. Med. J.*, 2:976.

VANDEPITTE, J. 1959. The incidence of haemoglobinoses in the Belgian Congo. *In* J. H. P. Jonxis and J. F. Delafresnaye (eds.), *Abnormal Haemoglobins.* Blackwell, Oxford.

VANDEPITTE, J., AND J. DELAISSE. 1957. Sicklémia et paludisme. *Ann. Soc. Belg. Méd. Trop.*, 37:703.

VOGEL, F., H. J. PETTENKOFER, AND W. HELMBOLD. 1960. Über die Populationsgenetik der ABO-Blutgruppen. 2. Mttlg: Genhaufigkeit und epidemische Erkravkungen. *Acta genet.*, Basel, 10:267.

WALKER, J. C. 1951. Genetics and plant pathology. *In* L. C. Dunn (ed.), *Genetics in the 20th Century.* Macmillan, New York.

WALTERS, J. H., AND L. J. B. CHWATT. 1956. Sickle-cell anaemia and falciparum malaria. *Tran. Roy. Soc. Trop. Med. Hyg.*, 50:51.

WIENER, A. S. 1942. The Rh factor and racial origins. *Science*, 96:407.

WILSON, T. 1961. Malaria and glucose-6-phosphate dehydrogenase. *Brit. Med. J.*, 2:246, 285.

WOOLF, B. 1955. On estimating the relation between blood groups and disease. *Ann. Human Genet.*, 19:251.

M. S. BARTLETT
Department of Statistics,
University College,
London, England

XV. BIOMETRY AND THEORETICAL BIOLOGY

PREFATORY REMARKS

The approximate coincidence in time of an obligation on my part to give a presidential address to the British region of the Biometric Society and an invitation to contribute to a memorial volume to J. B. S. Haldane made me, in this over-hectic world, consider whether I could reasonably cover both commitments simultaneously. Haldane was, after all, for some years Weldon Professor of Biometry at University College, London, and a great theoretical biologist—for example, with his pioneering contributions to the mathematical theory of evolution. While this somewhat superficial survey of my theme justifiably might have provoked Haldane's sarcasm, I can at least feel that he would not have remained indifferent.

I nearly used the title "Biometry or Theoretical Biology" with a question mark to note the possible antagonism between the two—I shall be commenting further on this point later—but the value of a fruitful marriage rather than a sterile separation is so obvious that it would be an insult to all of us to labor it unduly. There was a somewhat analogous situation in economics in the days when economic theory and economic statistics kept very much to themselves, and the new subject of econometrics was introduced, not as a replacement of economic theory, but with the object of developing and studying theories and quantitative models that could be tested and checked against observation.

In the same spirit we can distinguish the science of biometry (or biometrics) from the biological statistics or other measurements themselves by characterizing the former as concerned with making sense of the latter whenever possible *in a real biological sense*. It is perhaps advisable, in view of rather divergent opinions on the definition and scope of biometry, to spend a little longer on this; I have found it interesting to refer back to the remarks made by W. G. Cochran, myself, and others at the Second International Biometric Conference held at Geneva in 1949 (*see* Cochran, 1950; Bartlett, 1950). The variation in attitude is from, on the one side, biological statistics to, on the other, all quantitative biology, including theoretical biology. Let me quote one or two relevant passages:

> We may . . . think of biometry briefly as quantitative biology. One incidental point made to me by Professor Ashby is that it is convenient to exclude from our definition purely biological experimental techniques,—for example, techniques in preparing slides for the microscope to study all cell and tissue growth,—not because they are not concerned with biometry and measurement, but because they are better classified and included by the biologist as part of his general laboratory training, in contrast with the rest of biometry which relies, at any rate in part, on mathematical and statistical concepts. (Bartlett, 1950, p. 86.)

> As a representative of the Chicago group of mathematical biologists, I am grateful to Professor Cochran for his excellent survey of the aims and methods of mathematical biology and for his plea for a broad concept of biometrics so as to include these aims. I am likewise indebted to Professor Rasch for emphasizing the fact that quantitative biology should go beyond the business of fitting empirical curves to equations; that it should actively seek a *rationale* which would explain the emergence of quantitative data, distributions, etc. (A. Rapoport, discussion following Cochran, 1950, p. 83.)

My earlier remark about making sense of biological measurements and statistics indicates that I would go along with Professors Rasch and Rapoport in emphasizing this. Nevertheless, if in the last quotation any implication were intended that biometry should embrace the whole of mathematical biology, then this appears to me unacceptable; I separate the two just as I have separated econometrics from economic theory. Indeed, the whole point of my present discussion is to examine the relation between the two.

Biometrical and Statistical Methods

I should hardly need to remind biometricians of our statistical tools, but it may be as well to recapitulate the nature and scope of the methods which I have in mind. Obviously *all* these methods are potentially useful to the biometrician, but those with historical or obvious application to biology are the methods most important to mention. There is no doubt that if these are attached to the individuals who first developed or promulgated them, they must be associated in the main with Karl Pearson and R. A. Fisher; though the cumulative effect of other great British contemporaries of theirs, such as Francis Galton, W. S. Gosset, A. G. McKendrick and G. Udny Yule, must not be overlooked.

On the statistical side, it was Galton who first seriously studied correlation and regression and Karl Pearson who continued, with characteristic zeal, with the general study of populations and distributions in biology—univariate, multivariate and qualitative. With his study of univariate distributions may be associated his theoretical system of distribution functions; with multivariate, the method of principal components; and with qualitative, his chi square test. Fisher's statistical work I have surveyed in more detail elsewhere (Bartlett, 1965), but in view of its importance to biometry I must mention it again briefly. In the paper cited I divided Fisher's work in statistics into three lines: "The first of these three lines consisted of the spate of solutions of exact sampling distribution problems, for which Fisher's geometrical approach proved so powerful. The second was the development of a more general and self-contained set of principles of statistical inference, especially for estimation problems. The third was the emergence of a precise technique of experimental design and analysis." Fisher's general aim was to carve out a precise statistical methodology, applicable to small samples as well as large. In this aim he achieved a remarkable degree of success, the first line of work facilitating the provision of tables of exact significance levels; the second providing the machinery of maximum likelihood estimation and the concept of the statistical information available on a parameter from a sample; and the third, the whole modern technique of statistical experimentation—orthogonal and balanced designs and associated analysis, randomization and assessment of error, factorial design, and confounding. On more controversial issues, the relative logical status of various theoretical schools, of fiducial, confidence, or Bayesian intervals of error, and so on. I do not consider that these issues greatly affect the *use* of the basic methods and techniques just referred to, though they may broaden our outlook when we do use them.

As for further specific developments in statistical methods in biology, those listed below tend to be a somewhat random sample, and a reference to the issues of a journal such as *Biometrics* could no doubt remind one of items overlooked. On the distributional side, one thinks of distributional models of heterogeneity and contagion, the negative binomial of Greenwood and Yule (heterogeneity and accident-proneness) or of McKendrick (contagion), the logarithmic distribution of Fisher or the contagion distributions of Neyman. One thinks of developments in sampling, such as capture-recapture methods, or sequential sampling and its applicability to clinical trials. Incidentally, I distinguish medicine from biology, and, hence, medical statistics from biological statistics, but statistical techniques such as sequential design or bio-assay experimentation all may properly be included in biometry. There have been further developments in experimental design by Yates and others, or, in the study of response surfaces, by Box. On general sampling methods, a useful review has been given recently by Sukhatme (1966).

The analysis of time series is not of particular biological relevance, being more familiar in the physical or economic domain, but is of some importance in the study of animal populations and has potential application also in the study of electroencephalograph records.

With regard to fields of study, it is worth recalling J. B. S. Haldane's contribution to the discussion on Professor Cochran's paper (1959). Haldane listed animal demography, paleontology, and histology, referring in histology to cell counts in solid organs as well as in blood and in paleontology to the statistical estimation of evolutionary rates of change of measurements.

MATHEMATICAL AND THEORETICAL BIOLOGY

If we turn now to the development of theoretical biology, which is being given considerable encouragement and attention at the present time, especially in the United States, it again will be helpful to recall some of the pioneering contributions already made. It is, I think, generally agreed that mathematical and theoretical approaches to a science tend to assume more dominance as the science matures. This is because one cannot hope to formulate abstract and general principles that have proper relevance until a sufficient body of fact and empirical analysis has accumulated. Such formulations, thus, depend rather critically on the historical development of a science and will prove abortive if attempted prematurely. They also, of course, must await the outstanding men of science whose vision is broad enough to see the whole wood when it has developed rather than (or better, as well as) the individual trees.

Morowitz (1965) in a recent comprehensive survey has drawn attention to very early work by Borelli (seventeenth century) on the mechanics of animal motion, by von Helmholtz (nineteenth century) on the perception of light and sound, and, of course, by Mendel (nineteenth century), but he suggests that the modern era in theoretical biology can be dated from D'Arcy Thompson's work on growth and form in 1917. While not denying the importance of the latter in relation to the development of an *individual* organism, I think that Morowitz has overlooked the relevance to theoretical studies of biological *populations* of the work at the turn of the last century by biometricians, such as Galton and Karl Pearson. For example, Galton's theoretical discussion, in his *Natural Inheritance*, of the problem of extinction of surnames was a fascinating prelude to the role of the problem of survival of mutations in the theory of evolution. Such studies became of greater value when combined with the previously neglected work of

Mendel, and, once the science of genetics had become established, paved the way for the modern work of R. A. Fisher, J. B. S. Haldane, Sewall Wright, and others. Morowitz also omitted mentioning Charles Darwin, whom I also have, momentarily, overlooked just because of his great stature, and yet who certainly should be classified as a theoretical biologist as well as a naturalist.

Clearly Darwin's thesis of the evolutionary origin of species by the process of natural selection embodies a biological theory of the greatest power and depth, as its impact on society demonstrated. This work emphasizes the point that theoretical biology is not necessarily particularly mathematical, though usually the more detailed quantitative assessment that comes later requires mathematics. Theories can be built on observations that are simple and universal, such as the sky being dark at night (the universe cannot be infinite and everlasting and stationary) or a fire not usually making things colder (the Second Law of Thermodynamics).

In his article Morowitz divides theoretical biology into three general areas: formal theory, physical theory, and systems theory. Formal theory covers logical, e.g., mathematical, deductions from a set of assumptions or postulates. Such theory is an obvious concomitant of many sciences and in biology would include pure mathematical investigations into theoretical processes originally conceived as biological models, such as, say, the simple birth and death process. As an ancillary, such theory is often necessary, but biologists would rightly look askance if its importance were exaggerated; when we come to more general formal theory, such as Woodger's *The Axiomatic Method in Biology* (1937), the suspicion is overwhelming that such attempts are premature (for the reasons I have mentioned already).

The value of physical theory in biology, i.e., in biophysics, seems less controversial, and even systems theory, with its comparisons with servomechanisms, computers, communication systems, and the like, has proved stimulating to many biologists (for one recent intriguing article, *see* Michie and Longuet-Higgins, 1966). Even here however, one senses the danger of any excessive advocacy of one or another approach at the expense of the biology. The extensive work by Rashevsky and his Chicago school of mathematical biophysics, for example, imaginative as it is, has seemed too often ready to explore possibilities with inadequate discussion of how sensible or correct such possibilities are. This seems a pity, especially as this school has reached some striking conclusions, at times based on very abstract arguments of the formal variety. For example, in connection with the natural replacement of lost or injured organs, Rosen (1960; cf. Rashevsky, 1965) has proved that if an organism is represented by an oriented graph, with organs or components of the organism represented by points, inputs by directed lines to the points, and outputs by directed lines from the points, *then* it is impossible for every component to be re-establishable, provided the normal functioning of any component requires all the inputs that it receives. Such deductions are of theoretical interest, but their biological relevance is so dependent on the assumptions that very careful explanation and justification of these assumptions is necessary before we can take the conclusions seriously. The deductions are of the same type as von Neumann's celebrated proof that the universe cannot be crypto-deterministic because this is not allowed by the current principles of quantum mechanics. This "proof" carried more conviction because quantum mechanics already was, and is still, an accepted physical theory, but, of course, the snag even here is that his conclusion is not necessarily true because this theory is not "true," and, in fact, is already known, in spite of its great success and use, to have limitations.

Classification, like notation, is no more than a convenience, but I would prefer to envisage, as far as is practicable, the division of theoretical biology as bounded by the unit of study. Admittedly, any unit smaller than the whole can never act in isolation, but this difficulty is not peculiar to biology; there seem to be advantages in thinking in terms of a hierarchy of scales. In this way one proceeds naturally from the molecular biology level to the organization and functioning of a single cell, from there to the structure and functioning of parts of an organism, such as the muscles or the nervous system, thence to the structure and behavior of the entire organism, and, finally, to the statistical properties of whole populations. Of course, there will often be "disciplines" which appear to cut across such a classification, e.g., genetics with its ramifications from the molecular level to the phenotypic organism and on to genetic selection in populations; but this difficulty does not seem crucial, and the advantage of formulating one's classification in terms of biological units seems worth maintaining. In fact, the science of genetics represents an attempt to formulate biology in terms of a further set of convenient biological units, the genes, and the synthesis achieved in terms of them is not to be exploded by the realization that they are probably as much convenient fiction as physical atoms and must similarly be analyzed ultimately into still smaller structural units.

We may consequently, with Haldane (1964), reject Mayr's criticism (quoted by Haldane) when Mayr (1963) said: "The Mendelian was apt to compare the genetic contents of a population to a bag full of colored beans. Mutation was the exchange of one kind of bean for another. This conceptualization has been referred to as 'beanbag genetics.' Work in population and developmental genetics has shown, however, that the thinking of beanbag genetics is in many ways quite misleading. To consider genes as independent units is meaningless from the physiological as well as the evolutionary viewpoint."

One advantage of the hierarchical classification is that it avoids fruitless attempts to explain properties at any level in terms of detailed analysis at a lower level. This does not mean that we do not want to investigate how phenomena at any level are relying on organization below that level, which is different from saying that such further elucidation is necessary for explaining the phenomena in question. A well-known example in physics is the extent to which the macroscopic behavior of aggregates of atoms is independent of the microscopic behavior or detailed properties of the atoms making up these aggregates. This science of statistical mechanics is at the same time more satisfying than was the earlier, more formal axiomatic theory of thermodynamics, as it rationally explains principles, such as the Second Law of Thermodynamics, which would otherwise have to be taken as an empirical assumption based on observations. An analogous situation in epidemiology is the existence of threshold levels of susceptible populations, arising from the statistical nature of the system, and not having to be postulated either as an empirical fact, or, say, in terms of particular individuals in the population being susceptible and others not.

Another example is that of color in insects or animals. MacArthur (1965) asks why the (American) viceroy butterfly is orange, pointing out that, although we can consider this question on the biochemical level, the explanation at a different level is that it mimics a distasteful butterfly (the monarch). The second explanation has the advantage that it leads to successful prediction of a change in typical color in the viceroy butterfly with a change to an environment where another distasteful but browner butterfly (the queen) is prevalent.

Incidentally, MacArthur also raises problems not so far very much considered by population geneticists, as they arise, so to speak, on an even higher hierarchical plane. These concern the "fitness" of populations at a higher structural level than the survival of the fittest individuals. An example given is an ecological predator-prey relation. MacArthur argues that natural selection tends to promote greater instability in such relations and that the ultimate equilibrium will be a compromise between such natural selection and the extinction of population combinations that are too unstable. I did not find the details of his argument too clear, as I have shown (Bartlett, 1960) that the stability of such relations depends rather critically on age lags, which MacArthur apparently does not consider. How far MacArthur is correct in this particular context does not, however, affect the interest of the general questions that he raises.

The success of formal postulates which have proved important and apparently fundamental in other sciences, such as the one cited of the Second Law of Thermodynamics, or perhaps that even more remarkable one, the Principle of Least Action, is certainly a temptation to theoretical biologists. Before, however, undue premature theorizing, let us reflect on this last principle. It was formulated in the eighteenth century, in the days of Maupertuis, as an almost mystical postulate. Later it was realized that there were several equivalent postulates, so that it was sometimes more a matter of convenience than of necessity which one was used. Nevertheless, it still has to be admitted that the success of the principle in explaining both mechanical and electromagnetic phenomena is not fully understood, and one would like to have a deeper physical theory which would clarify this.

In biology the analogy with communication and control systems has led to the formulation of a Principle of Optimal Design (*see*, for example, Rashevsky, 1965). This is constructive in leading to a comparison of ideal and actual biological systems, with sometimes intriguing agreement (for example, the arterial system for the blood). Unless, however, we have an underlying theory to explain it, we must be on our guard not to make it inviolable. It was remarked a long time ago that the eye is a very efficient optical system of the lens variety. I cannot remember whether it could ideally be more efficient if the system were of the reflecting mirror variety, but the mechanism of the natural selection virtually dictated that the first type of optical system was evolved. Such situations have led to the modification of the principle to a Principle of Adequate Design, under given conditions. This promises to be more successful but, of course, is less predictive, for the stringency of the conditions to be specified leaves considerable latitude, and, to take the extreme case, if we specify the conditions too rigidly the predictive value of the principle would disappear.

Another attempt to formulate an optimum principle, in the field of natural selection, has been made by Kimura (1958). He showed, for example, that if *fitness a* is measured by the rate of increase of a genotypic population, and average fitness $\bar{a}$ by the mean of a over all genotypes, then natural selection changes gene frequencies n_i in such a way as to minimize the increase in $\bar{a}$, subject to the restriction

$$\sum_i \frac{(\delta n_i)^2}{n_i} = \tfrac{1}{2} V_g (\delta t)^2,$$

where V_g is the *genic variance*. This assumes the simple conditions of random mating, constant fitness of individual genotypes, and a single gene locus, conditions under which

$$V_g = 2\Sigma_i n_i d_i^2,$$

where d_i is the average

$$\frac{\Sigma_j a_{ij} P_{ij}}{n_i} - \bar{a},$$

a_{ij} being the net reproductive rate of the genotype (i,j) and P_{ij} its probability (for convenience of definition, $P_{ij} = \frac{1}{2}[P_{ij} + P_{ji}]$). Such simple conditions were extended by Kimura, so that with his more general theorem he could, with some justification, claim that it was "somewhat analogous to the principle of least action in physics and may be called the maximum principle in the genetic theory of natural selection. Whereas from the least action principle the laws of motion may be derived, we may from this theorem derive the rate of change in gene frequencies."

As with mechanical laws of motion, however, it is not clear whether Kimura's principle is a mathematically equivalent statement of the laws or whether it leads to greater insight into their scientific status.

The more direct comparison of the brain and central nervous system with a computer and communication system is one that has intrigued many workers, especially von Neumann. One warning conclusion, quoted by Morowitz (1965), was given by von Neumann: "whatever language the central nervous system is using, it is characterized by less logical and arithmetic depth than we are normally used to. . . . Thus logics and mathematics in the central nervous system when viewed as language, must structurally be different from those languages to which our common experience refers."

This warning only refers to one of the difficulties that face theoretical and mathematical biologists. Another was vividly put by Bernal (1965) when he referred to the historical and descriptive character of much biology, even today. He said:

> Biology, however, deals with descriptions and ordering of very special parts of the universe which we call life—even more particularly in these days, terrestial life. It is primarily a descriptive science, more like geography, dealing with the structure and working of a number of peculiarly organized entities, at a particular moment of time on a particular planet. Undoubtedly there should be a real and general biology but we can only just begin to glimpse it. A true biology in its full sense would be the study of the nature and activity of all

organized objects wherever they were to be found—on this planet, or others in the solar system, in other solar systems, in other galaxies—and at all times, future and past.

This is, of course, a very far-reaching and ambitious view of biology, but it is a very salutary counterblast to any more parochial attitude. The Darwinian theory of evolution was a landmark in unifying the study of biology; it gave rise, as I have already recalled, to quantitative studies developing the general genetic theory of natural selection. Epoch-making as these studies have been, we would do well to recall that they cover only a limited range of the evolutionary scale. Before the tidy scheme of gene stability with the occasional but accumulative natural selection of favorable mutations, there must have been a period when these genetic structures of genes and chromosomes themselves were being evolved. What is remarkable when we probe further to the molecular level is the complete basic unity of life. In particular, the genetic code appears from our present knowledge to be practically identical for all organisms. However, as Bernal (1965, p. 119) has noted:

> In life as we know it the nucleic acid replicating mechanism, whether it is DNA or RNA, is absolutely necessary to secure precise reproduction of molecules. . . . The precision and balance of the system is such that we can hardly imagine one part of it without all the others. Yet such complex harmony can hardly have evolved all at once as a complete system. Originally the same basic functions must have been carried out, though less efficiently, in other ways. At some time, molecular, but not necessarily organismal, reproduction must have depended on another kind of template than the nucleic acids because nucleic acids were not yet in existence.

And he goes on to suggest (p. 120):

> There may be better arrangements of molecules capable of even more economical, faster, or more intelligent life than anything we know of. However, we cannot more than suspect such possibilities until we can begin to understand the processes that gave rise to them. It would be possible in principle that nucleic acids could be built out of nucleotides other than the four or five that are actually used.

Biometry as the Control for Theoretical Biology

These vistas for biology are certainly challenging, but they are only approached step by step, and the role of biometry seems sufficiently clear—it is to act not only in a purely exploratory way but, as theoretical biology develops, to act also as a check and control of theory or surmise whenever possible. It is in this sense that we can approve the link of biometry with mathematical biology urged by Cochran, Rapoport, and

others. For this reason, I cannot entirely accept Dr. Pearce's remarks
(1965, p. 144): "The only way to find out how well an insect flies is to
observe it flying; the matter cannot be decided by static measurements
aided by reasoning. This is true in general; plants and animals are not
machines, fabricated from standard materials according to blueprints,
but living organisms developed by their own internal laws, which are
often unknown to the biologist."

Of course, these remarks are literally true, but their general import
should not be to oppose the trend to more theoretical biology, provided
it is not protected from the harsh reality of observation and experiment.
Some of the theoretical arguments on natural selection can have little
direct observational support because of their enormous time scale, though
observation should still be attempted whenever possible—for example,
Fisher attempted to find such support for his genetic theory of the evolution of dominance.

To turn to less general questions, in the future we may expect a rather
closer link than exists now between biometry and those aspects of theoretical biology that can be checked observationally, for example, by the
development of mathematical models that can be checked by statistical
observations. This movement is emphasized in the Symposium on
Stochastic Models in Medicine and Biology; among others, though, the
number of papers in this publication dealing with actual data is perhaps
relatively small (about four out of thirteen).

The greater use of mathematical and stochastic models, when combined
with the statistical analysis of biometrical data, has one consequence which
I have discussed before. This is the creation of new and often extremely
difficult problems of statistical analysis, especially in nonexperimental
situations where no replication, except perhaps in an extended and
correlative sense, is present. It is not my intention here to examine
these problems in detail, but I cite one or two illustrative cases. One
dilemma is that either a realistic, but intractable, model is set up or a
more manageable model that is too simplified to be correct; this dilemma
arises, for example, in the comparison of epidemiological models of
infectious diseases in a population and recorded statistics of incidence.

Sometimes the model is adequate and still reasonably simple, as, for
example, with simple Markov chain models of dependence. Where these
models relate to attributes, say, for discrete steps or time units, the
classical χ^2 test can be extended to check their goodness of fit. A fairly
simple geological example was given in my University College inaugural
lecture (1961). An even simpler one, as it is merely testing the null case of
complete independence, is of interest because of its field of application

(Williams *et al.*, 1961) and the need for extended tests may well arise in the same context.

In the case of more than one dimension, the analysis of dependence becomes, unfortunately, much more difficult to handle, one of the theoretical problems being the *consistent* specification of low-order dependence. Thus, in the case of a mosaic of presence and absence of a certain vegetation ground cover over a continuous area, I criticized the Markov dependence model used by Pielou (1965) for investigating the observed sampling properties over *line* transects as not necessarily consistent with any reasonable model in the *plane*. (Her model is, in fact, compatible with the areas cut off by random straight lines in a plane, but this is not a very plausible model in this context.)

The occasional use of stochastic models which are theoretically inconsistent or unattainable is certainly not confined to biologists, and it stresses that a fair knowledge of the mathematical theory of stochastic processes is sometimes needed to avoid this pitfall. In the early days of work on the theory of physical turbulence, impossible auto-correlation functions were sometimes assumed; even now in physical applications one can find a normal correlation function assumed in contexts where the complete determinism that it implies is incompatible with the randomness envisaged elsewhere in the model.

The problem of analysis with controlled and replicated experiments may seem more straightforward, and in some ways it is, because the replication usually permits accurate assessment or comparison of any particular features. It is, however, often not a difficult task to establish differences between different conditions or treatments. When the observations are of a complicated bilological process, such as Gause's experiments on prey-predator relations or Park's on competition between flour beetles (cf. Bartlett, 1960), the difficulty is to know how to summarize briefly and effectively the variable, and often very involved, results. It should be noticed that, in the case of possible extinction of one or another species due to an unstable interaction between the two species, it does not even follow that the replication permits the calculation of a sensible standard error for some features. (The use of a mean and standard error is pointless when the observations do not cluster around some central value.)

In such cases one of the more constructive procedures is to find a theoretical explanatory model for the observed behavior adequately describing the results. With complicated situations, further experimentation usually will be required, investigating specific aspects in more detail, as has occurred, for example, with Park's experiments. Such further experiments may permit more standard analyses, though with such biological material technical devices like transformations of the variables may be useful.

With more stable processes, such as learning behavior in psychological experiments, or electroencephalograph records in certain experiments, or the effect of drugs the problem of finding adequate models is still obviously important and must remain one of the long-term tasks. With sufficient ingenuity, the biometrician may discover more empirical functions of the observations which seem to summarize the results, and more study of this problem is needed; but they are less likely to be permanently useful to the biologist, unless they are consistent with some explanatory model or theory. Various forms of multivariate analysis, for example, when used in the analysis of experiments on animal growth, fall in this more empirical class of procedures.

REFERENCES

BARTLETT, M. S. 1950. Teaching and education in biometry. *Biometrics*, 6:85.
———. 1960. *Stochastic Population Models in Ecology and Epidemiology*. London.
———. 1961. *Probability, Statistics and Time*. Inaugural lecture, University College, London.
———. 1965. R. A. Fisher and the last fifty years of statistical methodology. *J. Amer. Statist. Ass.*, 60:395.
BERNAL, J. D. 1965. Molecular structure, biochemical function and evolution. *In* T. H. Waterman and H. J. Morowitz (eds.), *Theoretical and Mathematical Biology*. New York.
COCHRAN, W. G. 1950. The present status of biometry. *Biometrics*, 6:75.
DONALD, A. D., J. K. DINEEN, J. H. TURNER, AND B. M. WAGLAND. 1964. The dynamics of the host-parasite relationship. *Parasitology*, 54:527.
FISHER, R. A. 1930. *The Genetical Theory of Natural Selection*. Oxford.
GALTON, F. 1889. *Natural Inheritance*. London.
GURLAND, J. (ed.). 1964. *Stochastic Models in Medicine and Biology*. Univ. of Wisconsin Press, Madison, Wisconsin.
HALDANE, J. B. S. 1924. *A Mathematical Theory of Natural and Artificial Selection*. Part I. *Trans. Camb. Phil. Soc.*, 23:19.
———. 1964. A defense of beanbag genetics. *Perspect. Biol. Med.*, 7:343.
KIMURA, M. 1958. On the change of population fitness by natural selection. *Heredity*, 12:145.
KOSTITZIN, V. A. (1937). *Biologie Mathematique*. Librairie Armand Colin, Paris.
MACARTHUR, R. H. 1965. Ecological consequences of natural selection. *In* T. H. Waterman and H. J. Morowitz (eds.), *Theoretical and Mathematical Biology*. New York.
MCKENDRICK, A. G. 1926. Applications of mathematics to medical problems. *Proc. Edinburgh Math. Soc.*, 44:98.
MAYR, E. 1963. *Animal Species and Evolution*. Cambridge, Mass.
MICHIE, D., AND C. LONGUET-HIGGINS. 1966. Party game model of biological replication. *Nature*, 212:10.

MOROWITZ, H. J. 1965. The historical background. *In* T. H. Waterman and H. J. Morowitz (eds.), *Theoretical and Mathematical Biology*. New York.

NEUMANN, J. VON 1958. *The Computer and the Brain*. Yale University Press, New Haven, Conn.

PEARCE, S. C. 1965. The measurement of a living organism. *Biometric-Proaximetrie*, 6:143.

PIELOU, E. C. 1965. The concept of randomness in the patterns of mosaics. *Biometrics*, 4:908.

RASHEVSKY, N. 1938. *Mathematical Biophysics*. Chicago.

——. 1965. Models and mathematical principles in biology. *In* T. H. Waterman and H. J. Morowitz (eds.), *Theoretical and Mathematical Biology*. New York.

ROSEN, R. 1960. A relational theory of biological systems. *Bull. Math. Biophys.*, 20:245.

SUKHATME, P. V. 1966. Major developments in sampling theory and practice. *In* F. N. David (ed.), *Research Papers in Statistics*. New York.

THOMPSON, D'ARCY W. 1917. *On Growth and Form*. Cambridge.

WILLIAMS, J., J. B. CLEGG, AND M. O. MUTCH, 1961. Coincidence and protein structure. *J. Mol. Biol.*, 3:532.

WOODGER, J. H. 1937. *The Axiomatic Method in Biology*. Cambridge.

WRIGHT, S. 1931. Evolution in Mendelian populations. *Genetics*, 16:97.

SPECULATIVE AND SOCIAL BIOLOGY

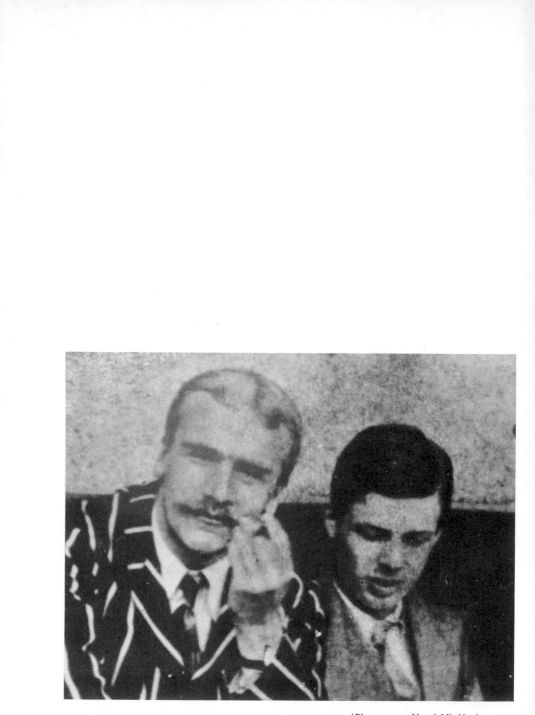

(Photo courtesy Naomi Mitchison)

J. B. S. Haldane (left) and Aldous Huxley, Oxford, 1916.

JOSHUA LEDERBERG
Stanford University Medical School,
Stanford, California

XVI. HALDANE'S BIOLOGY AND SOCIAL INSIGHT

Haldane was one of the most consistent exponents of the necessity for building a scientific outlook for the recognition and solution of the world's social problems. His irrepressible rationalism led him to a commitment to dialectical materialism as the best of available choices, but this commitment did not inhibit him from exercising his egregious critical faculties without hindrance. When he had to speak out against unscientific perversions of the rational society, he did so. Certainly, it was the ironic tragedy of his philosophical life that it was precisely in the field of genetics that authoritarian dogma in the Soviet Union perpetrated the worst travesties of pseudo-science under the leadership of Lysenko.

Even this conflict had its creative side, leading Haldane to look especially critically at the misapplications of Mendelian thinking to human affairs, in what might be regarded as a partial balancing of the sins of the western democracies against those of the communist dictatorship. On the negative side, the conflict tended to isolate Haldane from many of his closest intellectual confreres, particularly in the U.S.

Haldane's social commentary today may seem naively overoptimistic in places: let the scientific attitude merely have a proper trial, and all would be well with the world. Quite possibly, the USSR would be just the arena in which such a revolutionary development might have the best chance to become rooted. The world seems far more complicated today; a little science seems more likely to usher in the *Brave New World* than a Wells-Haldane form of utopia. It is perhaps more than a trivial coincidence that Haldane's most striking prophetic misjudgment had to do with the time it would take for the practical realization of atomic energy. This scientific catastrophe, more than any other, has exploded the peaceful dreams of social scientism.

Nevertheless, Haldane's insistent demand for the incorporation into politics of scientific thinking and of the actual facts of scientific reality is more relevant today than ever. His writings have already had a deeper impact on contemporary thought than is widely recognized, but most of them are (incomprehensibly!) out of print and not as well known as they should be to a contemporary generation.

My original intention had been to write a longer critical commentary on Haldane's prophetic writings. Its realization was inhibited by Haldane's own eloquence: what commentary could compete with his own words? I have, therefore, tried to prepare a special treat, a brief anthology of epigrams culled from his collected essays[1] (1932, Chatto and Windus, London). In doing this, I have applied only one bias—to look for the more universal insights and to relieve his own emphasis on dialectical materialism as the philosophical, or perhaps motivational, basis for his comments. This bias may make his commentary more significant to a wider readership. I doubt that he would ever have forgiven me for it.

The enemies of science alternately abuse its exponents for being deaf to moral considerations and for interfering in ethical problems which do not concern them. Both of these criticisms cannot be right.

Preventive medicine could be made into the moral equivalent of war. It is already so for a few people. A colleague of mine was recently translating a French paper on chemotherapy when he came upon the phrase "tué par l'ennemi" in reference to a deceased pharmacologist. "I suppose," he said, "that means that he died of an accidental infection." I undeceived him; the enemy in this case had been the German nation; but his attitude was typical of medical scientists to-day. "For we wrestle, not against flesh and blood, but against principalities, against powers, against the rulers of the darkness of this world." St. Paul thought that the world was largely ruled by demons. We know better to-day, and we demand the general adoption of the scientific point of view because in its absence human effort is so largely devoted to conflicts with fellow-men, in which one, if not both, of the disputants must inevitably suffer. It is only in times of disaster that the average man devotes a moment's thought to his real enemies, "the rulers of the darkness of this world" from bacteria to cyclones. Until humanity adopts the scientific point of view those enemies will not be conquered.

But until the scientific point of view is generally adopted, our civilization will continue to suffer from a fundamental disharmony. Its material basis is scientific, its intellectual framework is pre-scientific. The present state of the world suggests that unless a fairly vigorous attempt is made in the near future to remedy this disharmony, our particular type of civilization will undergo the fate of the cultures of the past.

[1] The following quotations (an abridgment of pp. 3–224 of *Science and Human Life*, by J. B. S. Haldane, copyrighted 1933 by Harper & Brothers; renewed 1961 by J. B. S. Haldane) are reprinted by permission of Harper & Row, Publishers. Acknowledgment is also made to the British publishers, Chatto & Windus, Ltd., who published the same book under the title, *The Inequality of Man and Other Essays* (1932).

Now we cannot at present control segregation, except to a small extent, but we can and do control heredity in animal and plant breeding, and could in human society if eugenics became a reality. That is why eugenics is at present the only possible way of improving the innate characters of man. But for all that, biology does not support the idea that the hereditary principle is a satisfactory method of choosing men or women to fill a post. Segregation sees to it that very few human characters breed true. The average degree of resemblance between father and son is too small to justify the waste of human potentialities which an hereditary aristocratic system entails. If human beings could be propagated by cutting, like apple trees, aristocracy would be biologically sound. England would presumably be governed by cuttings of Cromwell and Chatham; America, as I believe Bateson once suggested, by cuttings of Washington and Lincoln. But until the art of tissue culture has developed very considerably, such possibilities need not even be thought of.

It is, of course, irrational that each man's vote should possess equal value. But the alternatives so far tried or suggested are still less rational. They usually take the form of increasing the political power of those who are wealthy enough to be able to influence politics already. One eminently desirable reform would be the disfranchisement of persons over sixty-five years of age. The main effects of their votes will not appear during their lifetime; they would be useless in a civil war, and their political views depend on issues of a generation ago. In England our old men and women vote for a protective tariff because they were formerly opposed to Irish Home Rule, in America because their childish sympathies in the Civil War were for the North!

I like philosophers, and I believe that they fulfil a function of great importance. There are a very large number of questions with regard to which there is no satisfactory evidence, and it is important that they should be considered as open. Now agnosticism is an intellectual tight-rope which most people cannot tread for long.

"The materialist," [Eddington] says, " . . . must presumably hold the belief that his wife is a rather elaborate differential equation, but he is probably tactful enough not to obtrude this opinion in domestic life." I recently put this point to a happily married physicist of my acquaintance. He replied that he would not love his wife if he did not believe that she was a differential equation, or rather that her conduct obeyed one. He loves her because she has a definite character which renders her conduct intelligible even when it is surprising. And in this she certainly resembles a differential equation. There are dull differential equations just as there are dull wives.

If innate human diversity is an ineradicable fact, the ideal society is one in which as many types as possible can develop in accordance with their possibilities. So far every society has tended to idealize one particular type.

Moral indignation is regarded as out-of-date. It has its uses, but it is the finest known excuse for cruelty, just as cruelty is the best excuse for moral indignation. I regret to say that my bosom often swells with moral indignation against all kinds of people whom it would be more rational to pity for their conduct.

A certain fraction of human conduct is largely controllable by social pressure, and praise and blame are effective means of controlling it. They prevent a large number of bad actions. But they do not, as it seems to me, involve any particular view as to the freedom of the will. They are part of the environment which determines our actions. Every crime represents a failure of society to control a criminal, as well as a failure on the part of the criminal to respond to social control. We do not at present know enough of biology to alter the structure of the criminal's brain and mind; or to prevent potential criminals being born; we must take him as we find him, and attempt so to order society that he does not commit crime.

At present the principal clue to the spot where civilization began comes from an entirely unexpected source, namely, plant genetics. Civilization is based, not only on men but on plants and animals.

For example, maize, as compared with wheat or oats, is very poor in vitamin B2. Hence populations living mainly on maize get a skin disease called pellagra. This is probably one reason why the maize-civilizations of central America never reached the level of the wheat, barley, and rice civilizations of the old world.

Between 3000 B.C. and A.D. 1400 there were probably only four really important inventions, namely the general use of iron, paved roads, voting, and religious intolerance.

Christianity and other religions have, of course, on occasion been great weapons in the hands of moral reformers, but they have also been effectively used for the opposite purpose. To take an obvious example, slavery, and what is worse, slave raiding, still exist in Christian Abyssinia, the latter evil nowhere else.

The man who is probably the greatest living experimentalist once said to me that but for Galileo and men like him he would never have thought of using experiment rather than unaided observation and thought to search out the nature of things. If Galileo and a few more like-minded men had been burned alive at an early age we might very possibly still be living under a civilization not greatly different from that of the Middle Ages.

It is only in the last hundred years that civilization, after six thousand years, has begun to change all through. But to-day the external conditions of life in civilised communities differ more from those of 1829 than did the conditions of 1829 from those at the time of Noah's flood. And this change, the real world revolution, has only just begun. We have gone an immense way in improving and organizing production and communication; we have nearly abolished water-borne and insect-borne diseases, and that is about all. Science has not yet been applied to most human activities. It can be, and I hope will be, applied to all.

The world is, of course, full of alleged applications of science outside the realms of production and hygiene, but the vast majority of them show no trace of scientific method. Thus there are numberless systems of education which are supposed to be based on scientific child psychology. But they are usually applied to small groups of children, in many cases to the children of unusually intelligent parents, brought up in unusually intelligent homes. If such children later turn out to be more successful than the average, this proves nothing at all.

Who, then, have been the real world-revolutionaries, the men who have done such deeds that human life after them could never be the same as before? I think that the vast majority of them have been skilled manual workers who thought about their jobs. The very greatest of them are perhaps two men or women whose real names will remain forever unknown, but whom we may call Prometheus and Tiptolemus, the inventors of fire and agriculture. Prometheus, who was a Neanderthal man[1] with great brow ridges and no chin, discovered how to keep a fire going, and how to use it to such advantage that his successors were induced to imitate his practice. Probably some later genius discovered how to kindle a fire by rubbing sticks together, and I like to imagine that it was a woman who first presented her astonished but delighted husband with a cooked meal. Fire was a very ancient invention, made in the early part of the old Stone Age, but apparently seeds were first systematically sown not so very long before the dawn of history. The immediate result was to make possible a fairly dense and settled population in which civilization was able to develop.

Those intellectuals who have also been intelligent with their hands have mostly confined their writing to scientific and technical questions. Perhaps I

[1] Recent excavations in China suggest that the ape-man Sinanthropus possessed fire. Prometheus lived longer ago than I thought.

ought to do so myself. But when I look at history, I see it as man's attempt to solve the practical problem of living. The men who did most to solve it were not those who thought about it, or talked about it, or impressed their con- temporaries, but those who silently and efficiently got on with their work.

The great majority of us are quite capable of some kind of useful activity. The essential social problems of to-day, as they present themselves to a biologist, are to determine the abilities of different people, and to organize society so that the demand for various kinds of human ability should equal the supply.

There is plenty of room at the top. In biology we need men with a knowledge not only of the biological sciences, but of mathematics, physics, chemistry, and sociology. Without such supermen biology will break up into a group of isolated sciences divorced from one another, and from human life. Our needs in litera- ture are essentially similar.

Very few serious attempts . . . are made to portray society as a whole, which it is. And such attempts generally fail because of the immense reach required in a mind which is to do the kind of thing which H. G. Wells has occasionally accomplished.

We cannot expect nature to start improving our innate abilities once more. The usual fate of a species in the past has not been progress, but extermination, very often after deteriorating slowly through long periods. The animals and plants alive to-day are the descendants of the few species which have escaped this fate. There is no reason to suppose that man will escape it unless he makes an effort to do so. And we do not at present know how to make that effort. Doubtless complete idiots should be prevented from breeding, but the effort to eliminate all sorts of "unfit" human types is a very much more dubious proposition. When I hear people talking of the "elimination of the unfit" I am always reminded of the crowd who shouted at St. Paul, "Away with such a fellow from the earth, for it is not fit that he should live." St. Paul was eliminated, and very possibly would be to-day. Many of the "unfit" are unfit for society as it is to-day, but that is often society's fault. The attempt to prevent them from breeding really involves the appalling assumption that society as at present constituted is perfect, and that our only task is to fit man to it. That is why eugenists are generally conservative in their political opinions. It also goes a long way to explain the objection which many religious people feel for negative eugenics. They regard it as interference with God's will. I do not share this view, but still less do I regard the average medical board or bench of magistrates as qualified to direct the evolution of the human race.

Pictures of the future are myths, but myths have a very real influence in the present. Modern political ideas are very largely the creation of the Jewish prophets, who foresaw the new Jerusalem in the future, at a time when their contemporaries of other nations had no particular hopes for the betterment of humanity. History has certainly been very different from what Isaiah and Daniel believed it would be; but they helped to make it what it is, and perhaps they would not be altogether dissatisfied with it if they could live to-day. Our greatest living mythologist, Wells, is certainly influencing the history of the future, though probably in ways which he does not suspect.

The time will probably come when men in general accept the future evolution of their species as a probable fact, just as to-day they accept the idea of social and political progress. We cannot say how this idea will affect them. We can be sure that if it is accepted it will have vast effects. It is the business of mythologists to-day to present that idea. They cannot do so without combining creative imagination and biological knowledge.

Science impinges upon ethics in at least five different ways. In the first place, by its application it creates new ethical situations. Two hundred years ago the news of a famine in China created no duty for Englishmen. . . . To-day the telegraph and the steam-engine have made such action possible, and it becomes an ethical problem what action, if any, is right. Secondly, it may create new duties by pointing out previously unexpected consequences of our actions. We are probably divided as to the duty of vaccinating our children, and we may not all be of one mind as to whether a person likely to transmit club-foot or cataract to half his or her children should be compelled to abstain from parenthood.

Thirdly, science affects our whole ethical outlook by influencing our views as to the nature of the world—in fact, by supplanting mythology. One man may see men and animals as a great brotherhood of common ancestry. . . . Another will regard even the noblest aspects of human nature as products of a ruthless struggle for existence. . . . A third, impressed with the vanity of human efforts amid the vast indifference of the universe, will take refuge in a modified epicureanism. In all these attitudes and in many others there is at least some element of rightness. Fourthly . . . anthropology . . . is bound to have a profound effect . . . by showing that any given ethical code is only one of a number practised with equal conviction and almost equal success; finally, ethics may be profoundly affected by an adoption of the scientific point of view; that is to say, the attitude which men of science, in their professional capacity, adopt towards the world. This attitude includes a high (perhaps an unduly high) regard for truth, and a refusal to come to unjustifiable conclusions . . . agnosticism.

If the great aim of education is to know yourself, it is essential to begin at the beginning—namely, with anatomy and physiology. If an almost equally important aim is to promote human solidarity, it is in the realm of hygiene that this is most completely displayed. On the political and economic plane my neighbours' misfortune may be my advantage; in that of hygiene this is never so.

The usual course of study for would-be politicians is, I believe, history. I think that the study of history is somewhat fallacious owing to the enormous changes which have taken place in the last fifty years. For example, up till fifty years ago every State was based on the presupposition that most of the population would have to spend the greater part of their time in hard physical work. That is no longer the case. It seems to me that facts such as that make the lessons of history a little dubious in their application to modern problems.

Biology may not be taught to children seriously; that is to say, it may not be taught to them in connection with their own lives. Human physiology and genetics upset quite a number of our prejudices. The physiology of digestion, reproduction, and excretion are indecent; the physiology of the brain is irreligious. On the other hand, chemistry, physics and certain branches of botany have no immediate bearing on conduct, and therefore they do not come into conflict with any deep-seated prejudices, and are taught in schools. It has, moreover, been found that a good course of systematic botany, taught on the lines of Greek grammar, can immunize the average child against any further interest in science.

If the structure of society is such that the best stocks in it are being bred out, we must change that structure. If the rich limit their families it is, largely, I believe, for two reasons: they want to be able to leave money to their children and they want to be able to afford an expensive education for them. To my mind, the obvious moral to be drawn is that it would be a eugenic measure to abolish hereditary wealth, and have one, and only one, school system for all the population.

In the past it has been an historical function of religion to hold up before humanity a transcendental ideal, however imperfectly presented. If the only function of religion is to establish the Kingdom of God on earth, the Socialists say, "We can do it better than you." To-day it seems to me that transcendental ideals which take men out of the field of ordinary life are only active in the realms of science and art.

It is quite possible, I think, that as the ideals of pure science become more and more remote from those of the general public, science will tend to degenerate more and more into medical and engineering technology, just as art may degenerate into illustration and religion into ritual when they lose the vital spark.

Now I am not going for one moment to suggest that there is not a very grave danger for science in so close an association with the State. It may possibly be that as a result of that association science in Russia will undergo somewhat the same fate as overtook Christianity after its association with the State in the time of Constantine. It is possible that it may lead to dogmatism in science and to the suppression of opinions which run counter to official theories, but it has not yet done so.

Even now psychology is beginning to become scientific. I do not think that the results of scientific psychology are yet very clear, but if we start trying to take a scientific attitude about our own behaviour, looking at ourselves objectively, the first thing we do is to laugh, and that has an extremely good effect on our behaviour.

Even if man does not perish in this dramatic manner, there is no reason why civilization should not do so. All civilization apparently goes back to a common source less than ten thousand years ago, possibly in Egypt. It is a highly complicated invention which has probably been made only once. If it perished it might never be made again.

A modern world followed by revolutions might destroy it all over the planet. If weapons are as much improved in the next century as in the last, this will probably happen. But unless atomic energy can be tapped, which is wildly unlikely . . . the odds are slightly against such a catastrophic end of civilization.

If science is to improve man as it has improved his environment, the experimental method must be applied to him. It is quite likely that the attempt to do so will rouse such fierce opposition that science will again be persecuted as it has been in the past.

Again, if scientific psychology and eugenics are used as weapons by one side in a political struggle, their opponents, if successful, will stamp them out. I think that it is quite as likely as not that scientific research may ultimately be strangled in some such way as this before mankind has learnt to control its own evolution.

If so, evolution will take its course. And that course has generally been downwards. The majority of species have degenerated and become extinct, or, what is perhaps worse, gradually lost many of their functions. The ancestors of oysters and barnacles had heads. Snakes have lost their limbs and ostriches and penguins their power of flight. Man may just as easily lose his intelligence.

227

It is only a very few species that have developed into something higher. It is unlikely that man will do so unless he desires to and is prepared to pay the cost.

It was possible either to suppose that life had been supernaturally created on earth some millions of years ago, or that it had been brought to earth by a meteorite or by micro-organisms floating through interstellar space. But a large number, perhaps the majority, of biologists, believed, in spite of Pasteur, that at some time in the remote past life had originated on earth from dead matter as the result of natural processes.

It is probable that all organisms now alive are descended from one ancestor, for the following reason. Most of our structural molecules are asymmetrical, as shown by the fact that they rotate the plane of polarized light, and often form asymmetrical crystals. But of the two possible types of any such molecule, related to one another like a right and left boot, only one is found throughout living nature.

There is nothing, so far as we can see, in the nature of things to prevent the existence of looking-glass organisms built from molecules which are, so to say, the mirror-images of those in our own bodies. Many of the requisite molecules have already been made in the laboratory. If life had originated independently on several occasions, such organisms would probably exist. As they do not, this event probably occurred only once, or, more probably, the descendants of the first living organism rapidly evolved far enough to overwhelm any later competitors when these arrived on the scene.

It is doubtful whether any enzyme has been obtained quite pure. Nevertheless, I hope to live to see one made artificially.

Our social organization of to-day is so rudimentary that one feels justified in hoping that our present lives are very poor samples. There is no physical reason, so far as we know, why our humanity should not continue for thousands, perhaps millions, of millions of years more; and it is reasonable to hope that they will, on the whole, be happier than the present or past ages.

If, however, evolution continues, it is likely that in most of our past and future lives you and I have been or will be relatively feeble-minded throwbacks among a more perfect humanity.

As a man I am a biologist, and see the world from an angle which gives me an unaccustomed perspective, but not, I think, a wholly misleading one.

228

A survey of the beliefs which intelligent men in the past have held as certainties makes that sufficiently clear. One cannot order one's life without a set of beliefs of some kind. But the intellectually honest man must recognize the utterly provisional nature of his beliefs.

The psychological, even the intellectual, benefits of marriage, seem to me to be enormous. If a man has lived for some years in the closest intimacy with a woman, he learns to look at life from her point of view as well as his own. A man who cannot do this is like a man blind in one eye. He does not appreciate the solidity and depth of the world before him. The ideas I am putting before you here are largely my wife's, or at any rate, family ideas, rather than my own private productions.

Finally, I am a human being, a citizen of the world which applied science is daily unifying. My own profession of scientific research knows no frontiers and no colour bars. Japanese, Indians, and Chinese, as well as Europeans and Americans, are, or have been, among my colleagues. I am naturally in favour of any measures tending to unify humanity and prevent war. But my views as to the best methods of achieving these aims are not informed by sufficient knowledge to be worth stating. For the same reason I am saying nothing about economics.

We still have intellectual, aesthetic, and spiritual starvation, which to my mind are greater evils than any mere economic inequality. Until our educational system is so altered as to give a fair deal to every boy and girl who desires a first-rate education and is capable of benefiting by it, my political views are likely to remain, as they are now, on the left.

There is a worse evil than intellectual starvation, and that is the deliberate suppression of free thought and free speech. I rejoice to live in a free country where this evil, though it exists, is less serious than in most other countries.

I am a part of nature, and, like other natural objects, from a lightning flash to a mountain range, I shall last out my time and then finish. This prospect does not worry me, because some of my work will not die when I do so.

In this age of applied science it is gradually being realized in some circles that, if civilization is to continue, scientific thought must be applied to men as well as to nature. Hence the public is beginning to try to understand how scientific workers approach a problem. And here they are at once confronted with the curious but, as we shall see, quite intelligible inarticulateness of most scientific workers.

I am interested not only in the progress of science, but in trying to detect the still, small voice of common sense among the shouts of the anti-scientific and pseudo-scientific extremists.

Though not an adherent of any religion, I find religions an absorbing topic. They represent man's attempt to adjust himself intellectually and emotionally to the universe. The intellectual side of this effort interests me mainly because of its fantastic character. . . .

But the emotional side seems to me an altogether more serious affair. If science is not to leave a gap which will inevitably be filled with superstition, man must learn to feel himself a citizen of the universe as depicted by science. Fortunately I know that such a state of mind is possible.

I am less interested than the average person in politics because I am convinced that all the political principles of to-day are makeshifts, and will ultimately, though not in my time, be replaced by principles based on science.

Women interest me, for I am a normal man, but my interest in them is not mainly intellectual. . . . The average boy is something of a scientist, and an artist too. . . . a fairly bright boy is far more intelligent and far better company than the average adult. I am interested in our increasing knowledge of the child's mental processes, but even more in the attempts which are being made, in the face of ferocious opposition, to teach the child the subject which most children find the most fascinating of all, namely human biology. . . . The child represents the hope of humanity. We are not giving our children a fair deal. Many of those who could benefit most from higher education do not get it. Others are given more education than they either want or can assimilate. Hardly any are introduced to the scientific outlook until their minds have been so filled with pre-scientific ideas as to make scientific thought very difficult. I think that justice for children is even more important than justice for adults . . . as a biologist I realize that all men are different, and I do not offer them [my thoughts] as a pattern for others.

SHELDON C. REED
Dight Institute for Human Genetics,
University of Minnesota,
Minneapolis, Minnesota

XVII. EUGENICS TOMORROW

This tribute to J. B. S. Haldane is motivated by the great pleasure which I obtained from a short walk with him in Ithaca, New York, in 1932. I was an inconspicuous country boy, aged 21, and attending my first genetics congress. I was surprised and delighted that the world-renowned scientist, resplendent in his blue and white striped blazer, would bother to initiate a conversation with me. It is great moments such as these which influence a young man's future reactions.

Professor Haldane wrote numerous books and papers about eugenics, some of which will be mentioned as we proceed. By far the most interesting of them to me is a small book, *Daedalus; or Science and the Future,* written in 1923 when he was 31 years old. He was already an old man in the sense that he heard his first lecture on Mendelism at the age of eight and was working in practical genetics at nineteen. *Daedalus* was popular and stimulating; there were seven printings within the first year of its publication. The book owed its popularity to its imaginative and prophetic thoughts. The more specific predictions did not turn out to be correct, but some still may come to pass. His solution for the exhaustion of the British coal mines was a network of windmills producing electricity, and he stated that, "On thermodynamical grounds I do not much believe in the commercial possibility of induced radioactivity." It is his biological predictions, however, which interest us because they probably influenced H. J. Muller's very serious thoughts about the genetic future of man. Let me quote a few passages, out of context, from *Daedalus.*

> With regard to the application of biology to human life, the average prophet appears to content himself with considerable if rather rudimentary progress in medicine and surgery, some improvement in domestic plants and animals, and possibly the introduction of a little eugenics. The eugenic official, a compound, it would appear, of the policeman, the priest, and the procurer, is to hale us off at suitable intervals to the local temple of Venus Genetrix with a partner chosen, one gathers, by something of the nature of a glorified medical board. It is more likely, as we shall see, that the ends proposed by the eugenist will be attained in a very different manner.

Haldane perhaps exaggerated a little when he stated that every physical and chemical invention is a blasphemy, while the biological invention tends to begin as a perversion and end as a ritual supported by unquestioned beliefs and prejudices. He pointed out the "radical indecency" of milking cows, particularly when it is done electrically. He stated that, "The Hindus have recognized the special and physiological relation of man to the cow by making the latter animal holy." It is interesting that, at age 31, Haldane referred frequently to India, not to Canada, nor to any of the other young and developing countries, but to India—a subcontinent with a glittering past and a difficult future. It is probably fair to say that when the Haldanes retired to India and Hinduism it was a subconscious attempt to return to the glory of the pre-Muslim days or at least because of a nostalgia for past visits to India. Naturally, such a life-long interest in the past might have tended to dull his interest in the eugenics of tomorrow.

The *Daedalus* predictions were in the form of a myth, that is, an essay to be written by a rather stupid undergraduate 150 years hence. It starts thus:

> As early as the first decade of the twentieth century we find a conscious attempt at the application of biology to politics in the so-called eugenic movement. A number of earnest persons, having discovered the existence of biology, attempted to apply it in its then very crude condition to the production of a race of super-men, and in certain countries managed to carry a good deal of legislation. They appear to have managed to prevent the transmission of a good deal of syphilis, insanity, and the like, and they certainly succeeded in producing the most violent opposition and hatred amongst the classes whom they somewhat gratuitously regarded as undesirable parents. (There was even a rebellion in Nebraska.) However, they undoubtedly prepared public opinion for what was to come, and so far served a useful purpose. Far more important was the progress in medicine which practically abolished infectious diseases in those countries which were prepared to tolerate the requisite amount of state interference in private life, and finally, after the league's ordinance of 1958, all over the world; though owing to Hindu opposition, parts of India were still quite unhealthy up to 1980 or so.

To move on to quotes of greater imaginative power:

> It was in 1951 that Dupont and Schwarz produced the first ectogenic child. As early as 1901 Heape had transferred embryo rabbits from one female to another, in 1925 Haldane had grown embryonic rabbits in serum for ten days, but had failed to carry the process to its conclusion, and it was not till 1940 that Clark succeeded with the pig. Dupont and Schwarz obtained a fresh ovary from a woman who was the victim of an aeroplane accident, and kept it living in their medium for five years. They obtained several eggs from it and fertilized them successfully, but the problem of the nutrition and support of the

embryo was more difficult, and was only solved in the fourth year. Now that the technique is fully developed, we can take an ovary from a woman and keep it growing in a suitable fluid for as long as twenty years, producing a fresh ovum each month, of which 90 per cent can be fertilized, and the embryos grown successfully for nine months, and then brought out into the air. France was the first country to adopt ectogenesis officially, and by 1968 was producing 60,000 children annually by this method.

As we know, ectogenesis is now universal, and in this country less than 30 per cent of children are now born of woman. The effect on human psychology and social life of the separation of sexual love and reproduction which was begun in the nineteenth century and completed in the twentieth is by no means wholly satisfactory. The old family life had certainly a good deal to commend it, and although nowadays we bring on lactation in women by injection of placentin as a routine, we must admit that in certain respects our great grandparents had the advantage of us. On the other hand it is generally admitted that the effects of selection have more than counterbalanced these evils. The small proportion of men and women who are selected as ancestors for the next generation are so undoubtedly superior to the average that the advance in each generation in any single respect, from the increased output of first-class music to the decreased convictions for theft is very startling.

The problem of politics is to find institutions suitable to it. In the future perhaps it may be possible by selective breeding to change character as quickly as institutions.

Haldane did not claim originality for the above ideas, but he deserves great credit for having stated them. They must have been influential in molding present-day thought and in the acceptance of biological advances of the future.

In *Daedalus* we find a mild admiration for Marxism which later developed into a rather long friendship for the Soviet Union. *Heredity and Politics* was written in 1937 during the early stages of his flirtation with the political left. This book is in part a text on human genetics, in part a complaint about the American state laws which permit the sterilization of patients in mental institutions, and a discussion of the race problem. The most enjoyable parts of the book are the gems of expression which grace all of the good Professor's writings.

I might mention that Haldane's attitude toward sterilization seems to have been rather Victorian. To be sure, sterilization and old age are minor mortifications as both represent the loss of power. Sterilization, however, is a useful form of contraception, while old age and death are necessary in order to provide an opportunity for the young to mature. How would the sociologists cope with a society in which no one died? No doubt, in the near future most women will have two or three children and then request a hysterectomy or some equivalent technique in order to be spared the nuisance of the monthly period. Improvements in local anesthesia and in surgical techniques will remove the element of fear from the operation, and physicians no longer will be reluctant to provide assistance in turning off the reproductive flood.

There is no question but that Haldane had an excellent sense of social justice throughout his life, but the vivid imagination and prophetic skill found in *Daedalus* did not appear again. He gave no hint in *Heredity and Politics* that Great Britain would be at war with Hitler in less than two years from the time of his writing. The statement in *Heredity and Politics* (p. 186) that, "We shall not find that Mussolini has been very successful with his measures, and we wait to learn what success is achieved by Hitler's laws and propaganda after the initial excitement of the National Socialist Revolution has died down. . . . " does not imply that there were both biological and political crises already at hand.

Professor Haldane also was strangely unaffected by the world's greatest problem, that of the high birth rate. In *Heredity and Politics* (p. 114) he stated that, "It is generally believed that this country [England] will attain its maximum population about 1940. After that it will gradually decline." Apparently he was not thinking about the fact that there is no guarantee that the birth rate will fall in any country. We are here only because birth rates have exceeded death rates in the past. We are the living testimony to the success of natural selection for Darwinian fitness. One would have expected that Professor Haldane, one of the most brilliant students of natural selection and Darwinian fitness, would have had greater anxiety about this terrible pressure and its relation to the future of England. Even today, however, the leaders of Great Britain seem to be serenely unaware that their birth rate is their number one long-term problem.

The last part of *Heredity and Politics* is concerned with racial differences. Some of the differences between races are certainly genetic. These genetic differences are clearly of relatively recent evolutionary origin and related to geographic isolation. The eugenic importance of differences *within* a particular race is great, but the importance of genetic differences between races becomes less with the development of geographic emancipation. The Negro can now live as comfortably in Greenland as can the Eskimo. The disappearance of geographic isolation means the gradual loss of genetic racial differences, because there are no other completely effective barriers to genetic integration. The fact that genetic variation for "important" traits such as body size, intelligence, and personality is much greater within races than between races means that race differences are not of *eugenic* concern. Genetic race differences relate only indirectly to serious social differences, and these problems can be solved by social

234

EUGENICS TOMORROW

action. Such social differences could be resolved immediately by the elimination of a minority race, such as the Caucasian, by a majority race, such as the Mongoloid. This would be genocide but not eugenics. This solution is not recommended by the present writer partly because of the inhumanity involved and also because other social differences would arise promptly among the surviving mongoloids. Social perfection is probably even more difficult to achieve than is eugenic perfection.

Let me conclude my quotations from *Heredity and Politics* with one of Professor Haldane's statements (p. 193) which is the axiom upon which progress in eugenics must be based. He stated, "In the long run the application of biology to social problems must depend on the ideals of the community, and the possibility which its structure offers of realizing those ideals." The eugenics of tomorrow hardly will be recognized as such because, as is the case today, it will be part of the socially accepted structure. It will be a part of normal existence, not a crusade.

Let us return to the large threat to man's future which could prevent eugenic progress of any kind, that is, the problem of the birth rate. Gradually, people are beginning to realize that in the practical sense we are witnessing an extraordinarily serious excess of births over deaths. It is clear that the present rate of population growth cannot continue for very many generations and that our birth rate will have to be checked in various ways. One would hope that this will occur as the result of a universal attitude of responsible parenthood. We must not ignore the opposing pressure of the necessity for reproduction if the species is to exist. In almost all of man's past, the problem has been one of under-population, but now we must struggle with the much more difficult situation of overpopulation. We must now thwart the tremendous pressure of fertility which natural selection has provided us with such success. How can this delicate reproductive balance be achieved?

The secret of success lies in the changing of attitudes. It relates to that ugly word propaganda, though words with a softer sound are usually used. Propaganda is considered to be bad only by those who oppose the ideas which it disseminates. Those who approve of a slogan, such as "Prevent Forest Fires," do not worry about the fact that the slogan is propaganda. Hardly anyone is in favor of forest fires, and soon large families will be equally unfashionable. The small family propaganda has to be a little more subtle than that concerned with forest fires, but it is of much greater importance and the government has ever-increasing opportunities for influencing the subconscious.

In India the propaganda for smaller family sizes does not have to be especially delicate. The thousands of people whose only homes are the sidewalks of Calcutta know that something is wrong. It is estimated that

415,000 sterilizations were performed in 1965 and that about 550,000 intrauterine devices were inserted in the same year in India. This is a small beginning toward a reproductive balance, and there is no guarantee of eventual success. But there is hope!

In the United States it is not likely that people can be entreated successfully to have smaller families because of the world population problem. It is probable, however, that the government will introduce propaganda, somewhat more subtle than a meat-ax, which will suggest that the small family is the only way of life, not because the government says so, but because your friends, relatives, and neighbors say so. The childless family will have to continue to have a poor image to prevent extinction of the species, while the one- or two-child family must become the fashionable size; otherwise, the death rate must go up if a population catastrophe is to be averted. At present in the United States, large families are often an intentional bid for prestige (proof of virility), or the result of sloth in regard to birth control, or the price of the failure to use such techniques. In the future a couple can anticipate that they will be considered either ignorant or careless if they have a large family. This attitude is already rather prevalent and can be expected to spread. The drop in family sizes will be slower in rural areas where children can still be utilized as agricultural workers than in others. Social pressure is a powerful force and can be expected to assist in curbing the birth rate in both literate and nonliterate societies.

It is easy to see that there can be no intelligent control of man's evolution (eugenics) until a substantial proportion of a population voluntarily regulates its family size, and does so deliberately. Fortunately, this situation exists in all technologically developed countries today, and to a significant degree. Consequently, the stage is set for a conscious eugenic advance. Furthermore, the tools are at hand to make the advance possible. Artificial insemination, or semi-adoption as it is sometimes called, invites the substitution of eugenically selected sperm when the husband is sterile. Muller has argued repeatedly for the initiation of sperm banks so that couples could select a famous personality of the past as their donor. No progress has been made in actually establishing the banks, but the technique of semi-adoption is in routine use, and thousands of women have accepted it in order that they might give birth to children and at the same time keep their otherwise successful marriage intact. It should be mentioned that those who have needed and obtained radical technical assistance, such as semi-adoption or sterilization, are deeply grateful for the opportunity and seldom regret their decision. Thus, it is rather gratuitous of those who have no need for such minor medical changes to deny them to those who need them. It is the same as throwing a stone to the starving, instead of bread.

Problems center around determining who should be invited to contribute to the sperm banks or to provide tissue cells for the mitotic reproduction of identities after the death of the original person. One would expect much less demand for replicas of Hitler or Stalin in the future than in the past. What would the world do with 10,000 virtuous George Washingtons? These celebrated genotypes would behave very differently in their new environments, so it would probably be safe to try out a small number of them. Leaving frivolity aside, it seems more sensible to use sperm from successful persons in the many thousands of artificial inseminations which occur today than donations collected in a random fashion.

Other techniques already are available or could be developed quickly if man became really excited about his genetic future. In the eugenics of tomorrow, couples may rear test-tube babies instead of reproducing their own genes. This may seem unlikely but there is no point in knocking it until we have tried it!

There are other techniques which hold great promise, but which are not likely to be available for many years. One might in future years be able to inject a chemical into the body of a person carrying the gene for phenylketonuria and cause this gene to change back to the chemical configuration of the normal gene in every cell of his body, including the gonads. Only about one person in 50 carries the recessive gene for phenylketonuria, but the list of deleterious mutant genes is so horribly long that each one of us carries perhaps three or four definitely undesirable genes which should be changed back to the normal by such directed mutation. Also, by genetic surgery, it is conceivable that a chromosome might be inserted in the egg cell in place of the chromosome bearing the undesired gene. The ideas mentioned in this paragraph will not be elaborated upon because they have so little likelihood of being applicable in the near future.

We are thrust back, therefore to the basis from which eugenics has always operated, that of differential reproduction. Some people have more children than do others. The manipulation of human reproduction so that the average genotype is improved is eugenic, but, if genotypes are impaired, the social manipulation is dysgenic. Geneticists seem to be largely unaware of the great amount of social manipulation of reproduction that occurs all the time. It is my estimate that about 500,000 persons of reproductive age are in mental institutions, prisons, or hospitals on any

SHELDON C. REED

one day in the United States. Several million persons must spend some part of their reproductive life in such institutions, which results in prevention of reproduction at those times. This restriction of reproduction could prevent the transmission of some desirable genes and therefore be dysgenic, but the net effect probably will be a greater restriction of undesirable gene transmission and so turn out to be eugenic. This eugenic result would have only a small effect on the gene frequencies in each generation, but no one should expect to obtain the perfect genotype in all people in one generation. Furthermore, there is no single perfect genotype. Considerable genetic variation is necessary for the good of the species.

Unquestionably, several techniques in use now result in differential reproduction. There are not only the reproductive restrictions resulting from residence in institutions but also voluntary termination of reproduction by persons who carry genes resulting in gross defects of many kinds. Let me recite one of the many such instances from my genetic counseling experiences. A young woman and her boyfriend came to me for assistance. She had osteogenesis imperfecta (broken bone disease) and he had achondroplasia (dwarfism). Both traits depend upon a single, though different, dominant gene for their expression. They were both little people who seemed to be compatible and fitted for each other, except for their reproductive dilemma. One would expect one-quarter of their children to be normal, one-half to display one trait or the other, and one-quarter to have both traits. There is no description of one person with both traits in the literature, so the prospects of viewing such a child were rather titillating. The couple had come to me for support of the woman's request that she receive permanent contraception, as she realized that her chances of having all normal children were small. Her request resulted in a letter from me to her physician strongly supporting her need for help. The physician vacillated and prescribed the "pill." She had difficulties from side effects of the pill and discontinued using it, with the husband using a contraceptive, sometimes. She became pregnant, but medical curiosity was thwarted as she had a macerated miscarriage which was in such poor condition that nothing could be learned from it. A second pleading letter from me to her physician was followed by a tubal ligation and the story ends.

One practical comment may be helpful. In almost all cases where permanent contraception is desired by the couple, it turns out, from my experience, that it is the wife who will go through with the red tape and surmount the other barriers until an operation is performed. Wives usually will place the family well-being ahead of their desire to reproduce, if the risks are about 25 per cent or greater of having a child with a severe defect.

238

It should be noted that in addition to the practice of negative eugenics, which is a more or less accepted part of our culture, as no one wants to produce a child with a severe abnormality, there is some practice of positive eugenics, particularly at the federal governmental and university levels. From these sources come loans, scholarships, dependency allowances, and other inducements to college students to have children. It should be mentioned, however, that the military service legislation is probably dysgenic, because all males with severe genetic handicaps are excused from service. We will presume that in the eugenics of tomorrow military service will not be necessary; no doubt Professor Haldane would agree with this aspiration, which is impossible of attainment at this moment.

How can we clarify the eugenic goals which we would like to achieve by tomorrow? Tomorrow may be as long as 1,000 years from now, because the length of the human generation is so long. Obviously, it is urgent that the population rampage be slowed down within the next few generations, or better, in the next few years. Eugenic progress is less urgent, though those who think that a problem can be ignored because it is not urgent are irresponsible and betray their posterity. As Muller once said, "We are but the genes' way of making more genes!" The corollary follows that we should strive to make the best genes we can and that procrastination will be expensive.

What are the obstacles to clarification of eugenic goals?

Probably the greatest one is the necessity for genetic variability and the likelihood that some of the variability depends upon polymorphic gene loci, such as those for some of the blood groups. Let us consider obesity-thinness, an important polygenic trait. It is clear that there are extremes of both fatness and thinness which prevent the reproduction and survival of the person. It is well known that extremely obese persons have a short life expectancy. The extremely thin people probably are more susceptible than are others to tuberculosis and presumably to other ailments. It is entirely reasonable to assume that there is genetic selection against both the extremes of fatness and thinness though no good evidence on this point is known to me. If one desired to select toward *either* fatness or thinness, as a part of the common behavior pattern, excellent progress could be made in 1,000 years or less. It is the heterogeneous middle of the range of fatness-thinness, however, which is widely accepted as average and "normal" as well as desirable. Assortative mating, and other factors, tend to retard the genetic progress of the population toward the average value for fatness-thinness, but it is likely that social pressure will bring about greater uniformity for this trait in the health-oriented society of tomorrow. In the matter of shortness-tallness, social pressure toward tallness seems to exist, and a look at the Scandinavians or the Watusi indicates how successful genetic selection has been and could be for this trait. The problem of insufficient food supply however, suggests an upper limit to body size which would be tolerated by the culture. Even today, life is difficult for the tallest as well as the shortest people, but probably selection will occur for larger size and more impressive physiques than exist at present for some time to come.

Practically all graded traits seem to be undesirable at the two extremes of the continuum, even personality traits such as extraversion and intro-version being poorly adapted at the extremes and thought of as mentally abnormal. To what extent are these nonadaptive personality types a "segregational" load and to what degree a "mutational" load? We should know some answers to this question as an aid to our eugenics program of tomorrow. The problem of the relative importance of segregational load, that is, the continuous production of poorly adapted homozygotes as the price we pay for the desirable over-dominant heterozygotes, com-pared with the rare undesirable homozygote due to mutation pressure alone is intellectually very exciting today. The eugenics program of tomorrow certainly will be successful in reducing the frequency of un-desirable homozygotes from both segregational and mutational loads to some extent. Even the wildest hopes for genetic surgery and other future eugenic techniques, however, cannot envision anything near 100 per cent success in application. We can never arrive at the goal of genetic perfec-tion, partly because the goal probably will move about. Nevertheless, the nature of man's mind no doubt will remain enough as it is now so that pursuit of the goal will never cease. Those who object to eugenic attempts do not seem to understand that this quest for genetic improvement is a basic drive. It is a fundamental part of the process of natural selection and could be stopped only by the extinction of our species. It will continue no matter how frequent and disastrous are the mistakes we make along the way. None of the eugenic techniques so far contemplated could result in complete genetic homozygosity, which is fortunate, as it gives future generations the opportunity to correct the mistakes of previous ones.

The contemplation of the quantitative conditions, such as extraversion-introversion and fatness-thinness, which give viability at the mass of middle values but lethality at both extremes undoubtedly reduces eugenic ardor. Haldane's ambivalent attitude toward eugenics no doubt stemmed from his comprehension of the difficulty of eliminating both ends of the continuum for common traits and his realization that, on the other hand, very large immediate gains could be obtained by environmental manipu-lation through political change. The appropriate blend of anarchy and authority which will bring about the optimum social state still remains to be discovered.

There is one collection of characteristics, namely, intelligence, which though heterogeneous, is grossly measurable. The curve produced by the measurements of intelligence is similar to that for fatness-thinness and other common traits. The persons at the lower extreme of the intelligence measurements are poorly adapted as over half of those with apparent subnormal intelligence die without having reproduced. The persons at the upper extreme of the intelligence curve behave very differently from those at the lower end. Those with the highest measured intelligence almost always have one or more children. This differential reproductive behavior seems to be slightly positively eugenic at present and certainly has been during the last several million years when man has developed the largest cerebral hemisphere of any species. Reasons suggesting that human intelligence probably is still evolving, genetically, are given in my paper in the September, 1965, issue of the *American Scientist*. It is possible also that the evolution of desirable personality characteristics is still in progress. On the other hand, traits such as fatness-thinness do not seem to be appreciably different in man from what they are in other mammals. They seem to be in a permanently balanced polygenic system; for the physical traits, the average is the most desirable and the reduction of assortative mating probably would result in a tendency toward a greater proportion of the population having the average degree of expression of the trait than now do. The average amount of body fat (or height), however, could be shifted eugenically toward either extreme as society changed its preference for fatter or leaner people. Naturally, the short-term changes would be induced environmentally, but genetic changes would follow if the same preference were maintained for several thousand years.

There probably are conditions other than intelligence which do not handicap persons at one extreme of the curve in adaptation to the environment and for which eugenic selection would be beneficial. For the immediate future the major eugenic goal might well be the improvement of intelligence. The studies of Terman and his associates on the intelligence of the offspring of gifted persons showed only a moderate regression toward the average intelligence in these offspring, indicating that a significant gain in the genetic basis for intelligence is possible if society wishes to make such a gain, which fundamentally it must. The compulsion toward greater intelligence than now prevails is simply that a decrease in intelligence toward the level of other mammalian species is an unacceptable alternative. It is unlikely that man's intelligence will stay just as it is now, though in a world population of over three billion persons the genetic basis for intelligence will not change greatly in any single generation—with or without any reasonable eugenics program.

Finally, let me introduce a few farfetched speculations concerning presently imaginable eugenic products of the distant future some several thousand years from now. It seems reasonable to think that directed mutations could be produced which would broaden the range of reaction of a person to many kinds of stimuli. It should be advantageous for each of our descendants to perceive both longer and shorter wave lengths of both light and sound. Perhaps special sense organs will develop to warn of the presence of radioactive material. Bats have sonar and some fishes emit electrical signals. Perhaps man will evolve some useful form of long-distance communication—a kind of selective and strengthened extra-sensory perception, this taking the place of some of his machines. Could color perception of distant objects, similar to color television, come about in some way? What unknown personality types have yet to appear as a result of intentional genetic changes? All this is fiction now, but everyone is aware that much of the science fiction of one hundred years ago is reality today. Who knows what is possible for human evolution when *eugenic* selection becomes more important than natural selection in population dynamics?

We come to the end of this appreciation of Professor Haldane with the realization that future world population behavior is the actual key to the eugenics of tomorrow. Unless birth rates are lowered in relation to death rates, one can foresee only a chaotic future in which man will have even less control over his heredity and evolution than he has at present. At best, none of the techniques so far envisioned by Haldane, Muller, Lederberg, and others could cause much change in one generation in the heredity of a world of well over three billion people. Nonetheless, the mind of man compels him to try to improve his genotype, and the improvement of the genetic basis for intelligence seems both the most advantageous and most promising goal to work toward at this time. While perfection is unobtainable, the rewards from small gains will be great.

REFERENCES

HALDANE, J. B. S. 1924. *Daedalus; or Science and the Future*. E. P. Dutton and Co., New York.

———. 1938. *Heredity and Politics*. W. W. Norton and Co., New York.

———. 1942. *New Paths in Genetics*. Harper, New York.

———. 1955. The prospects of eugenics. First Woodhull Lecture. The Royal Institution of London.

———. 1963. The implications of genetics for human society. *Proc. XI Int. Congr. Genet.*, 2:xci–cii.

———. 1965. The proper social applications of the knowledge of human genetics. *In* M. Goldsmith and A. Mackay (eds.), *Science of Science*. Science of Science Foundation, London.

MULLER, H. J. 1965. *In* T. M. Sonneborn (ed.), *The Control of Human Heredity and Evolution*. Macmillan, New York.

ARTHUR C. CLARKE
47–5, Gregory's Road,
Colombo 7, Ceylon

XVIII. HALDANE AND SPACE

Professor J. B. S. Haldane was perhaps the most brilliant scientific popularizer of his generation; starting in 1924 with *Daedalus; or Science and the Future*, he must have delighted and instructed millions of readers. Unlike his equally famous contemporaries, Jeans and Eddington, he covered a vast range of subjects. Biology, astronomy, physiology, military affairs, mathematics, theology, philosophy, literature, politics—he tackled them all. He also wrote a workmanlike *novella*, *The Gold Makers*, and a charming tale for children, *My Friend Mr. Leakey*.

Although some are naturally dated by the progress of science, most of Haldane's scores of essays—they appeared in such varied places as *Harper's Magazine*, the *Saturday Evening Post*, the *Strand Magazine*, the *Spectator*, the *Daily Express*, the *St. Louis Post-Dispatch*, and, of course, the *Daily Worker*—may still be read with great profit. Some of the volumes in which they were reprinted, such as *Possible Worlds* (1927) or *The Inequality of Man* (1932), now may be difficult to obtain. However, one of Haldane's most famous essays, "On Being the Right Size," is readily available in James Newman's *The World of Mathematics* (Vol. 2). It is a perfect example of his lucidity and the breadth of his interests.

So far as I can recall, I was first attracted to Haldane's writings by the element of extrapolation they contained. He obviously was sympathetic to science-fiction and astronautics; indeed, I have just discovered this paragraph in his very first book, *Daedalus*: "I should have liked had time allowed to have added my quota to the speculations which have been made with regard to inter-planetary communication. Whether this is possible I can form no conjecture; that it will be attempted I have no doubt whatever."

It was through space flight that I made my first, and somewhat alarming, encounter with Professor Haldane. In 1951 as chairman of the British Interplanetary Society, I invited him to give our organization a paper on the biological aspects of space flight. Despite very short notice (the lecture was a substitute for one by Professor J. D. Bernal, which had to be postponed), Haldane at once agreed to step into the breach.

He and Helen Spurway duly arrived at the Caxton Hall, Westminster, in one of the most decrepit cars I have ever seen; it appeared to be held together largely by rust. When I greeted him at the top of the steps and reached out to take his hat, he insisted on retaining it for sanitary reasons. The cat, he explained, had just used it for an unauthorized purpose— though he put the matter more pithily, if you will excuse the pun.

After this not very auspicious beginning, the lecture was a great success (1). It dealt with three problems: how men would live in space-ships, how they would live on other planets, and what sort of life they might find there. In 1951 these were not subjects with which many reputable scientists cared to be associated, and Haldane himself had sometimes adopted a rather conservative attitude toward space flight. In his remarkable essay "The Last Judgement" (in *Possible Worlds*), he set the first landing on Mars in the year 9,723,841 and an expedition to Venus "half a million years later." This demonstrates, once again, how hard it is for even the most farsighted scientist to anticipate the future. Haldane hardly could have believed, in 1927, that he would live to see the Apollo project and to participate himself in state-sponsored conferences on exobiology.

Though it has naturally been superseded in many respects, Haldane's 1951 paper still contained some ideas still of interest. He must have been one of the first to point out the dangers of solar flares and to suggest that space voyages should be made during periods of minimum solar activity. With his tongue firmly in his cheek, he suggested that we should take seriously the hypothesis that life has a supernatural origin—from which he concluded that, as there are 400,000 species of beetles on this planet, but only 8,000 species of animal, "the Creator, if he exists, has a special preference for beetles, and so we might be more likely to meet them than any other type of animal on a planet that would support life."

After the lecture, we took Haldane and Spurway to dinner at the Arts Theatre Club, and of the sparkling conversation that doubtless ensued I remember only one item. This, however, involves such a striking and melancholy coincidence that it is worth recording.

Presumably we had been discussing problems of respiration, for Haldane expressed the belief that, in the right circumstances, animals could "breathe" water. One of his reasons for believing this was the observation that it is extremely difficult to drown newborn mice; it seems that their lungs are still capable of extracting oxygen from water. Haldane then made the sadly prophetic statement: "If I knew that I was dying of cancer, I'd like to make this experiment. It would probably be rather painful. . . ."

Now, of course, Klystra has demonstrated water breathing with animals up to the size of dogs, but Haldane had been thinking of this as far back as 1951.

Our paths did not cross again for almost ten years, when we had both migrated to the East. In November, 1960, the Ceylon Association for the Advancement of Science invited Haldane to Colombo to address its annual meeting, and it was characteristic of him that on arrival he immediately abandoned the official hotel in favor of a modest Indian (and vegetarian) hostel in a less fashionable suburb of the city.

I debated for a considerable time before calling on him. In the intervening years, I had heard rumors of his ferocity—some reports of his behavior to journalists made him sound similar to Conan Doyle's Professor Challenger—and I had no idea whether he remembered our last encounter, still less whether I was *persona grata*. Nevertheless, quaking slightly, with my partner Mike Wilson to give me moral and (if necessary) physical support, I called at his hotel and sent up my card.

His first words when he arrived on the scene, dressed in his white gown and looking as a Hindu patriarch would, were not very reassuring. "Oh, my god!" was distinctly discouraging, and a real or feigned deafness made any further communication appear hopeless. I was about to leave with as little fuss as possible when I suddenly realized that, far from being exasperated at the intrusion, he genuinely was glad to see me. I was not so surprised to discover that he had read most of my books, for Haldane, of course, had read *everything*.

Within a couple of hours the Haldanes had arrived at my house, where the Professor leaped upon my technical library like a starving man. Later in the afternoon we took him on tour of Colombo's excellent zoo, not knowing that he was suffering from a spinal injury that must have caused him great discomfort. When this subsequently was discovered, he apologized for any absentmindedness, adding that a fractured vertebra was not all that important as "I have learned to ignore certain types of sensory input."

A few days later, the Wilsons and myself invited the Haldanes and their Indian colleagues (Drs. Davis and Dronamraju) to dinner at our house. After this length of time, I can remember only two fragments of small talk. At one point, the Haldanes were demolishing reputations with such gusto that I felt constrained to remark "That's what I like about science—the way it rises above personalities." And when the conversation turned, via unidentified flying objects, to atmospheric electricity, I asked the Professor: "Is it true that when he had a research station on Pike's

Peak, your father did some work on ball lightning?" He answered at once, "No, ball lightning did some work on *him*."

After the dinner, we screened Mike Wilson's underwater movie, *Beneath the Seas of Ceylon* (2), showing the behavior of the teeming population of the Great Basses Reef, and, in particular, recording the intelligence of a family of black groupers (*Epinephelus fuscoguttatus*). The spectacle of these giant fish co-operating as movie extras impressed Haldane so much that he frequently gave vent to a surprisingly schoolboyish "Golly!"—a term which, for all its *naïveté*, expresses the sense of wonder that is the hallmark of the great scientist.

We never met again—but our real acquaintance had started and continued in subsequent correspondence. In April, 1962, I received a pressing invitation to stay with the Haldanes, opening with a rather ambiguous compliment: "Allow me to congratulate you on the Kalinga Prize. Personally I should also like to see you awarded a prize for theology, as you are one of the very few living persons who has written anything original about God. You have in fact written several mutually incompatible things . . . if you had stuck to one theological hypothesis you might be a serious public danger."

To my lasting regret, I was unable to accept Haldane's hospitality as I had contrived to get myself almost completely paralyzed, and it was some months before I was able to walk again. And when I finally got to the Kalinga ceremony, it was in New Delhi, not Orissa, so I was farther away from the Professor than if I had stayed in Ceylon.

Thereafter, my slow convalescence and a series of other problems prevented a rendezvous, but we continued to correspond hopefully. Haldane's letters, usually handwritten, often ran to 1000 words and were so full of ideas as his agile mind jumped from one subject to another that they were both good fun and hard reading. It was obvious that he took great pride in the team he had built up around him at Bhubaneswar; as he put it: "I seem to have taken the lid off some young men, and they are making really fantastic discoveries."

A few extracts will serve to give the flavor of that final correspondence, covering the period April 12, 1962, to January 8, 1964:

> I want to talk to you seriously about the soul and all that.
>
> You have been listening to the apiary in Professor J. B. S. Haldane's bonnet.
>
> It is clear that a gibbon, and still more a prehensile-tailed South American monkey (or a man-sized version of one) is much better pre-adapted than *H. sap* for low gravitational fields . . . we might get back these lost appendages by intranuclear grafting. We should then find it natural to count up to 210 (10

246

fingers) × (10 fingers + 10 toes + 1 tail). This would be a better base than 10 (being 2 × 3 × 5 × 7) and a slight improvement either in cerebral organisation or teaching methods would enable people to learn the necessary multiplication table.

I suspect the hymenoptera and isoptera are the best hope for studying non-human technology. My wife, for reasons of her own, regards the diptera as Top animals.

I have been thinking about cosmonautics (i.e., going to Alpha Centauri and further). It seems to me that there are two possibilities. (1) It is practicable to reach speeds of the order of ½ that of light. (2) To avoid too highly energetic collisions with dust clouds, it is not practicable to exceed about 1,000 km/sec. which is near the upper bound of relative stellar velocities in our neighborhood.

As there are probably a lot of animal species in the galaxy with a technology more advanced than ours, but they don't seem to visit our planet often, I suggest that (2) is the more probable. If (1) is more correct, the voyages would mainly be undertaken at speeds near that of light. . . .

An intelligent species is pre-adapted for interstellar travel if (a) it is very long-lived or reproduces clonally, so that the crew will have the same set of personalities after the numerous generations needed to travel long distances, and (b) it is accustomed to a very large gravitational field. If white dwarfs cool down, and life evolves on them, their inhabitants, though nearly two-dimensional, could be boosted with an acceleration which would flatten you and me. Has this point been made? If not, it is a present for you.

The last letter I received from Haldane was written from University College Hospital on January 8, 1964, and characteristically it linked his final illness with the subject of astronautics. After describing his present plight after his colostomy he remarked "I (and a million other surgical cases) would be quite satisfied with lunar surface gravitation (1/6g). A few would no doubt be better in free fall. . . ."

The same letter reverted to our earlier discussion of interstellar flight. During his visit to the United States, Haldane met Carl Sagan, who had given him his stimulating paper on direct contact between galactic civilizations (3). This obviously inspired these speculations: "I suggest the following hypotheses. Interstellar travel occurs on a vast scale. 'Cosmic rays' are merely the exhaust of rockets. The rocketeers do not often visit us for any of several reasons. They may think we are nasty chaps. They may mostly be social arthropods, uncertain how to help members of a different phylum to evolve or behave. And so on."

The length, cheerfulness, and intellectual energy of this letter completely deceived me. Haldane always had seemed indestructible, and I continued to plan for our meeting in Orissa.

ARTHUR C. CLARKE

It was a great shock to hear of his death a few months later and to realize that communication had at last broken with the finest intellect it has ever been my privilege to know.

REFERENCES

1. SLATER, A. E. 1951. Biological problems of space flight. A report of Professor Haldane's lecture to the Society on April 7, 1951. *J. Brit. Interplanetary Soc.*, 10 (July 4, 1951):154–58.
2. CLARKE, ARTHUR C., AND MIKE WILSON. 1961. *Indian Ocean Adventure.* Harper.
3. SAGAN, CARL. 1963. Direct contact among galactic civilisations by relativistic interstellar spaceflight. *Planetary Space Sci.*, 11:485–98.

ORIGIN OF LIFE

N. W. PIRIE
Biochemistry Department,
Rothamsted Experimental Station,
Harpenden, Herts., England

XIX. THE DEVELOPMENT OF HALDANE'S OUTLOOK ON THE NATURE AND ORIGINS OF LIFE

Until the seventeenth century the origin of life did not seem to be a serious scientific problem. Observation was often casual and little use was made of controls or even of deliberate experiment. Then, increasing knowledge of the stages in development of the smaller animals and plants made suspect the old casual assumption that maggots and putrefaction appeared automatically in aging organic matter. Homer knew (*Iliad*, xix) that maggots would not develop if flies were excluded, but this knowledge was not put on an experimental basis until 1668 when Redi described the practical method we still use for excluding flies from food with gauze, which allows access of air. This was a period of general skepticism. Though Harvey did not use the phrase *Omne vivum ex ovo* commonly attributed to him, it sums up, as the designer of the frontispiece to his *De Generatione Animalium* realized, his point of view. Similar points of view were expressed by Boyle, Leeuwenhoek, and many others.

Opinion became more fluid in the eighteenth century. Although vast advances were made in anatomy, physiology, and biological classification, discussion on the origin of life tended to be metaphysical and nonexperimental. The explanation lies in part in the crudity of the criteria that had to be used for recognizing an organism: they amounted to little more than the presence or absence of spontaneous movement. This is a legacy from language. The Bible speaks of the quick and the dead, and even scientific language separates oviparous from viviparous animals. Scientists seem to agree generally with the original inhabitants of Australia who use the word "bilabong," which means literally "dead water," for backwaters and other parts of a stream that are not flowing.

The next advance, again, came from the domestic arts. In 1810 Appert published his book *L'Art de Conserver, Pendant Plusieurs Années, Toutes les Substances Animales et Végétales*, and his methods of food preservation by heating and sealing quickly became the basis of worldwide industry. The scientific basis for this practical activity was established 50 years later by Pasteur, and the problem of the origin of life gained formal recognition. It was discussed copiously by Pasteur, Engels, Huxley, Tyndall, Schaefer, and others and treated somewhat cavalierly by Darwin, who remarked in a letter: "It is mere rubbish thinking at present of the origin of life. One might as well think of the origin of matter."

These writers agreed on one issue: there was no reason to think that any experiment had ever demonstrated the appearance of an organism in an initially sterile medium, but they all believed it possible that this could happen and probable that it had happened in the early stages of earth's development. As Pasteur put it, "La génération spontanée, je la cherche sans la découvrir depuis vingt ans. Non, je ne la juge pas impossible." The century closed with an animated exchange of letters in *Nature* on the significance of steroisomerism in argument about the origins of life; I have discussed this elsewhere (Pirie, 1959).

Interest lapsed at the beginning of this century, and the statements made in many textbooks were both foolish and inaccurate. Pasteur was commonly said to have demonstrated the impossibility of spontaneous generation, and Arrhenius revived Liebig and Kelvin's old idea that one must assume that life had come here from elsewhere—thus merely transferring the problem. Darwin and his contemporaries simply had assumed that organic matter would gradually be synthesized from the simple carbon compounds and minerals on a sterile earth; a great advance was made when Haldane (1929) described a plausible mechanism. Herbert Spencer suggested that most, or even all, atmospheric oxygen had been made by green plants. Haldane pointed out that, if the probiotic world were anaerobic, any complex molecules that were generated would be more stable than they tend to be in the presence of oxygen and that there would be no ozone in the atmosphere. Ozone absorbs ultraviolet light strongly, so that only a small proportion of that present in sunlight now gets through to us. Before there was free oxygen in the atmosphere, much more ultraviolet light would have got through, and it was already well known to be a powerful agent promoting synthesis. From this he concluded that the primitive ocean would have "the consistency of hot dilute soup," so that any organism that did manage to appear would have abundant food. He went on to argue that they must have depended, as embryos and many bactcria do, on fermentation, that is to say, on getting energy by catalyzing reactions within and between molecules that do not involve their oxidation. This is a logical necessity for life in an anaerobic environment, but it is difficult to envisage the types of reaction that might have been involved and that would not already have been brought about by the postulated intense ultraviolet radiation acting for very long periods.

It seems more probable that then, as now, life, if it arose in this way, depended on the flux of solar energy. An extensive summary of this paper appeared in *Nature* in 1928 and Haldane included it in *The Inequality of Man*, a collection of essays published in 1932. As a result, these ideas became widely known, among biochemists at any rate. They soon gained, and have retained, general acceptance in principle. Haldane commented (1954, 1963*b*) that their acceptance in both the U.S. and the U.S.S.R. caused him some perturbation because of his mistrust for orthodoxy.

Interest in this paper centered around the plausible mechanism suggested for the nonvital synthesis of complex organic molecules. The paper also contains some very interesting speculations on the nature of viruses and genes and the suggestion that they may be considered fragments of organisms that, though unable to reproduce in normal culture media, could do so in the specialized environment of a cell. Haldane also suggested that somewhat similar half-organisms originally may have come together and, by co-operation, built up the prototype of a free-living organism. At that date, few of those studying either viruses or genetics were sufficiently accustomed to biochemical modes of thought to grasp the significance of these suggestions. Briefly, while discussing these issues, and more fully in a later (1936) paper, he analyzed the effect of molecular size on the concept of reproduction. Haldane pointed out that, if genes were thought of as large molecules, they would not grow and then divide as do cells, but, by a process analogous to crystallization, a sister gene would be built near the original. He used the word "sister" rather than "daughter" because "modern physical concepts suggest that no series of observations could determine with complete certainty which of a pair of 'sister' genes is the model and which the copy, though they could, I think, make a statement on the subject highly probable. . . ." As Fitzgerald made Omar Khayyam say: "Who *is* the Potter, pray, and who the Pot?"

The origins of life were not discussed in Haldane's *The Marxist Philosophy and the Sciences* (1938), but some attention was given in that book to our criteria for calling something an organism and to the nature of replication, or reproduction. The accepted organisms can multiply in an inert environment, but he suggested that viruses, which need a host for their multiplication, may persuade the host to copy them "as, for example, a limerick persuades a man to repeat it." This book adumbrated the idea to which he returned in later articles (1944, 1945) that, in thinking about the chemical processes involved in the origins of life, we may be in error if we think in terms of contemporary chemistry exclusively.

Starting from the observation that there is a "red shift" in the light from galaxies that is roughly proportional to their distance from us, and accepting the idea that this is a Doppler effect and that the universe is expanding, he extended Milne's deduction that this would entail a change with time in the nature of some chemical reactions. Haldane argued (1944, 1945) that the ratio of the rates of inter- and intra-molecular reactions would alter, and calculated that in pre-Cambrian times the rate at which energy could be liberated by a system resembling present-day muscle would have been so slow that a land animal would scarcely have been able to crawl. In simpler organisms the main factor influencing the maintenance of metabolism in a cell is diffusion; he suggested that cellular life had to await a time when changing chemistry had made possible the liberation of energy at a sufficient rate to maintain the necessary internal environment. In 1947 he told me that ideas involving changes with time in physical and chemical constants were now becoming unfashionable, and he repeated this in a later article (1954). The idea that our form of life could arise only when the universe had evolved a chemistry suited to it, is intriguing and would go far, as Haldane (1938) pointed out, to resolve the at-first-sight improbable congruity between vital requirements and the chemistry of such simple substances as water and carbon dioxide which worried L. J. Henderson so much. The possibility of such changes should be borne in mind but judgment may, for the moment, be suspended.

If, as Erasmus, Darwin thought

> Without parents by spontaneous birth
> Rise the first specks of animated earth. (*Temple of Nature*, 1, lines 247–48)

it should be possible to calculate the probability of the appearance of a degree of complexity and activity that could justify the use of the term "living." Using different assumptions, Haldane made this calculation several times (1952, 1954, 1964). In the first article he estimated that an ocean containing a variety of organic molecules would by pure chance probably meet specifications calling for between 50 and 200 "bits"[1] in 10^9 years and that a bacteriophage contained about 100 bits. His conclusion is quoted for the characteristic phrasing: "If Brahma, though not eternal, has a time scale of about 10^{15} of our own, his easiest method of creating intelligent beings like ourselves might be to leave a few planets at a suitable distance from their suns for 2×10^9 years, as we light a match with confidence that one of a large number of random events will usually

[1] A "bit" is the unit of information or of choice between two equally probable alternatives. Thus the selection of one object, or course of action, from among four, requires two "bits," from among eight, four "bits," and so on. It can also be regarded as a unit of negative entropy.

set off a chain of reactions. This is not intended as an argument for Theism, but merely as a plea for precision in the discussion of that hypothesis." The last article made the appearance of life seem less probable. Even one enzyme of the present day type would need 100 bits, and he suggested that 5000 would be needed for an artificial organism.

The disparity between these two estimates depends primarily on the capacities demanded of an organism. Haldane partly resolved this by enlarging (1953, 1954) on his earlier suggestion that organisms about which there could be no equivocation may have arisen by the concrescence of two or more simpler sub-vital units capable of only a brief existence in the free state. This suggestion implies the independent appearance of systems with a quasi-vital degree of complexity, and Haldane was one of the first to write of the origins of life instead of using the more usual singular. He had argued, however, in earlier articles that the uniformity with which organisms use molecules of one stereoisomeric type, e.g., the L amino acids, to the exclusion of the other, was evidence that there had been a single origin. This argument was again stressed in 1958, but in 1960, after the demonstration that in certain nuclear reactions parity is not conserved, so that some chiral selectiveness is present in atoms themselves, he pointed out that this phenomenon might explain the observed biological uniformity.

The apparent immense improbability of the spontaneous appearance of life can be resolved in various other ways. A probability states no more than the number of trials you *expect* to make to get the required result; you may need many more—or many less. If we were not here now the issue would not be under discussion. The required result can only be stated if we know the parameters of life; all we know are the parameters of our type of life, and there may be others. Some may not even depend on carbon as their primary element.

The idea of alternative ways of living has a natural attraction for the imaginative and can be completely sterile if the principles of chemistry and physics are not kept firmly in mind. Haldane suggested (1954), as others had done, that metaphosphates may at first have filled the role that adenosine triphosphate fills now and (1957) that when adenosine triphosphate appeared it may have brought about phosphorylations on surfaces of a different nature from the enzymes now used. He also suggested that life could exist in ammonia and other nonaqueous environments. Similar suggestions were made by others, and it would be unprofitable to try to assign precedence.

Many microorganisms 0.5–1.0 μm in diameter are known; a few members of a rather ill-defined group, classed together as Mycoplasmataceae, have only a tenth of that diameter. The viruses are very much smaller but cannot be included in the group of "living" organisms because their multiplication is absolutely dependent on the activity of a host—there is no reason to think that they do more than divert host metabolism into anomalous channels that lead to the production of more virus. The apparent absence of organisms with diameters less than about 100 nm may be the result of the inadequacy of our techniques of recognition, but if it is real it raises a very interesting question: What is it that sets a lower limit to the size of organisms able to multiply without the co-operation of a larger organism? Haldane discussed this problem in the paper that he contributed to the meeting celebrating his father's centenary (1963*a*). Starting with the proposition that quantal events have no details, that is to say, that they are spread without parts throughout the space and time in which they occur, he considered the extent to which separate quantal events will overlap. With the rapid events taking place in an atom, overlap is rare, but he argued that there would be significant overlap with the slower and less energetic events in a cell. The basic principle is that the extension in time of a quantal event is inversely proportional to its energy, and the less the energy the greater the extension in space—as is well known with electromagnetic radiation. He suggested that independent life is a quality that can emerge only when many juxtaposed processes, considered as quantal events, can "interact" because of this overlapping. The argument is somewhat nebulous because our habits of thought are attuned to matter in bulk and not to atoms and quanta, but he argued that his suggestion was not more metaphysical than the conventional explanation of the phase change from gas to liquid. In the former the molecules interact very little; in the latter they interact thoroughly.

A similar line of thought runs through three other papers (1956, 1963*b*, 1964) which examine, in the light of quantum physics, Spinoza's idea that there may be mind-like correlates in "other modes of being." He argued that, if thought processes are small-energy events, they may be essentially delocalized in the brain; this is what animal experiments and human injury suggest. The argument was intricate and it ramified in many directions, such as the interpretation of intracellular structure and the mechanism of telepathy, if it should prove necessary to accept that. The suggestion most relevant to this discussion is that "thought" may exist in the dense matter of a white dwarf star. It may be impossible to visualize thought without a thinker to communicate with, but if any such system should be recognized we could not begrudge it the title "living" merely because it is constructed from unconventional material.

One of the consequences of the Copernican revolution, which moved earth from the center of the universe to a subsidiary position, was to rob human beings of their apparently privileged position as the most advanced type of organism. We are now beginning to worry about the possibility that we may contaminate other planets. This is commendable. It is of more immediate and mundane importance, however, to take care, if astronauts are being returned to earth from some other planet, that they do not bring contaminants back with them. If there are alien forms of life, or xenobionts, with a completely different form of metabolism from our own chthonobionts, they are likely to be poorly adapted to this environment and are not likely to be troublesome; but if they should have a similar constitution and metabolism, either because this is the only one possible, or, as Haldane (1954) suggested, because organisms from a common source were deliberately scattered around the universe, an introduction could be catastrophic. Although evolution is likely to have followed different, though comparable, courses in different environments, the end products may be similar enough to be pathogens on one another.

Haldane did not, so far as I know, express firm opinions in writing on the validity of the suggestion that there is life on Mars, but in conversation (1929) he said that Phobos and Deimos seemed better evidence for it than the so-called canals. These satellites are so small and they are so near the parent body that it seemed to him possible that they had been made by intelligent creatures. This suggestion was also made by Manhattan (1953).

Haldane wrote about the nature and origins of life for 35 years and put forward at least one novel idea in every article. He often did this because he was more aware than most biologists of current developments in physical theory and immediately explored the biological consequences that would be entailed if the conclusions being propounded in physics proved to be well founded. The problem was defined in broad outline by Pasteur, Huxley, and Tyndall; Haldane gave it a concrete biochemical form. Many laboratories are now engaged in the study of the types of molecule that are formed in environments similar to those we postulate on the probiotic earth, and we may soon expect astronauts to bring back information on the past or present state of biology elsewhere. Their work will be facilitated and their ideas clarified if they read Haldane carefully. It will be still further facilitated if, emulating him, they strive to keep all the possibilities simultaneously in mind, even if they assign different probabilities to them. Nothing inhibits research so much as the premature assumption that we know the general framework within which phenomena take place.

REFERENCES

HALDANE, J. B. S. 1929. The origin of life. *Rationalist Ann.*, p. 3.
―――. 1936. Some principles of causal analysis in genetics. *Erkenntnis*, 6:346.
―――. 1938. *The Marxist Philosophy and the Sciences*. G. Allen and Unwin, London.
―――. 1944. Radioactivity and the origin of life in Milne's cosmology. *Nature*, 153:555.
―――. 1945. A new theory of the past. *Amer. Sci.*, 33:129.
―――. 1952. The mechanical chess-player. *Brit. J. Phil. Sci.*, 3:189.
―――. 1953. Foreword to Evolution. *Symp. Soc. Exp. Biol.*, 7:ix.
―――. 1954. The origins of life. *New Biol.*, 16:12.
―――. 1956. Time in biology. *Sci. Progress*, 175:385.
―――. 1957. Genesis of life, p. 287. *In* D. R. Bates (ed.), *The Planet Earth*. Pergamon Press. London.
―――. 1958. *The Unity and Diversity of Life*. Pub. Div., Min. Inf. Broadcasting, Govt. of India, Delhi.
―――. 1960. Pasteur and cosmic asymmetry. *Nature*, 185:87.
―――. 1963a. A possible development of J. S. Haldane's views on the relation between quantum mechanics and biology, p. 103. *In* D. J. C. Cunningham and B. B. Lloyd (eds.), *The Regulation of Human Respiration*. Blackwell, Oxford.
―――. 1963b. Life and mind as physical realities. *Science Survey B*, p. 224. Penguin Books, Harmondsworth, Middlesex.
―――. 1964. Data needed for a blueprint of the first organism, p. 11. *In* S. W. Fox (ed.), *The Origins of Prebiological Systems and Their Molecular Matrices*. Academic Press, New York.
MANHATTAN, A. 1953. The bewildering mystery of Mars. *Rationalist Ann.*, p. 67.
PIRIE, N. W. 1959. The position of steroisomerism in argument about the origins of life. J. C. Bose Memorial Volume. *Trans. Bose Inst.*, 22:111.

A. I. OPARIN
A. N. Bach Institute of Biochemistry,
The Academy of Sciences of the U.S.S.R.,
Moscow, U.S.S.R.

XX. HALDANE AND THE PROBLEMS OF THE ORIGIN OF LIFE[1]

Haldane, exceptionally versatile as a scientist, paid particular attention to the problem of the origin of life. His first works on this problem already had appeared by the latter 1920's, and almost at the end of his life he again gave a general account of this subject at the Conference on the Origin of Prebiological Systems in Florida at the end of 1963.[2]

The broad development of research into the origin of life, therefore, is associated continuously with the illustrious memory of Haldane.

We cannot in our time directly uncover the beginning of life on our Earth, because this process in the past had a unilaterally directed, unrepeatable character. We also are deprived of the possibility of artificially reproducing it in full as it happened on our planet, because this process took millions of years. We can objectively illustrate the outstanding events of this process, however, discovering them in nature (not only on Earth but also on other objects in the Universe), if the conditions are preserved here which existed in the epoch preceding the appearance of life. Equally, we can, by artificially reproducing these conditions in the laboratory, imitate the prebiological systems existing at the time of the origin of life. Finally, the study of primitive protoplasmic structures and the first stages of metabolism in contemporary lower organisms, particularly in bacteria and blue-green algae, helps us understand the beginnings of life. This research is useful in helping to explain the course of the evolution of metabolism and of its earliest stages, which arose in the very process of the establishment of life.

Using all of the information obtained about the different stages of evolution, we can hope to reproduce artificially the whole process of the development of life, by consciously substituting for the long natural evolution a deliberate combination of the processes which formerly appeared as successive links in the evolutionary chain.

[1] Translation of the original Russian manuscript by Richard Harris.
[2] S. W. Fox (ed.), *The Origins of Prebiological Systems*. Academic Press, New York, p. 11.

Underlying the beginning of life on our Earth (and perhaps on other heavenly bodies) is the process of the evolution of carbon compounds. It can be divided provisionally into three stages: (1) The beginning of the simplest organic substances (hydrocarbons) and their nearest derivatives. (2) The beginning of the "primeval broth"—the solution in water of varied and complicated organic substances, monomers, and polymers. (3) The beginning of complicated multimolecular open systems, serving as initial developments for the formation of the first living substances.

The first stage of the evolution of carbon compounds—the abiogenetic development of the simplest organic substances—is extremely widely diffused in the Cosmos. It is now complete and can be discovered in widely varied objects in the universe. This stage is accessible to a known degree, therefore, to our immediate study, and in the future our knowledge of this stage will be established more fully in proportion to the penetration of man into the Cosmos.

Immediately, it is true that, of all non-earthly objects, we can directly investigate chemically and mineralogically only meteorites (carbonaceous chondrites). In connection with other heavenly bodies, our work is based only on spectroscopic and other indirect data. Here and now it is best to reckon that the main mass of hydrocarbons appeared on the surface of the Earth during the formation of its crust and the development of the secondarily renewed atmosphere and hydrosphere. In addition, now as in the past, our planet is always being "fed" by simple organic substances from meteorites and comets, as are the Moon and Mars.

The second stage of the evolution of organic materials is revealed at the present time in the numerous model experiments in abiogenetic synthesis in laboratory conditions, which imitate the conditions once existing on the surface of the Earth. Here research naturally starts from the contemporary belief that the chemical potencies of methane or of another organic substance are invariable, whether in the past or present, whether in the primary or secondary atmosphere of the earth, or in the contemporary chemist's retort. By consciously reproducing the conditions of the pre-biological epoch, therefore, we are justified in expecting results on the basis of which we can judge the events of the distant past.

The experiments referred to give a solid base to the possibility of the development at a defined period in the history of our planet of the so-called primeval broth, that is, the aqueous solution of various organic substances including such complicated and biologically important polymers as polypeptides and polynucleotides. It is true that, in contrast to contemporary albumens, they would have possessed only a very simple, accidentally arranged disposition of monomers in their chains of polymers.

Of course, much in the study of this stage of evolution still remains unclear and demands further research. In particular, it is possible to argue about the general or local concentration of the primeval broth, about the presence in it of this or that compound, and so on; but, in principle, the question of the primitive abiogenetic development of the aqueous solution of organic substances on the still lifeless Earth can be regarded as settled.

A different, much more complicated, matter arises with the third, more amenable, stage of evolution—with the formation of prebiological and biological systems.

Life is not diffused in space as were the materials of the primeval broth. It is represented by systems made up of discrete organisms spatially separate from the surrounding external medium, but interacting with this medium according to the type of open system. The stability of systems of this sort and the length of their existence are determined not by immutability and tranquillity but, on the contrary, by the constancy of the change in materials, by the regular synthesis and dissolution of these materials, and by establishment of biological metabolism.

On the basis of data now at our disposal, we cannot see the feasibility of the direct development of every kind of living system from the primitive mixture of organic substances; nor can we observe or artificially reproduce development of such living systems, either in relation to whole cells or to separate organelles.

The breach existing between the primeval broth and the most primitive living systems could be filled in the course of natural evolution only by way of a long development. A gradual improvement of organisms must be assumed, with some systems much simpler than the organisms of the prebiological systems capable of forming themselves in the primeval broth, producing themselves from it in the form of basic individual systems, mutually interacting, however, both chemically and genetically, with the external medium surrounding them. It is possible not only to imagine such a self-filtering system but, in fact, to obtain a very large number and variety of such systems. In particular, it is pertinent here to mention S. Fox's microsphere or coacervate drops. These last seem to us especially suitable as models, though they are far from being the only possible ones for the reproduction of the phenomena which took place in the primeval broth.

Their formation does not require the presence of polymers possessing strongly determined intramolecular organizations such as contemporary albumens or nucleic acids. As is shown by experiments in our laboratory, coacervate drops can be formed by a simple mixing of solutions of unspecific or monotonously constructed polypeptides and polynucleotides.

The only important thing is the dimension of the molecule. With the simultaneous synthesis of the polymers indicated, as soon as the determined degree of polymerization is reached in the resulting solution, coacervate drops invariably are formed.

Thus, the creation of coacervates in the primeval broth appear to have provided a direct means for the development of high-molecular primitive polymers. The improvement of the intramolecular structure of the latter in the process of further evolution must have occurred not simply in the solution, but precisely in the multimolecular systems indicated.

Polymers form in the coacervate drops in a very concentrated form (50 per cent or more) even when the drops come from a very dilute solution. In addition, the drops are capable of selectively absorbing various low molecular substances from the surrounding broth. Even if some of these substances are capable of catalytically speeding up the reactions taking place in the drops, the drops change into open systems, interacting in a specific way in the external medium.

In our model experiments, by inserting into the drops various simple and complex catalysts (organic substances and nonorganic salts), we produced in the coacervate drops the reactions of oxide reduction, synthesis and dissolution of polymers, and so on. In some cases we used ferments as catalysts, although, of course, ferments cannot have been in the primeval broth, but their use was advantageous in the laboratory work and, therefore, we thought it permissible to utilize them.

As an example, I introduce the scheme of one of our experiments. The drop is represented in the scheme by a square contour, consisting of a polynucleotide and a histon and including in itself the ferment in the solution containing AP.

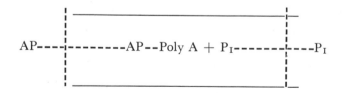

Entering the drop from the external medium, AP polymerizes, forming all new and new portions of the polynucleotide (Poly A). For its part, the drop grows in size and weight, and the nonorganic phosphorus is liberated into the external medium. We produced more complicated schemes of metabolic flow in the coacervates, in which not one but several different reactions were produced and in which a quicker or slower growth of the drops, or even their dissolution, was brought about.

Open and multimolecular systems endowed with primitive metabolism, similar to our models, must have been easily produced in the primeval broth, as a result of the inclusion in the coacervate drops of various organic and nonorganic catalysts from the external medium. The systems of this sort growing in size and weight (provisionally we will call them protobionts) must in the conditions of the primeval broth have grown and then crumbled under the influence of external mechanical forces (for example, wash or the impact of waves) like the crushing of drops of emulsion when it is shaken.

The protobionts produced in this diaster preserved permanently to a known degree the character of their interaction with the external medium, all the time absorbing from the external medium specific catalysts and so preserving permanently the relationship of the speed and mutual adjustment of the reactions taking place in them. Of course, such permanency was very incomplete compared with the capacity of contemporary organisms for reproducing themselves. On this basis it was already possible to produce what may be called a "rivalry" between the protobionts in the quickness of growth and of multiplication. We can assume here an original prebiological selection.

We have succeeded in demonstrating the possibility of such "selection" in model experiments with coacervates. For this, a complex of catalysts was included in one drop, leading, in the given conditions of the external medium, to a comparatively quick synthesis of the polymers and the expansion of all the systems as a whole. On the other hand, in other drops the catalytic complex was less complete. In the first sort of drops quick growth occurred, but the second sort suppressed growth. Comparable biochemical research into the metabolism of the most primitive contemporary organisms allows us to imagine the subsequent path of evolutionary development, a path produced as a result of the aforementioned prebiological selection on the way to the beginning of life.

Of course, between our models and even the most primitive living substances there still lies a great gulf, and it is precisely the filling of this gulf that must form the principal content of the prospective work on the origin of life to be undertaken in the very near future.

The formation of the bases of biological metabolism and cellular structure in the process of the development of life demanded many, many hundred million years, perhaps half of all the time during which life has existed on the Earth. If we clearly imagine the whole magnitude of that evolution, how naïve do those hopeless experiments now appear which were carried out so recently in attempts to reproduce artificially the spontaneous self-production of life in decaying matter and existing organic substances. Only by discovering the ways by which living substances were formed in the process of the evolution of matter under natural conditions can we hope to produce them artificially, not by that tortuous path of Nature, but in a relatively short period, consciously assembling in our laboratories the necessary conditions and the indispensable sequence of events, substituting for natural selection the deliberate combination of materials, systems, and processes. This way leads us hopefully towards the realization of the solemn aim of mankind—to the artificial synthesis of life.

The successes achieved permit us to look on synthesis of such life as not such a distant prospect.

PHYSIOLOGY AND EMBRYOLOGY

ALBERT R. BEHNKE
San Francisco, California, and
RALPH W. BRAUER
Wrightsville Marine Bio-Medical Laboratory,
Wilmington, North Carolina

XXI. PHYSIOLOGIC INVESTIGATIONS IN DIVING AND INHALATION OF GASES

Perhaps no scientist has ever been better endowed by heritage, natural gifts, and training than J. B. S. Haldane to pursue studies in diving physiology and the effects of inhalation of gases. His investigations in applied and basic physiology, although only a small part of his published scientific endeavor, have had worldwide influence, because of the qualities of leadership and certain attributes centering in his ability to resolve a problem into essentials, to separate relevant from irrelevant, to employ simple means in brilliantly conceived tests, to make critical observations based upon an intimate knowledge of experimental conditions, and to express his results with mathematical precision.

It was the realistic problems in diving physiology of World War II, however, that provided the impetus for Haldane's notable contributions to the British naval war effort. Unfortunately, much of this work some twenty-five years after completion is in restricted archives so that a complete account of his achievements is not possible.

Professor Haldane's interest in problems related to underwater physiology was manifest early in his career. In 1922–23, he was one of the authors of a series of papers dealing with electrolyte and carbohydrate metabolism. These papers (1, 2) reflected many of the characteristics of his later work. Tests were performed exclusively on human subjects. Simple methods were employed to produce drastic changes in the physicochemical state of the subjects which many investigators would not choose to replicate. A compression chamber was used as a flexible and important tool for research. Notably, Haldane served as subject-investigator: "Since these experiments are extremely uncomfortable, I have unfortunately not been able to confirm my observations by those of other experimenters." This penchant for somewhat heroic experiments that combined subject with investigator was highly rewarding, because Haldane's rigid scientific discipline allowed him to make detailed and accurate observations according to protocol and also concerning the

267

numerous seemingly incidental subjective reactions which in many cases have formed important points of departure for subsequent studies.

An example of the scope and depth of Haldane's analysis of a biological problem was his early study of the toxic effects of carbon monoxide (3). In 1895 J. S. Haldane reported his classical experiments (4) which have provided a continuing stimulus to present accelerated developments in hyperbaric medicine, namely, that at three atmospheres dissolved oxygen transported by the blood could satisfy the metabolic requirements of the rat when hemoglobin was excluded as a carrier by reason of saturation with carbon monoxide. There was little or no follow-up of this dramatic finding until 1927, when J. B. S. Haldane investigated the role of carbon monoxide as a tissue poison. He found, as did his father, that mammals can live on oxygen dissolved in their blood at high pressures when almost all of their hemoglobin is combined with carbon monoxide at a partial pressure that does not exceed one atmosphere. It remained, however, for J. B. S. Haldane to demonstrate that the addition of more than one atmosphere of carbon monoxide, despite adequate transport of oxygen in solution, affected some substance in their tissues which caused the death of the animals. Haldane's thorough investigation called for examination of such diverse specimens as cress seed, moths, and rats. His advanced and facile use of mathematics enabled him to describe the kinetics of CO poisoning of enzymes within the context of basic formulations postulated by Michaelis and Warburg. In his physiologic contributions, Haldane consistently supported his superb critical observations with requisite physical-chemical data and appropriate mathematical analysis. This early series of experiments was apparently left to itself for over a decade while Haldane turned his primary attention to problems of high altitude physiology and numerous other matters.

During this period Haldane had not neglected his earlier interests. In a brief review of the field of underwater physiology written in 1941 (6), Case and Haldane listed six principal problem areas: mechanical effects, nitrogen intoxication, oxygen intoxication, aftereffects of carbon dioxide, bubble formation during decompression, and cold. Comparison of this series of topics with those covered during a recent international symposium on the same subject (7) reveals that to a very large extent these topics have remained the key areas of concern.

INVESTIGATION OF OXYGEN TOLERANCE LEVELS

Oxygen inhalation by underwater demolition and salvage teams was a matter of vital importance during World War II. Previously, medical officers of the U.S. Navy had determined tolerance limits for the inhalation of oxygen in the dry chamber and by divers during decompression at rest (8). More than 500 decompressions on oxygen beginning at the 60-foot level had been made prior to 1943, and a routine had been established for inhalation of oxygen as the prime therapeutic adjuvant in the treatment of decompression sickness. The inhalation of oxygen by divers "on the bottom," however, was another matter, since exercise was known to reduce drastically tolerance to oxygen. Professor Haldane, as advisor and himself a subject, ably served the distinguished group of diving and medical officers with surgeon Lieutenant-Commander Donald in charge. There followed one of the most exhaustive programs of diving experiments ever attempted in which more than 1,000 dives in water were carried out at toxic levels to water depths of 90 feet.

Some indication of the scope of these crucial physiologic studies and the problems involved is apparent from the contents of a letter dated May 7, 1943, in reply to an earlier communication:

DEAR DR. BEHNKE:

I had hoped to send you a full report on our own work but I am told that this had better go through official channels. So will you please get moving at your end to expedite proper contact. Meanwhile, I comment on some points in your memorandum for which I thank you very warmly.

Regarding sensitivity to oxygen, we have tested 28 naval subjects in air (i.e., in the dry tank) at 90 feet, breathing from a "Salvus" apparatus with a flow of about 2 liters per minute at one atmosphere, CO_2 being absorbed by soda lime. The times varied from 6 to 90 minutes. The average was 28.8, the median, 22. The coefficient of variation was 77 percent. Only the best quarter lasted over 45 minutes. The tests rarely ended in a convulsion, but always with face twitching or some well marked symptom. We cannot predict who will be tough. Thus, the second place in our records (not included in the above total) is held by a rather unathletic woman (ARB: Dr. Spurway who subsequently became his wife). We opine that your two subjects would last about an hour at 90 feet and thus fall into our toughest quarter.

We find it very hard to believe that CO_2 is responsible for the difference between performance in the wet and dry. Our experience is that both at 60 and 90 feet, a given man lasts about 4 times as long in the dry as in the wet. The CO_2 percentage used in one type of suit averaged about 0.1%, in another, about 0.2%, but never rose to 0.5 percent. We do not find that partial pressures under about 3% lower oxygen tolerance appreciably. Thus today I breathed 99.27% O_2 + 0.73% CO_2 in the dry chamber through non-return valves at 90 feet. My face twitched after 12 minutes. My last five similar tests with pure O_2 lasted 13, 10, 9, 9½, and 12 minutes. So my tolerance was not lowered by a partial pressure of 2.7% CO_2 (effective). I think that the effect begins around 3-4% judging by rather few experiments.

We are inclined to think that you are erring on the dangerous side regarding the breathing of pure oxygen underwater. We have had several convulsions in under 30 minutes at 40 feet, and one at 35 feet. One can generally pick out several subjects in the dry, but tolerance may vary enormously. Thus in the course of a year, Dr. Spurway and I have had the following experiences. We both started with tolerances of over 35 minutes at 90 feet in the dry. We both had convulsions in other tests. Her tolerance fell so low that she convulsed after 13 minutes in the dry at 90 feet, while I had symptoms after $10\frac{1}{2}$ minutes. Since then her tolerance has gradually risen to over 80 minutes, while mine went up to 32, but has fallen to a steady level around ten.

We therefore think that for 100% safety from convulsions you must aim at a pretty low partial pressure of oxygen, not more than two atmospheres absolute, though many people can last 30 or even 60 minutes in diving suits at 3 atmospheres absolute.

It was on this basis that we chose 45% oxygen mixtures for the special suit which Lt. Hoffman will describe to you. The Tables worked out for it are based on actual experience, but not as yet quite enough of this. We originally intended to draw up Tables on the following basis. The partial pressure in the helmet was calculated when the diver was using one liter of oxygen per minute. The corresponding equivalent depth was then calculated, i.e., the depth where a diver on air would get the same partial pressure of nitrogen. We found that we could decompress much quicker than this without bends. This is probably due to two causes. The British decompression Tables for depths up to 120 feet and times up to one hour err, in anything, on the safe side (for greater depths or longer times are not safe). And the additional oxygen cuts down circulation, and therefore absorption of nitrogen. We shall only be able to assess this factor when we have done a lot more control decompressions on air to compare with decompressions on mixtures. These are underway.

The statement in the letter that for 100 per cent safety one must aim at a partial pressure of oxygen of not more than two atmospheres absolute has been repeatedly confirmed and represents today the upper limit for work under water during the course of oxygen inhalation. The employment of oxygen-nitrogen mixtures in recent years has been exploited as a notable advance in diving without the need for decompression, as reported by an Italian group headed by Dr. Pellegrini (9). The problem of greater oxygen toxicity in the wet suit (at rest), emphatically recognized by Haldane, compared with dry chamber conditions remains to be solved.

INERT GAS NARCOSIS

In Haldane's day it seems fair to say that working depths in excess of 200 feet called for exceptional skill and technical capability; depths down to 400 feet achieved by Haldane and his co-workers approached the record depths then conceivable. Today, while a great deal of underwater work is still conducted at depths not much in excess of 200 feet, work dives in the 400- to 500-foot range are performed by commercial divers; in the near future routine work by means of "excursion" diving will be feasible (10). In line with this progress, maximum diving depths under investigation point to 1000 feet, although greater depths cannot be excluded. The specific restrictions to attainment of greater depths are the narcosis and the more recently uncovered muscular tremors and convulsive phenomena of gas physiologically inert at normal pressure (11, 12, 13, 14).

Professor Haldane was at first skeptical of reports of impairment in compressed air as a manifestation of the narcotic action of nitrogen described some thirty years ago (15, 16). Together with E. M. Case (6), he conducted a systematic investigation with himself, of course, as a subject together with a sufficient number of co-workers to ensure validity of findings. Helium, hydrogen, nitrogen, and even argon mixtures with oxygen were inhaled under conditions that called for arithmetic and other tests of cerebral function. All facets of the pressurized environment were explored, however. A case of pneumothorax, for example, was reported in a colleague who showed, on radiologic examination, lung cysts, a condition subsequently that has given rise to some of the most serious cases of decompression sickness in tunnel workers. Such diverse matters as odontalgia were recognized as effects of hyperbaric pressure variation and Haldane himself provided a tooth to confirm this finding.

In one noteworthy phase of the tests, the effect of cold was evaluated: "EMC and JBSH lay inside the pressure chamber in a bath containing water and large amounts of broken ice," according to a prosaic record.

During the course of inhalation of gases at various pressures, Case and Haldane reported the interesting observation that oxygen and nitrogen at sufficiently high pressures affected the sensation of taste; the taste threshold for oxygen was stated to lie below 6 atm and that for nitrogen, below 8 atm on half of the subjects tested. "It is clearly inaccurate to describe a gas as inodorous and tasteless. On the contrary most all gases may be expected to display these properties at sufficiently high pressures, just as they liquefy at sufficiently low temperatures. Whether man can survive the pressure under which, say, hydrogen develops a taste or smell is, of course, as yet unknown" (117).

With reference to reactions under pressure, it was stated that the arithmetic was worse at 8.6 atm; Case made ten mistakes out of twenty, and Haldane made nineteen out of twenty-one compared with normal values of three and five mistakes out of twenty, respectively. On decompression there was almost always an immediate feeling of subjective improvement when the pressure was reduced to five atm. "I feel normal again," "Erholt sich alles," and, "My god, I'm sober," are typical of the entries. A further notation brings our attention again to the reactions of a phenomenal person. "One subject, H. Spurway, though subjectively affected, was so resistant that her arithmetical performance was actually slightly improved at a pressure corresponding to 250 feet (8.6 atm)."

During the intervening years, although the study of inert gases has expanded to a remarkable degree, there has not been an investigator such as Haldane, who surely would have relished the opportunity to breathe hydrogen-oxygen mixtures at the newer, greater depths in excess of 500 feet. Studies of helium-oxygen mixtures have enabled man to approach the 1000-foot level without clear-cut evidence of anesthesia, but with the discovery of the strange neuromotor disturbances previously alluded to. Animal experiments have led to the suggestion that the neuromotor phenomena may, in fact, prove to be prodromal to much more severe fasciculations and outright convulsions which occur in helium-oxygen atmospheres at tremendous pressures. It is even plausible to attribute these effects to the action of high hydrostatic pressures upon excitable tissues rather than to specific pharmacologic effects of any inert gas.

Work with hydrogen and helium using new mixed gas extrapolation techniques has established for the first time definite values for the ratio of anesthetic potencies of both these gases to nitrogen (12). Hydrogen was found to be approximately two and one-half times more potent as an anesthetic than helium, and helium, in turn, proved slightly less than one-half as potent as nitrogen. Independent confirmation of this latter figure by totally different methodology lends additional support to the values obtained. As a result of these tests, the place of hydrogen among potentially useful diving gases appears clearly fixed within the range of depths between 300 and 700 feet dictated by explosive properties when mixed with oxygen (300 feet and less) and by anesthetic properties of hydrogen at depths in excess of 700 feet.

One may now better appreciate the implications of Haldane's conclusion during the course of experiments conducted with Case, namely, that he was not in a position to compare the physiological effects of helium and hydrogen: "To do so it would be necessary to carry out experiments at 20–30 atm where one or both of them may have an effect." Haldane particularly would have been intrigued by the current elucidation of basic mechanisms underlying the action of inert gases, since he was not satisfied with a simple explanation that centered in lipid solubility.

Effects of Carbon Dioxide

The controversial role of CO_2 in the etiology of oxygen poisoning and inert gas narcosis persists to the present day. Symptoms and reactions have been attributed to carbon dioxide by investigators, who, in the main, have not themselves worked in pressure chambers and inhaled various gas mixtures in which CO_2 is a component. It has been a contribution essentially of the subject-investigator to resolve conflicting ideas on the basis of consistent experience and accurate observation. Haldane's statements in a letter to the *British Medical Journal* in 1947 (18) succinctly summarized his position which is in accord with Behnke's experience.

Sir:

May I venture to doubt Sir Leonard Hill's theory (June 21, p. 900) that oxygen convulsions and nitrogen and argon narcosis are both due to carbon dioxide accumulation? Subjectively and objectively the symptoms of the two conditions are utterly different. I have never experienced or observed confusion or euphoria before an oxygen convulsion. Confusion is universal and euphoria common in nitrogen narcosis. Carbon dioxide enhances both oxygen and nitrogen poisoning. The obvious explanation of this fact is that it causes cerebral vasodilatation, and thus facilitates absorption of other gases by the brain. I hope shortly to publish data which may help to clear this question up.

With regard to questions of priority raised in his letter, the Official Secrets Act makes a full discussion illegal . . . so long as publication is restricted it is impossible to assign credit objectively, and controversy can lead nowhere.

Perhaps no investigator was better qualified than Haldane to analyze the effects of carbon dioxide and the role played by elevated CO_2 concentration in the sunken Thetis. Following this catastrophe an intensive, though brief, investigation was made in the effort to simulate conditions responsible for the loss of 104 of 108 persons who were aboard. In the report by Alexander *et al.* (19), one learns that Haldane, again as a subject-investigator, was placed in a test compartment. He slept intermittently from 12:30 to 8:30 A.M. when the CO_2 concentration reached 5.1 per cent. Panting was severe, but there was no distress. At 10:50 the CO_2 had reached 5.8 per cent; panting was severe, there was slight headache, photophobia, and transient nausea. At noon, respirations were forty-four per minute, but the pulse rate was only sixty compared with a normal figure of about seventy-five. At 12:40, the CO_2 had risen to 6.6 per cent; there was slight confusion, though the headache was not severe and there was no vomiting. Haldane left the chamber and put on a Davis escape apparatus. After two to three minutes he removed the mouthpiece in order to vomit, which he did at intervals, bringing up a pint of clear fluid. He had not eaten or ingested fluids during the previous sixteen hours in order to parallel conditions in the submarine.

In 1948 Haldane in his report on human life and death at high pressures in connection with submarine escape (20) enunciated a cardinal principle in preventive medicine that should be on the desk of every medical administrator:

> The main physiological problem to be tackled in planning escape from submarines at depths of 100 feet or more is how to steer, so to speak, between the Scylla of nitrogen poisoning and 'bends,' and the Charybdis of oxygen poisoning. ... I am convinced that physiologists have been far too negligent in investigating the limits of human existence, or at least of human consciousness. Physicists often find that mathematicians have already provided them with methods which they need for a theoretical account of their findings. It would be well if physiologists were to investigate the effect of abnormal conditions on human beings, before, rather than after, these conditions have killed numerous people, whether in war or in industry.

In 1949 the United States Medical Research Institute and the Naval Medical Center at Bethesda, Maryland, were honored to have Professor J. B. S. Haldane as a distinguished lecturer. Those of us privileged to know him cherish his memory, and all of us who have been or are engaged in naval investigation have been sustained by his dedicated, profound, and courageous contributions to our basic knowledge and to the solution of our practical problems. We shall continue to practice his Golden Rule of medical experimentation, "To test on ourselves first that which we would have others do."

References

1. HALDANE, J. B. S., V. B. WIGGLESWORTH, AND C. E. WOODSON. 1924. The effect of reaction changes on human inorganic metabolism. *Proc. Roy. Soc. Lond., B.* 24:1.
2. HALDANE, J. B. S., V. B. WIGGLESWORTH, AND C. E. WOODSON. 1924. The effect of reaction changes on human carbohydrate metabolism. *Proc. Roy. Soc. Lond., B.* 24:15.
3. HALDANE, J. B. S. 1927. Carbon monoxide as a tissue poison. *Biochem. J.* 21:1068.
4. HALDANE, J. S. 1895. The relation of the action of carbonic oxide to oxygen tension. *J. Physiol.* 18:201.
5. BOEREMA, I., *et al.* 1959. Life without blood. Arch. Chir. Neerl. 11:70.
6. CASE, E. M., AND J. B. S. HALDANE. 1941. Human physiology under high pressure. I. Effects of nitrogen, carbon dioxide, and cold. *J. Hyg.* 41:225.
7. LAMBERTSEN, C. J (ed.). 1967, *Proceedings of the Third Symposium on Underwater Physiology.* Williams and Wilkins Co., Baltimore.
8. BEHNKE, A. R., AND T. L. WILLMON. 1939. U.S.S. Squalus; medical aspects of the rescue and salvage operations and the use of oxygen in deep-sea diving. *U.S. Nav. Med. Bull.* 37:629.

9. PELLEGRINI, L. 1965. *In The Undersea Challenge.* 2d World Congr. Underwater Activities. Brit. Sub-Aqua Club Pub., London.
10. KRASBERG, A. R. 1967. Saturation diving: vertical excursion techniques, p. 345. *In The New Thrust Seaward.* Marine Technol. Soc. Washington, D.C.
11. BRAUER, R. W., R. O. WAY, AND R. A. Perry. 1967. Narcotic effects of helium and hydrogen in mice and hyperexcitability phenomena at simulated depths of 1500 to 4000 feet of sea water. *Fed. Proc.* 26:720.
12. BRAUER, R. W. 1967. R. A. Fink (ed.), *In Toxic Effects of Anesthetic Agents; a Symposium.* Williams and Wilkins Co., Baltimore.
13. MILLER, K. W., W. D. PATON, W. B. STRETT, AND E. B. SMITH. 1967. Animals at very high pressures of helium and neon. *Science* 157:97.
14. BENNETT, P. B. 1966. *The Aetiology of Compressed Air Intoxication and Inert Gas Narcosis.* Int. Ser. Monogr. Pure Appl. Biol. Zool. Div. Vol. 31. Pergamon Press, Oxford.
15. BEHNKE, A. R., AND O. D. YARBROUGH. 1939. Respiratory resistance, oil-water solubility, and mental effects of argon compared with helium and nitrogen. *Amer. J. Physiol.* 126:409.
16. BEHNKE, A. R., R. M. THOMPSON, AND E. P. MOTLEY. 1935. Psychological effects of breathing air at 4 atmospheres. *Amer. J. Physiol.* 112:554.
17. CASE, E. M., AND J. B. S. HALDANE. 1941. Tastes of oxygen and nitrogen at high pressures. *Nature* 148:84.
18. HALDANE, J. B. S. 1947. Letter to the editor. *Brit. Med. J.* 2:226.
19. ALEXANDER, W., P. DUFF, J. B. S. HALDANE, G. IVES, AND D. RENTON. 1939. After effects of exposure of men to carbon dioxide. *Lancet* 2:419.
20. HALDANE, J. B. S. 1941. Human life and death at increased pressures. *Nature* 148:458.

JOSEPH NEEDHAM
Gonville and Caius College,
University of Cambridge,
Cambridge, England

XXII. ORGANIZER PHENOMENA AFTER FOUR DECADES: A RETROSPECT AND PROSPECT

The paper here following was designed as an introduction to the reprint of the book *Biochemistry and Morphogenesis* which the Cambridge University Press is about to make. Here it has been by their kindness made available as a contribution to the memorial volume for John Burdon Sanderson Haldane. Haldane was my immediate predecessor as Sir William Dunn Reader in Biochemistry at Cambridge, in the laboratory founded and presided over by our great teacher and friend Sir Frederick Gowland Hopkins. For nearly a decade Haldane was an outstanding source of inspiration and provocative stimulus to all his colleagues and students— one of those who did most to give the place and the period its unforgettable brilliance. Experimental work on eggs and embryos in those days had benefit from his pipe-puffing criticism; his Johnsonian dicta at tea and tea-club talks sharpened many ideas in the writing of *Chemical Embryology*. Then, in the same year, 1933, he departed permanently for London, and we, with C. H. Waddington, for that period in Berlin which started for us the fusion of biochemistry and *Entwicklungsmechanik*. This is the subject of the present retrospect and prospect. Many occasions later on gave opportunity for meeting, and Haldane's conversion to Indian culture had the deepest sympathy and appreciation of one who had become, as it were, an honorary Chinese. Now I am honored indeed in contributing this paper to the ancestral altar of so old a friend.

The problems of differentiation, determination, and embryonic induction occupy today a central position in the forum of wider discourse on biological informational theory in all its aspects, the control of protein replication by nuclein compounds organized in the genome and the general ultrastructure of cells and metazoan organisms. At the beginning of World War II, this was not yet the case. Nevertheless, *Biochemistry and Morphogenesis* (1942), though centering upon a survey of the efforts made during the previous decade to elucidate the chemical nature of the "organizers" or "morphogenetic hormones," covered a very wide field of causal biology because the implications of these interactions were seen to be so far-reaching. At the same time it was designed to bring *Chemical Embryology* (Needham, 1931) up to date in the process. Hence, its three movements, opening with the raw materials and nutrition of embryos, ending with metabolism and ultrastructure, while the central *andante moderato* was devoted to the stimuli of morphogenesis and histogenesis from the biochemical point of view. One feature still giving value to the book, perhaps, is the critical study of the classical principles and terminology of experimental morphology (*Entwicklungsmechanik*) which its writing involved; perhaps it was the first time that a biochemist had struggled with the concepts of that field of biology so rich in philosophical difficulties. The earlier book had appeared indeed at an unexpectedly appropriate time, the year just before that in which the stability of the primary organizer (the dorsal lip of the blastopore in the amphibian embryo) to boiling and other forms of protein denaturation had been demonstrated conclusively, first by the German and then by the British school. Hence, the well-definable, if tantalizing, period which followed.

The intellectual climate of biology in 1965 is so completely different from what it was twenty-five years ago that there would be little point in any attempt to revise *Biochemistry and Morphogenesis*, even if I were in a position to do so. It is better left alone to continue to function for some decades to come as a background *mise-en-scène* for readers of contemporary books on morphogenesis. Besides, advances cannot be made along the whole front of biology all the time, and since the book ranges over many sorts of inquiry, some of the questions which were put before 1942 and have since been forgotten may prove stimulating to those who can reinterpret them and rephrase them in terms congruent with the ideas and techniques of today and tomorrow. I may, I think, make so bold as to offer the book to modern readers as a work in some sense parallel or ancillary to the classical book of H. Spemann, *Embryonic Development and Induction* (1938).

Whoever wishes to be acquainted with the present position in this subject must first read *Primary Embryonic Induction* by L. Saxén and S. Toivonen (1962), an indispensable book which concentrates closely on the biochemistry of the primary morphogenetic stimuli of amphibian development, summarizing the brilliant results of the Finnish and Japanese schools, to which I shall later refer. A counterpart to this is the interesting lecture series in 1962 of my own collaborator of many years, C. H. Waddington, "New Patterns in Genetics and Development," a further exploration of the now extremely "hot" borderline between hereditary transmission, biochemistry, and causal morphology, along the path adumbrated earlier in his small monographs on the *Epigenetics of Birds* (1952) and especially *Organisers and Genes* (1940). The most recent book works out the new approach to the basic problems of embryonic development, inquiring into the control of what genes become dominatingly active in what cells at what times. Seekers of light in these regions will also be well advised to read Waddington's *Principles of Embryology* (1956) which, ranging widely through the phyla in a comparative manner, provides orientation to the work of the Swedish, Swiss, and Italian schools on echinoderm, and "mosaic" invertebrate development. Books primarily in the *Entwicklungsmechanik* tradition also worthy of mention here are those of F. E. Lehmann, *Einführung in die physiologischen Embryologie* (1945), and A. M. Dalcq, *Introduction to General Embryology* (1952). Since I consider it unfortunate that Western workers neglect so much the work of Easterners I would also note the *Cercetări de Embriologie Experimentală* of B. Menkes (1958), and B. P. Tokin's *Regeneratsia i Somaticheskie Embryogenese* (1959).

More important for those who are as interested in the chemical as in the morphological aspects of ontogenesis are the writings of my old friend Jean Brachet, to whom, more perhaps than to any other man, is due credit for laying the foundations of our contemporary understanding of the role of ribonucleic acid in controlling the synthesis of specific proteins by the embryo and all that that implies. Witness his "Le Role Physiologique et Morphogénétique du Noyau" (1938). His *Embryologie Chimique* (1944) was a treatise somewhat parallel to *Biochemistry and Morphogenesis* and written at almost the same time, though under the infinitely worse conditions of occupied Belgium. Its emphases are different and complementary. Brachet continued his exposition in the later *Biochemistry of Development* (1960), hardly less useful today than the books of Saxén and Toivonen and Waddington, already mentioned.

Since the first publication of *Biochemistry and Morphogenesis*, the upsurge in the sciences of physico-chemical embryology and experimental morphology has necessitated the foundation of half a dozen specialized journals, several new review journals, and the publication of the proceedings of a number of symposia, some small and others on the grand scale. Among these last, I would mention two in particular, the *Analysis of Development* (1955), edited by B. H. Willier *et al.*, and *A Symposium on the Chemical Basis of Development* (1958), edited by W. D. McElroy and Bentley Glass. These would be required reading for anyone wishing to know what has happened in many of the topics discussed in *Biochemistry and Morphogenesis*. Among the smaller symposia, one might single out three, two of which were held in 1962. *Cytodifferentiation and Macro-molecular Synthesis* (Locke, 1963) was the twenty-first of a long series held under the auspices of the (American) Society for the Study of Development and Growth, to the first of which, held at North Truro, Massachusetts, in 1939 (in the days when these publications rejoiced in the auspicious name of *Growth Supplements*), I made a contribution at a focal point in time which I shall refer to again in a moment. The second, *Induktion und Morphogenese* (Klenk, 1963), was the thirteenth colloquium of the Gesellschaft für physiologischen Chemie (in itself, perhaps, a significant fact), and memorable for the contributions by Tiedemann and Zilliken, which will be mentioned further below. The third, *Biological Organisation, Cellular and Sub-Cellular* (held in 1957), was a lively Unesco-sponsored symposium edited by C. H. Waddington (1959). Finally, I should like to refer to a type of publication usual in the history of science but not until very lately undertaken in ontogenetic fields, the source book. We now have the *Foundations of Experimental Embryology* (1964), edited by B. H. Willier and Jane Oppenheimer, a volume which reproduces a number of original papers from Wilhelm Roux to Johannes Holtfreter—excellent reading, warmly recommended. Alone, the classical paper of Otto Warburg on the respiratory changes at echinoderm fertilization might better have been withheld for inclusion in a parallel source book (which will become more obviously necessary every year and imperative twenty years from now) on physico-chemical embryology.

In all this, I have said nothing about books which are mainly practical guides to technique readily found by those working in the field, and for the most part I have confined my remarks to publications since the first appearance of *Biochemistry and Morphogenesis* in 1942. My object was to limn a view of the modern scientific literature which assumes a knowledge of the contents of *Biochemistry and Morphogenesis*. I turn now to speak very briefly about the vicissitudes of our knowledge of induction phenomena during the past twenty-five years.

Here a central place is still occupied by the analysis of the primary induction of the vertebrate neural axis, for on the success of this all understanding of "dependent differentiation" itself still depends. After the first fundamental discovery in 1932 that the neutral inductor effect was stable to physico-chemical denaturing agents, its elucidation was thought of as a problem in a new kind of endocrinology. Grave difficulties were introduced, however, by the second fundamental discovery made by my old friend Holtfreter in 1933 and 1934 (without doubt the greatest living representative of the German *Entwicklungsmechanik* tradition) that in certain circumstances the inductor property could be awakened in tissues which did not normally show it and that the ventral ectoderm (the only reaction system upon which the inducing property could be tested) was one of these. Hence the concept of "indirect induction" set forth in my short review at the Growth Symposium of 1939 and in some detail in *Biochemistry and Morphogenesis* during World War II. Hence, the situation that all the purified chemical substances which had been tested (some of which had proved very effective in neural evocation) might be, and probably were, acting as indirect inductors, no light being thrown by them, disappointingly, on the nature of the naturally occurring substances.

After World War II, Holtfreter, while demonstrating that under conditions of true normality no ventral ectoderm can ever spontaneously neuralize in culture, developed the concept of "sublethal cytolysis" or "subcytolysis" (1944 to 1948), still generally acceptable, a condition in which the tissue's own neural inductor is liberated. This process is now often called "autoneuralization." There followed, during the late forties and early fifties, a widespread tendency, especially marked among those of primarily zoological and morphological expertise, to retire to that celebrated last redoubt of baffled biological thinking, the "unspecific stimulus." Even Holtfreter himself sometimes seemed to approve of these proceedings. Parthenogenetic fertilization, often in those days appealed to, constitutes no real parallel. One cannot, in fact, put all the weight upon competence or reactivity, basic though its importance is, and though no doubt it too can and will be investigated physico-chemically and ultrastructurally. Every biological phenomenon has its Yang and Yin aspect, the stimulus side and the reaction side, as was fully recognized in *Biochemistry and Morphogenesis* (cf. pp. 112ff., 670, 682). My faith then was, however, that we ought to be able to make great progress by pursuing biochemically the *Wirkstoffe* of organizers, and I felt (as I still do) that this intimate connection between metabolism and organic form was the bridge of the sages for which von Baer and Roux had earnestly sought. The analogy of induction with virus infection has been attributed to me (probably because of what I wrote about homoiogenetic induction and neoplasmic propagation on pp. 267ff. in *Biochemistry and Morphogenesis*), but that was never our main idea; we always thought primarily in endocrinological terms. In any case, those who continued to adhere to the view that a specific biochemical stimulus passes during the induction process (such as Brachet and myself) found in due course that the tide turned.

The tactical checkpoint was overcome by an unexpected armored column—the study of regional specificity (the "headness" or "tailness" of the primary organizer) combined with the use of adult tissues, generally of other species (i.e., heterogenous), as inductors. This line of work, begun in Berlin before the war by Chuang Hsiao-Hui at Holtfreter's suggestion, and also in Helsinki by Toivonen (cf. pp. 279 ff., *Biochemistry and Morphogenesis*), led soon to results of great importance in Finland and Japan, which are still continuing. This was the third phase of discovery. In a long series of papers from the end of the forties onward, Toivonen and his collaborators established that inductions carried out in the newt by tissues such as the liver and kidney of the guinea pig, were qualitatively varied. Some gave primarily or exclusively archencephalic inductions (forebrain, eye, lens, nasal placodes, balancers), others only rhombencephalic (deuterocephalic) inductions (mid- or hindbrain, ear-vesicles), others again only spinocaudal inductions (neural tubes with notochord, muscle somites, tails, fins, pronephros, blood, and limb-buds). If the hypothesis of specific inductor substances is rejected, such very different regional effects would require as many different types of specific sublethal cytolysis for their explanation, a possibility much more difficult to credit, if not, indeed, ruled out on Ockham's Principle. The point was well put by Kuusi, one of Toivonen's collaborators, in 1951: "How can two tissues," she said, "treated in exactly the same way with alcohol, bring about two entirely different reactions in the competent ectoderm if they only work by means of cytolysis? One would have to assume two different kinds of cytolysis." A one-to-one correlation is a very different thing logically from a many-to-one situation; the tissue no longer gives the same answer to all questions but a different one to each.

Rejection of the concept of specific inductor substances also makes a wealth of findings unnecessarily enigmatic, e.g., the regularly repeatable changes in inductive effects which accompany various treatments of the inductor proteins. For example, in Kohonen's work with progressive heat-denaturation of mouse spleen protein, the "meso-hormic" inductor disappears first, then the "rhombo-hormic" property, during which time the "archi-hormic" principle appears and greatly increases, only to disappear itself in due course. Differences in the state of the heterogenous inductors are also important; for example, Engländer and his collaborators, following Toivonen, found long ago, using liver, that the hunger of the donor animal progressively decreases the rhombo-hormic and increases the archi-hormic effects. Broadly speaking, the archi-hormic inductor has turned out to be rather thermostable, while the others are highly thermolabile. Today the generalization seems well justified that the rhombo-hormic, spino-hormic, and meso-hormic inductors take precedence if they exist in a tissue; only during their destruction does the archi-hormic property come into predominance. Some believe, therefore, that they are its chemical precursors.

In 1953(*b*) Toivonen made what is assuredly the fourth fundamental experiment in this field. Stimulated by the observation of Levander and Lacroix that an alcohol extract of adult bone can, when injected into muscle, induce there cartilage and bone cells, he found that alcohol-denatured bone marrow would act in the newt as a pure mesodermal (meso-hormic) inductor. After implantation, notochord, fins, limb-buds, myotomes, pronephros, mesenchyme, and blood, with proctodaeal and anal openings, all appeared; but not a single characteristic neural cell, still less brain parts or cords, no inchoate neural vesicles, and not even neural palisades or plates. Such specificity points inescapably to direct, rather than indirect, induction. This discovery justified, as it were, the much more tentative earlier work of Fujii and Okada, who had obtained weak mesodermal inductions with amphibian skin. In both cases, if these heterogenous adult inductors were heat-denatured the archi-hormic property of neural induction appeared, and rose to a maximum with duration of boiling before disappearing. Kuusi, however, found that urca-denatured bone marrow proteins do not lose their meso-hormic property. There are now reports that purely endodermal structures (a recognizable pharynx, stomach, intestine, etc.) also have an inductor. Yamada has evidence of this from bone marrow, and it is being studied in rat liver by Wang Ya-Hui, Tsêng Mi-Pai, and their colleagues in China. It would be impossible here to mention more than a minute part of the wealth of work now going on in these fields, and the reader must be referred to the books and reviews already cited.

The great advances thus far sketched led to the possibility of "reconstructing" in some sense an entire embryo by combining the action of the archi-hormic and meso-hormic inductors on competent tissue, and this was successfully effected by the Finns in 1955 and the Japanese in 1959. Such "syncretistic" wholes were later produced with much quantitative delicacy and adjustment after the Finnish school had discovered the feasibility of using suspensions of cervical carcinoma (HeLa) cells cultured under different conditions so as to become archi-hormic and spino-hormic, respectively. They could also show that the normal sequence of induction of competent ectoderm may be reversed, so that the meso-hormic action precedes the archi-hormic—further striking evidence of the existence of different and independent active chemical agents. In 1958 at the Baltimore Symposium, Holtfreter, discussing a contribution by Yamada, addressed him as follows:

> The saving grace of your endeavors lies, I believe, in the fact that your various preparations not only neuralise the ectoderm explants—as many slightly damaging shock treatments would do—but that some of them bring about mesodermal and even endodermal transformations. . . . Whatever the chemical

nature of your inductive preparations may be, they produce *qualitatively* different results. One may infer indeed that in normal development too the different structures are induced by different inductive agents. Comparable to the ubiquitous auxins, the very substances of the embryonic inductors may indeed occur throughout the organic world.

An entirely new epoch opened in the mid-fifties when the Japanese school, led by Yamada Tuneo, began the fractionation of the active proteins obtained from heterogenous tissues giving regionally specific inductor effects. A beginning had been made somewhat earlier in this direction by the Finnish school but with less clear-cut results. It soon became apparent, however, especially in the work of Hayashi Yujiro and Takata Kenzo, that the specific activity of the archi-hormic and spino-hormic inductors resides in the ribonucleoproteins; but it seems to be in the protein moiety rather than the nucleic acid itself. Various methods of further separation of ribonucleoprotein fractions give distinct effects, e.g., the archi-hormic property on the one hand or a strong rhombo-hormic action on the other. Similarly, the new German school, led by H. Tiedemann, has succeeded in preparing from the same chick embryo tissue, by chromatographic and other methods, different protein and ribonucleoprotein fractions with quite different regional-specific and germ-layer inductor properties. Similar results are being obtained independently by the Japanese. The mesodermal inductor (e.g., from bone marrow) has proved with fair certainty to be a protein but not a ribo-nucleoprotein, and the same appears to be true of the endodermal inductor now being studied by the Chinese school (Chuang Hsiao-Hui and Wang Ya-Hui).

Of course we are still only at the beginning. There is as yet no assurance that all the heterogenous sets of spino-hormic or archi-hormic ribonucleo-protein inductors are chemically identical, nor do we know whether any of them are chemically the same as those which appear in the cells of the developing amphibian embryo itself. A fascinating field of work lies ahead in the not too far distant future when the biochemical techniques for handling proteins and ribonucleoproteins become sufficiently delicate to permit really penetrating fractionations from these embryos. Yamada, who has been able to produce many beautiful inductions by the use of a new technique which permits the testing of subcellular components of amphibian embryo germ-layers in the fresh state, is already hot on this trail. The activity of all the inductor types, it appears, is to be found in the various kinds of microsomes and ribosomes—a conclusion which extends and justifies the pioneer work of Brachet, who, over twenty years ago, obtained neural inductions by implanting pellets of protein rich in ribonucleic acid prepared from gastrula homogenates. One looks forward to the coming decades with the liveliest expectations. At the same time investigators will be attacking the problem of the sites of action of the various inductors in the reacting cells, and how the activities of the genes, especially in protein synthesis, are affected by them.

When purified chemical fractions, however, even of heterogenous adult inductors, exclusively and consistently perform operations of high specificity, such as inducing recognizable portions of the cephalo-caudal axis, or recognizable mesodermal and endodermal structures and organs, it is impossible, or more correctly, gratuitous, to believe that they are only unmasking intrinsic specific inductors in each case. "Auto-mesodermalization" and even "auto-endodermalization" are now on the *tapis*, but they will not affect the strength of these arguments. The more specificity experimental fractions show, the more improbable indirect induction, as an explanation of their action, becomes.

One is therefore obliged to consider the probability, as Saxén and Toivonen do, that there are at least two, perhaps three, and possibly more, chemically distinct agents capable of inducing not only regionally different parts of the central nervous system but also a wide variety of different tissues and organs with a very considerable measure of morphological form. When all the secondary and tertiary induction processes are taken into account, there must be twenty or thirty such agents. This was precisely the standpoint taken in *Biochemistry and Morphogenesis*, and the result in principle foreseen (pp. 176ff., 205ff., 278ff., 290ff.). At that time I was much inclined to believe (cf. p. 186), on the ground of quantitative dosage experiments, that substances of steroid and polycyclic hydrocarbon type, rather than proteins, acted as direct inductors. Though this is no part of present-day views, it would be ill-advised to deny that the lipids and steroids play a role in induction, for if not prosthetic groups, they may all too probably be involved in the diffusion and absorption of the inductor proteins through the cells and cell walls. I should like to see what happens in the next half-century before writing off the evocative autoneuralization (assuming that is what it is) produced by the hydrocarbons at very low concentrations as a phenomenon without significance. Our original observations of neural cells, and even neural tubes, evoked by extracts of embryos and tissues in organic solvents, recently have been confirmed once again by Hayashi, although of course the effects are feeble compared to the well-organized and recognizable structures, tissues, and organs now obtainable with the aid of specific protein inductors.

There has been a tendency to misinterpret some of this relatively modern history. Saxén and Toivonen have spoken aptly in terms of the exciting twenties, the optimistic but confusing thirties, the depressed and inactive forties, and, finally, the fifties, filled with new faith, new enterprise, and a renewed impression of an opening door. When they say of the thirties, however, that "after some years, the teams abandoned their task, no decisive results having been obtained," and that "enthusiasm died," it gives the impression that the pioneers of the biochemical study of morphogenic stimuli dropped the subject in despair for purely intrinsic reasons. Waddington also says (1962*a*): "All those of us who discovered 'unnatural evocation' very quickly dropped the subject and went on to something else; Brachet to his most productive work on the relation between RNA and protein synthesis, Needham to the energy-producing metabolism of the regions of the gastrula, and I to the control of tissue differentiation in *Drosophila* by systems of genes." And in his review of Saxén and Toivonen's book (1963) he remarked: "Most of the workers who had started with the biochemical approach, and found themselves gazing down into these impenetrable depths, thought discretion the better part of valour and turned their attention to other possibly more manageable problems." This, however, is not quite the whole story. One must not overlook the external social factors which operate in the history of science. The British school before World War II could never succeed in obtaining adequate financial assistance for these researches, which, in spite of their necessarily time-consuming nature, had to be carried on unaided in the interstices of university teaching and administration. The *technische Assistenten*, who had contributed so much to the German tradition, and the pilot plant necessary for working up large amounts of material, were both conspicuous by their absence. It was obligatory, therefore, to choose problems which did not need large-scale experiments, either in chemical preparations or morphological operations; furthermore, biochemical techniques were far less refined than they are now. Then there was World War II itself, which scattered embryologists and biochemists to the winds from China to Peru, almost completely destroying the great German school of *Entwicklungsmechanik*. Perhaps in a way the discouragement of the forties was only one aspect of the general depression in the biological sciences which World War II brought about.

Before all this came upon us, I stated the fundamental difficulty of "indirect induction," or what is now called auto-neuralization, with considerable clarity (cf. *Biochemistry and Morphogenesis*, pp. 165, 168ff., 174, 180ff., and especially p. 182, pages which could almost have been written at the present day). Indeed, the term "masked inductor" is still employed a good deal. It gives me now great satisfaction to recall that my colleagues and I were the first to recognize the process of unmasking an inductor within living competent ectodermal tissue in our work of 1936 on the methylene blue effect (p. 189). Our collaborators extended it to other vital dyes. Shen Shih-Chang and the rest of us knew very well that our arguments about the minimal dosage of the chemical agents applied (p. 183) could not be convincing proof of direct induction, but we felt that they were the best that could be done as the storm clouds of nazism and fascism descended upon us. The very year of the appearance of *Biochemistry and Morphogenesis* was that in which I left for China. After the war, for some years I gave up sending out reprints of my small review of 1939, because the general outlook seemed so hostile to its approach, but in the light of present-day knowledge I think there is not much wrong with it, and it now constitutes an interesting historical document.

The first of all the biochemical theories of embryonic induction was contained in the thoughts which Waddington and I put forward in the thirties on "evocation" and "individuation" (*see Biochemistry and Morphogenesis*, pp. 125, 188, 271ff., 683ff.). Looking back now, I think we were perhaps unduly influenced at that time by the field concept, which so far may not have proved as fertile heuristically in biology as it did long ago in physics, but when one compares these ideas with those of subsequent writers, such as Nieuwkoop with his "activation-transformation" theory, the resemblance is quite considerable. One might also say that the individuation part of our conception corresponded to some extent with the play of the mesodermalizing factor in the two-gradient theory of Saxén and Toivonen, though it included more, and more is still needed. The term "evocator" itself continues to be useful and, indeed, is still in use.

In sum, the center of debate at the present time is perhaps the question of just how much information the inductor brings into the competent cell; on this point the extreme "reaction-mechanicians" and the extreme "hormo-chemists" (if I may coin two new party labels) stand at the Yin and Yang poles of an ideological field of force. There are those who like to speak of a "nonspecific cue acting on cells primed with information," but can any really effective cue be nonspecific? How could any normal development be guaranteed if the embryonic reactivities were not guarded from chance releases?

Today the prevailing view about competent embryonic cells is that their genetic equipment contains (in principle) all the instructions that they need, but some of its information is, as it were, restricted, in the form of sealed orders. The envelopes of these can only be opened by the use of special kinds of scissors, and the inductor agents are precisely these scissors; or, in plain language (if that is the word for it), some of the operon genes which have to perform essential functions in directing the synthesis of particular proteins and enzymes at particular stages of development are themselves inhibited by substances produced by other genes, the regulators or repressors. These are the mechanisms upon which the inductor molecules act, lifting the intrinsic inhibitions, and turning "can't" into "can and will." Very often, as in primary induction or in later tissue interactions, they pass from one germ layer to another; but, as the phenomenon of indirect induction shows, there must be situations where the processes of metabolism can release them from a masked or bound condition in competent cells themselves, so as to release in turn the chromosomal operon from its bondage to the repressor. Normally the pre-established harmony of the embryonic life pattern keeps the inductor molecules and the inhibitory genome mechanisms well apart. The induction process is, as it were, the harrowing of the frozen hell of incapacity and immobility which takes place over and over again in every individual ontogenesis. Grobstein has given an interesting chart of the various theoretical possibilities of inductor molecule action vis-à-vis operons and repressors.

It is said that the idea of genes as messages is no older than a paper by H. Kalmus in 1950, but the speculations of Schrödinger in 1944 had recognized the chromosomes as a molecular script in code containing a specification of development. Since then, embryologists have enjoyed working out the obvious consequences of this idea in terms of the classical antinomy of epigenesis and preformation (Dalcq; Raven; Nieuwkoop; 1953–63). Meanwhile, efforts are being made to apply information theories derived from communication engineering to the genetic control of embryonic cells. It is proposed that biochemists should speak of semantophore (meaningful) molecules or semantides (DNA and RNA), episemantic molecules (specific proteins and enzymes), and asemantic molecules (absorbed food materials, vitamins, inorganic ions, and such), a terminology stimulating, at least, if telling us little that we did not know already (Zuckerkandl and Pauling). The very restricted participation of asemantic molecules in embryonic development, for instance, recalls the discussions of former times on cleidoic vs. non-cleidoic eggs (*Biochemistry and Morphogenesis*, pp. 33ff.).

In a recent retrospective address Medawar (1965) remarked that "the underlying assumption of Spemann's organizer theory (though not then so expressed) was that we should look to the chemical properties of the inductive agent [not to the genes] to find out why the amino-acid sequence of one enzyme or organ-specific protein should differ from the amino-acid sequence of another." Calling this the theory of the "instructive stimulus," he said that it has "gone the way of the philosopher's stone, an agent dimly akin to it in certain ways." From the standpoint of one who was there, this is a fine example of how not to write the history of science. The subjects of historical discourse do not often have an opportunity to rise up and protest, but in this case Medawar's words in brackets above put ideas into our heads that simply were not there in the thirties. If anyone had asked us at that time whether we looked upon the primary inductor as something which affected the genome of the competent tissue or as something which itself contributed instructions analogous to those of the genome, we would have said that we did not have the faintest notion. We saw only a stimulus and a reaction. Many long years had yet to pass before anything was known of messenger RNA. If this can happen within two generations, how fortunate it is that Harvey and Hippocrates have not had to read all the anachronisms that later historians have fathered upon them, to say nothing of Suśruta and Ko Hung in civilizations still more remote and long ago. Having thus erected his man of straw, Medawar cut him to pieces with suitable song and dance, concluding that an inductive stimulus must be "an agent that selects or activates one set of genetically encoded instructions rather than another." Nobody would want to question this formulation today, but nobody would have wanted to deny it thirty years ago—nobody had gotten around to thinking in such terms.

Looking back now, there was, I think, a certain hesitation in chemico-embryological circles in those days at ascribing too much to the genes. I remember often saying in lectures that "the genes certainly determine whether an organism has brown eyes or blue eyes, but do they really settle whether it has a liver or a hepatopancreas?" This point was put in *Biochemistry and Morphogenesis* (p. 351; cf. pp. 340ff., especially p. 418, where gene messenger action within the single cell was compared explicitly with diffusible inductor action across cell boundaries). We were not sure in those days that "the specific, generic, and even class characters of organisms" (in the taxonomic sense), with all their profound differences in fundamental bodily pattern and function, could be attributed entirely to their genetic equipment without cytoplasmic responsibility; and, if everyone nowadays accepts this, is it not an act of faith rather than a proven scientific doctrine? If indeed it is true, one still has to admit that "informostats," or genomes, fall into sixteen remarkably distinct stability states, the classical phyla of the animal kingdom. In any case, people are now eagerly pursuing the correlation of the molecular differences found in comparative biochemistry and phylogeny with the coding of the genomes which produced them. The search for ancestors

289

is coming back into fashion, but these will be protein chain patterns and nucleic acid codings rather than the hypothetical beasts and missing links of early Darwinian days. Chemical paleogenetics may perhaps do more than comparative morphology could to justify the history of living things to man.

We must return, however, to inductors. Some have hoped to clarify their thoughts by comparing inductor phenomena in metazoan embryos with the phenomena of enzyme induction in micro-organisms. Already before the end in 1948 of the life's work of the great Cambridge pioneer of chemical microbiology, Marjory Stephenson, much interest was being taken in adaptive enzymes, as they were then called, which the presence of the appropriate substrate would stimulate the cells to synthesize. The phenomenon had first been recognized by H. Karström in Finland in 1930. By common consent, the workers in the adaptive enzyme field developed a terminology modelled on that of experimental embryology, and how far it has been possible to go since the enzymic studies have been combined with microbial genetics is a matter of common knowledge; yet it remains gravely doubtful whether there is valid analogy between the two types of induction. The most refreshing discussion of this which I have seen is by H. Holtzer, who expressed just such doubts, writing, however, from the viewpoint of one who is a confirmed reaction-mechanician and an enemy to all unduly sanguine hormo-chemists. Yet in the very same Mosbach colloquium, his lecture was followed by the brilliant report of Zilliken on the isolation and purification of a substance from the spinal cord and notochord able to carry out the induction of cartilage, which those structures normally perform on the competent somites and which no other stimulus yet found is capable of effecting. This initiation of chondrogenesis was precisely the process which Holtzer himself had described in an important series of papers. The substance turns out to be a nucleotide-polypeptide containing carbohydrate and neuraminic acid, with a molecular weight of ± 6000. Whatever an inductor may do to the metabolism or the genes of the competent cells in which it acts, this substance of Zilliken's seems to any biochemist to deserve the name, yet Holtzer was loth indeed to admit its importance, using arguments which to me, I confess, seem extremely weak. Here one may perhaps hazard an *opinio conciliatrix* in the divergence between the reaction-mechanicians and the hormo-chemists. If the latter are so deeply interested in the exact chemical structure of inductor substances, it is not from any dilettante interest in organic formulas as such, but rather because a knowledge of it would assuredly give the most precious of clues to the nature of those genetic and enzymic mechanisms in the competent

290

cells which are affected by the entry of the inductor molecule, i.e., the very reaction mechanisms which lead to the further differentiation.

The chondrogenesis episode reminds us what a fascinating field lies open now in the biochemistry of the "secondary organizers" and the "eidogens," e.g., the induction of the lens by the eyecup, or of the tympanic membrane by its underlying ring of cartilage, or of the tubules of the salivary glands formed when their mesoderm acts upon their epithelium. It is perhaps surprising that more attention has not been given to the biochemical study of these inductors, for, so far as I am aware, none of the reacting tissues has ever been shown to contain the inductor in masked form. The dilemma of indirect induction does not, therefore, arise. In all this work an important part will certainly be played by the new techniques of disaggregation and reaggregation, whereby cells of different tissues and germ layers can be separated, shuffled, and combined at will, so as to demonstrate all kinds of affinities, repulsions, and inductive interactions—techniques which had not been developed when *Biochemistry and Morphogenesis* was written.

However the sixteenth or seventeenth centuries may look as we screw up our eyes to discern them through the distorting heat haze of time, it is certain that in the nineteenth and twentieth we can make out a great tendency for fashions in biological research. Thus, Wilhelm His tells us that in his day (1888) embryologists were so deeply occupied in the search for ancestors, according to Darwinian interpretations of the recapitulation theory, that they were entirely unwilling to give any attention to the physico-chemical processes whereby the cells, germ layers, and tissues of individual embryos perform their miracles of infoldings and outfoldings, fusions and perforations, crescences and excrescences, in the formation of the frame and organs of the developed body. In a famous passage His wrote:

> My own attempts to introduce some elementary mechanical or physiological concepts into embryology have not been generally agreed to by morphologists. To one it seemed ridiculous to speak of the elasticity of the germinal layers; another thought that, by such considerations, we "put the cart before the horse"; and one more recent author states that we have better things to do in embryology than to discuss tensions of germinal layers and similar questions, since all explanations must of necessity be of a phylogenetic nature. . . . The present fashion requires that even the smallest and most indifferent enquiry must be dressed in a phylogenetic costume, and while in former centuries authors professed to read in every natural detail some intention of the *creator mundi*, modern scientists have the aspiration to pick out from every occasional observation a fragment of the ancestral history of the living world.

291

The position was somewhat analogous when my *Chemical Embryology* was published in 1931, for Drieschian vitalism was then still in fashion. My volumes evoked a vigorous polemic from the veteran comparative embryologist, E. W. McBride (1932), a great mystagogue of the life force:

> We have to ask ourselves the question what prospect these (physico-chemical) data present of enabling us to resolve the problem of the nature of development, and we have regretfully to confess that the answer is, practically none. If, as we believe, it is more and more becoming evident that development in the sense, not of increase in size, but of differentiation, is due to a series of alterations in growth caused by emanations from the living nuclei, then even if, as is very probable, these emanations have material substrates, the quantity of these is out of all proportion small in relation to the magnitude of the effects they produce, and they will not be discoverable in the chemical analysis of the dead egg. After all, chemical analysis applied to eggs (and embryos) is an example of exact methods applied to inexact data. In a word, chemical embryology is not embryology, it is merely a branch of chemistry.

To this I replied that we were left to infer that morphological embryology was an example of inexact methods applied to inexact data. McBride also greeted organizer phenomena as a great support for vitalism. He said:

> These fragments can be grafted into the flank of a second embryo in a position where normally only ordinary skin would be formed, and they alter the whole development of the surrounding tissues, so that a second nerve-cord is formed in this abnormal position. This influence, as Spemann determined by experiment, proceeds from the nuclei of the "organiser", but only so long as these are alive. Now the only interpretation which, it seems to us, can be placed on these results is that all the nuclei of the embryo form a harmonic equipotential system; that in each nucleus slumber the capacities necessary to develop a whole animal, and that the portion of the powers which come into play is determined by the influences reaching each particular nucleus from its neighbours.

Only a month or two after he had written these words, the German school demonstrated the heat stability of the archi-hormic inductor of the dorsal lip of the blastopore. Thus, my delineation of the new field of chemical embryology was understood as an attack upon the prevailing biological fashion which averred that regulation proved the existence of "entelechy," and that biochemistry could have nothing to say about the problems of embryonic development, differentiation, and determination.

My reply contested, along the usual lines, the idea that biochemistry was only the study of dead cells and organisms, reproached as more truly thanatology the innumerable serial sections which McBride had spent his life looking at, and also pointed out that chemical embryology was still in its infancy because just at the time when embryos are most interesting they are also then most minute. As the text of the book itself (His, 1888) had said: "Let no entelechy congratulate itself upon its immunity from biochemistry on these grounds, for if one thing has characterized the recent history of that science more than any other, it is the ever-increasing delicacy of its methods." Revolutionary concepts were required, I went on, to aid the integration of the mass of accurate physico-chemical knowledge which was then developing with the vast body of morpho- logical information which also had been acquired. Animal form extends from crude anatomy at one end to subatomic physics at the other, and the chemist who studies the special configuration of the molecules of a living organism is co-operating with the zoologist who studies the special arrangements of its limbs or its blood. Both are collaborating with the embryologist, the physiologist, and the biochemist, who take into account not space only, but space-time, and examine the history of a living organ- ism at all levels of its organization. The task of uniting morphology and biochemistry was, I concluded, one of the most difficult in science at the time, but it must be mastered for otherwise "the substance and the mode of organisation of the substance will for ever remain separated in our thought, one science studying the constituents without knowing how they are joined together in actuality, the other studying the joining, but the joining of nothing in particular" (McBride, 1932).

A similar point was recently made by Waddington in the conclusion to his *New Patterns in Genetics and Development*. When he was a young man, he said, the prevailing fashion (not that it ever pertained in Cambridge, alas) was that of classical *Entwicklungsmechanik* stemming through Hans Spemann and Otto Mangold from Wilhelm Roux, an experimental morphology and embryology which in spite of all its tremendous achievement left little room for biochemistry, on the one hand, or genetics, on the other. Throughout the thirties, Waddington joined with us in Cambridge in work which was among the first to put a biochemical accent into the language of experimental embryology; thereafter, and since, in Edin- burgh, he has given to it the genetic idiom also. Now, he says, the great successes which have attended the X-ray analysis of macromolecules, the actual and conceptual chemical analysis of genome coding, together with the study of its control activities unravelled in the relatively simple systems of micro-organisms, have given biochemistry a new and fashion- able name, molecular biology. Again, the pendulum has swung too far in one particular direction, however, and what is palpably missing from the current movement is embryology, metazoan embryology as we know it today—the problems of induction, differentiation, genotropic substances, competence, cellular ultrastructure, histogenesis, and morphogenesis in general. Such phenomena cannot be safely neglected even in a first approximation. Waddington is abundantly right in saying that, after the breakthroughs which have been achieved in biochemistry and genetics, the next breakthrough we need is in fundamental embryology. I should like to express the hope that the reprinting of *Biochemistry and Morphogenesis*, by assisting the thought of those who wish to appreciate conveniently the point which had been reached by the beginning of World War II, may form some part of the background scenery of the stage upon which the long-awaited heroic virtuoso of molecular embryology will resolve the perennial enigma of morphogenesis. If this is messianism, it is an expectation which was also that of Karl Ernst von Baer more than 130 years ago. In 1828 he wrote (I:xxii): "I should be satisfied if it were considered my contribution to have shown that the type of organisation determines the manner of development. Other people to come will be honoured for their accomplishments. But victory will go to that fortunate man who relates the formative forces of the animal body to the common energy or the life destiny of the universe. The tree from which his cradle will be hewn has not yet germinated." Or, if you like, in those words of Francis Bacon which I used at the beginning of *Chemical Embryology*: "So have I been content to tune the instruments of the muses, that they may play that have better hands."

REFERENCES

BAER, K. E. VON. 1828, 1837. *Ueber Entwicklungsgeschichte der Thiere; Beobachtung und Reflexion.* Bornträger: Königsberg. 2 vol.

BAUTZMANN, H., J. HOLTFRETER, H. SPEMANN, AND O. MANGOLD. 1932. *Naturwiss.* 20:971.

BEATTY, R. A., S. DE JONG, AND, M. A. ZIELIŃSKI. 1939. (indirect induction by vital dyes) *J. Exp. Biol.*, 16:150.

BRACHET, J. 1938. Le Role physiologique et morphogénétique du noyau, *Act. Sci. Ind.*, no. 698. Herrmann: Paris.

———. 1943. (inductive action of ribonucleoproteins) *Bull. Acad. Belg.* (Cl. Sci.) 5e Sér., 29:707.

———. 1944. *Embryologie chimique.* Desser: Liége (Masson: Paris). (Eng. transl., Interscience: New York, London, 1950).

———. 1947. Nucleic acids in the cell and the embryo, *Symp. Soc. Exp. Biol.*, 1:207.

———. 1960. *The Biochemistry of Development.* Pergamon: London and New York.

BRACHET, J., T. KUUSI, AND S. GOTHIÉ. 1952. *Arch. Biol.*, 63:429.

CHUANG HSIAO-HUI. 1963. (heterogenous meso-hormic and endo-hormic inductor) *Acta Biol. Exp. Sinica.*, 8:370.

DALCQ, A. M. 1952. *Introduction to General Embryology.* Paris. (Eng. transl., Oxford Univ. Press: Oxford.)

———. 1953. Préformation et epigénèse dans leur acception actuelle, *Bull. Cl. Sci. Acad. Roy. Belg.*, 5e Sér., 39:1128.

De Haan, R. L., and J. D. Ebert. 1964. Morphogenesis, *Ann. Rev. Physiol.*, 26:15.

Englander, H., A. G. Johnen, and W. Vahs. 1953. *Experientia*, 9:100.

Fujii, T. 1941. *J. Fac. Sci. Tokyo Imp. Univ.*, 5:425.

———. 1944. *J. Fac. Sci. Tokyo Imp. Univ.*, 6:451.

Gebhardt, D. O. E., and P. D. Nieuwkoop. 1964. The influence of lithium on the competence of the ectoderm in *Amblystoma mexicanum*, *J. Embryol. Exp. Morphol.*, 12:317.

Grobstein, C. 1953a. (salivary gland and kidney tissue inductors or eidogens) *J. Exp. Zool.*, 124:383.

———. 1953b. *Science*, 118:52.

———. 1953c. *Nature*, 172:869.

———. 1955a. *J. Exp. Zool.*, 130:319.

———. 1955b. In, D. Rudnick (ed.), *Aspects of Synthesis and Order in Growth.* Princeton Univ. Press: Princeton, N.J., p. 233.

———. 1956. *Exp. Cell Res.*, 10:424.

———. 1963. In, M. Locke (ed.), *Cytodifferentiation and Macromolecular Synthesis.* Academic Press: New York and London, p. 1.

Hayashi, Y. 1956. (archi-hormic ribonucleoprotein inductor) *Embryologia*, 1:57.

———. 1959. (organic solvents and ribonucleoprotein fractions) *Devel. Biol.*, 1:343.

Hayashi, Y., and K. Takata. 1958. (fractionation of ribonucleoprotein inductors) *Embryologia*, 4:149.

His, W. 1888. *Proc. Roy. Soc. Edinburgh*, 15:287. (See also Picken.)

Holtfreter, J. 1933a. (denatured and heterogenous inductors) *Arch. Entwicklungsmech.*, 128:584.

———. 1933b. *Naturwiss.* 21:766.

———. 1934. *Arch. Entwicklungsmech.*, 132:225, 307.

———. 1944. (sub-lethal cytolysis and indirect induction) *J. Exp. Zool.*, 95:307.

———. 1945. (sub-lethal cytolysis and indirect induction) *J. Exp. Zool.*, 98:161.

———. 1946a. (sub-lethal cytolysis and indirect induction) *J. Exp. Zool.*, 101:355.

———. 1946b. (sub-lethal cytolysis and indirect induction) *J. Exp. Zool.*, 102:51.

———. 1946c. (sub-lethal cytolysis and indirect induction) *J. Exp. Zool.*, 103:81.

———. 1947. (sub-lethal cytolysis and indirect induction) *J. Exp. Zool.*, 106:197.

———. 1948. (sub-lethal cytolysis and indirect induction) *Symp. Soc. Exp. Biol.*, 2:17.

———. 1951. Some aspects of embryonic induction (Northampton Symposium), *Growth* (Suppl.), 10:117.

———. 1958. In, W. D. McElroy and B. Glass (eds.), *Chemical Basis of Development.* The Johns Hopkins Press: Baltimore, p. 255.

Holtzer, H. 1961. (chondrogenetic induction in somites). In, D. Rudnick (ed.), *Synthesis of Molecular and Cellular Structure.* Ronald: New York.

———. 1963. Comments on Induction during Cell Differentiation. In, E. Klenk (ed.), *Induktion und Morphogenese.* Springer: Berlin, p. 127.

Jacobs, W. P. 1959. What substance normally controls a given biological process? I. Formulation of some rules, *Devel. Biol.*, 1:527.

Kalmus, H. 1950. A cybernetical aspect of genetics, *J. Hered.*, 41:19.

Karstrøm, H. 1930. Ü. d. Enzymbildung in Bakterien. Inaugural Dissertation. Helsinki.

KAWAKAMI, I. AND K. YAMANA. 1959. (syncretistic inductions) *Mem. Fac. Sci. Kyushu Univ., E*, 2:171.

KAWAKAMI, I., IYEIRI, AND N. SASAKI. 1960. (chick embryo inductor fractions) *J. Exp. Zool.*, 144:33.

KLENK, E. (ed.) 1963. *Induktion und Morphogenese.* 13th Colloquium Gesellschaft fur physiologischen Chemie. Springer: Berlin.

KOHONEN, J. 1963. *Ann. Zool. Soc. Zool. Bot. Fennicae Vanamo*, Vol. 25, No. 3.

KUUSI, T. 1951. *Ann. Zool. Soc. Zool. Bot. Fennicae Vanamo*, Vol. 14, No. 4.

———. 1953. *Arch. Biol.*, 64:189.

———. 1961. (urea denaturation of meso-hormic inductor) *Acta Embryol. Morphol. Exp.*, 4:18.

LACROIX, P. 1947. *J. Bone Joint Surg.*, 29:292.

LEHMANN, F. E. 1945. *Einführung in die physiologischen Embryologie.* Birkhäuser: Basel.

LEVANDER, G. 1938. *Surg. Gyn. Obstet.*, 67:705.

LOCKE, M. (ed.) 1963. *Cytodifferentiation and Macromolecular Synthesis.* 21st Symp. Soc. Stud. Devel. Growth. Academic Press: New York and London.

MCBRIDE, E. W. 1932. New studies in chemical embryology, *Discovery*, 12:94.

MCELROY, W. D., AND B. GLASS (eds.). 1958. *Chemical Basis of Development.* The Johns Hopkins Press: Baltimore.

MEDAWAR, P. 1965. A biological retrospect, *Nature*, 207:1327.

MENKES, B. 1958. Cercetări de Embriologie Experimentală. *Acad. Sci., Bucarest.*

NEEDHAM, J. 1931. *Chemical Embryology.* Cambridge Univ. Press: Cambridge, 3 vols.

———. 1932. Embryology: exact or inexact? *Discovery*, 12:157.

———. 1938. Review of *Embryonic Development and Induction*, by H. Spemann, *Camb. Rev.* 59:33.

———. 1939a. Biochemical aspects of organiser phenomena, *Growth*, 3 (Suppl.) 1:45.

———. 1939b. Review of *Embryonic Development and Induction*, by H. Spemann, *Nature*, 143:44.

———. 1951a. Review of *Chemical Embryology*, by J. Brachet, for *Arch. Biochem.* (not printed).

———. 1951b. Biochemical Aspects of Form and Growth, in, L. L. Whyte (ed.), *Aspects of Form.* Lund Humphries: London, p. 77.

———. 1955. Development physiology, *Ann. Rev. Physiol.*, 17:37.

NIEUWKOOP, P. D. 1955a. *Exp. Cell Res.* (Suppl.), 3:262.

———. 1955b. *Rev. Suisse Zool.*, 62:367.

———. 1962. The "organisation centre"; I. Induction and determination, *Acta Biotheoret.*, 16:57.

NIEUWKOOP, P. D., et al. 1952. *J. Exp. Zool.*, 120:1.

———. 1955. *Proc. Kon. Ned. Akad. Wetenschappen C.*, 58:219, 356.

OKADA, Y. K. 1948. *Proc. Jap Acad.*, 24(10):22.

OPPENHEIMER, J. M. 1963. K. E. von Baer's beginning insights into causal-analytical relationships during development, *Devel. Biol.*, 7:11.

PICKEN, L. 1956. The date of Wilhelm His, *Nature*, 178:1162.

RAVEN, C. P. 1958. Information versus preformation in embryonic development, *Arch. Neerlandaises Zool.*, 13 (Suppl.):185.

SAXÉN, L. AND S. TOIVONEN. 1961. (two-gradient hypothesis) *F. Embryol. Exp. Morphol.*, 9:514.

———. 1962. *Primary Embryonic Induction.* Logos Academic: London.

Schrödinger, E. 1944. *What Is Life?* Cambridge Univ. Press: Cambridge, pp. 19 ff., 61ff., and 68.

Shen, Shih-Chang. 1939. (induction with water-soluble carcinogen at very low concentrations) *J. Exp. Biol.*, 16:143.

Spemann, H. 1938. *Embryonic Development and Induction.* Yale Univ. Press: New Haven, Connecticut. (Of historical interest are my two reviews of this book in *Nature*, 1939, 143:44 and in *Cambridge Review*, 1938, 59:33.)

Tiedemann, H. 1963. Biochemische Untersuchungen ü. die Induktionsstoffe . . . ." In, E. Klenk (ed.), *Induktion und Morphogenese.* Springer: Berlin, p. 177.

Tiedemann, H., K. Kesselring, V. Becker, and H. Tiedemann. 1962. *Devel. Biol.* 4:214.

Toivonen, S. 1949. (specificity of heterogenous inductors) *Arch. Soc. Zool. Bot. Fennicae Vanamo,* 4:28.

———. 1950. (specificity of heterogenous inductors) *Rev. Suisse de Zool.,* 57:41.

———. 1951. (specificity of heterogenous inductors) *Arch. Soc. Zool. Bot. Fennicae Vanamo,* 6:63.

———. 1950. (specificity of heterogenous inductors) *Rev. Suisse de Zool.,* 57:41.

———. 1952. (specificity of heterogenous inductors) *Experientia,* 8:120.

———. 1953a. (meso-hormic inductor) *Arch. Soc. Zool. Bot. Fennicae Vanamo,* 7:113.

———. 1953b. (meso-hormic inductor) *J. Embryol. and Exp. Morphol.,* 1:97.

———. 1954. (meso-hormic inductor) *J. Embryol. and Exp. Morphol.,* 2:239.

———. 1958. (meso-hormic inductor) *J. Embryol. and Exp. Morphol.,* 6:479.

———. 1961. (sequence change) *Experientia,* 17:87.

Toivonen, S., and T. Kuusi. 1948. *Ann. Zool. Soc. Zool. Bot. Fennicae Vanamo,* vol. 13, no. 3.

Toivonen, S., and L. Saxén. 1955a. (syncretistic inductions) *Exp. Cell Res.* (Suppl.) 3:346.

———. 1955b. (syncretistic inductions) *Ann. Acad. Sci. Fennicae,* Ser. A, vol. 4, no. 30.

Tokin, B. P. 1959. *Regeneratsia i Somaticheskie Embryogenese.* Univ. Press: Leningrad. (This entirely ignores the work of the Finnish and Japanese schools.)

Tsêng, Mi-Pai. 1963. *Acta Biol. Exp. Sinica.,* 8:230.

Waddington, C. H. 1933. *Nature,* 131:275.

———. 1934. *J. Exp. Biol.* 11:218.

———. 1940. *Organisers and Genes.* Cambridge Univ. Press: Cambridge.

———. 1952. *Epigenetics of Birds.* Cambridge Univ. Press: Cambridge.

———. 1956. *Principles of Embryology.* G. Allen & Unwin: London.

———. 1962a. *New Patterns in Genetics and Development.* Columbia Univ. Press: New York and London.

———. 1962b. The Nature and Importance of Developmental Biology. In *The Scientific Basis of Medicine, Annual Reviews,* p. 1.

———. 1963. Two cheers for the organiser, Review of *Primary Embryonic Induction,* by L. Saxén and S. Toivonen, *Nature,* 198:42.

Waddington, C. H. (ed.). 1959. *Biological Organisation, Cellular and Sub-Cellular.* Pergamon: London.

Waddington, C. H., and J. Needham. 1936. (evocation, individuation, and competence) *Proc. Kon. Akad. Wetensch. Amsterdam,* 39:887.

Waddington, C. H., J. Needham, and J. Brachet. 1936. (indirect induction by vital dyes) *Proc. Roy. Soc. Lond.,* B., 120:173.

WANG, YA-HUI, MO HUI-YING, AND SHENG CHIEH-I. 1963. *Acta Biol. Exp. Sinica*, 8:356.

WIENER, N. 1948. *Cybernetics*. Wiley: New York.

WILLIER, B. H., P. A. WEISS, AND V. HAMBURGER (eds.). 1955. *Analysis of Development*. Saunders: Philadelphia and London.

WILLIER, B. H., AND J. M. OPPENHEIMER (eds.). 1964. *Foundations of Experimental Embryology*. Prentice-Hall: Englewood Cliffs, New Jersey.

YAMADA, T. 1958a. Embryonic Induction, In, W. D. McElroy and B. Glass (eds.), *Chemical Basis of Development*, The Johns Hopkins Press, Baltimore, p. 217.

———. 1958b. (ribonucleoprotein inductors) *Experientia*, 14:81.

———. 1959. (heat treatment of meso-hormic inductor) *Embryologia*, 4:175.

———. 1961. A chemical approach to the problem of the organiser, *Adv. Morphogen.*, 1:1.

———. 1962. (electron microscopic studies) *J. Cell. Comp. Physiol.*, (Suppl.) 60:49.

YAMADA, T., AND K. TAKATA. 1955. (rhombo-hormic and spino-hormic ribonucleoprotein inductor) *J. Exp. Zool.*, 128:291.

———. 1956. *Embroyologia*, 1:69.

———. 1961. (new culture technique) *Devel. Biol.*, 3:411.

ZILLIKEN, F. 1963. Der Chondrogene Faktor aus Hühnerembryonen. In, E. Klenk (eds.), *Induktion und Morphogenese*. Springer: Berlin, p. 144.

ZUCKERKANDL, E., AND L. PAULING. 1965. Les bases chimiques d'une phylogénie moléculaire, *Atomes*, 20(227):339.

APPENDICES

NAOMI MITCHISON
Carradale, Scotland

APPENDIX A

BEGINNINGS

The earliest memory I have is of a dark square above me, the hood of my pram, and then, coming under it, something bright for me to reach for and grip, which I identify as my brother's long gold curls. As the fashion for children then allowed, he kept his curls until he went to school.

There were just the two of us and, naturally, we had a very strong love-hate relationship. For a couple of years we were at the same school, fellow Dragons, though he was much senior, already writing Latin verses and being groomed for an Eton scholarship, but breaking off to have glorious fights with other boys. He kept inventing for me a fascinating saga of the doings of a similar group who were called,—oh, so wittily, it always started us off on shrieks of laughter!—the Wagons. It must have been of the wham-socko variety, but that was before the days of comics, so we had to get them out of our heads.

I trailed after my brother and his big friends, climbed inefficiently, watched the trail of gunpowder being laid, and had my eyebrows singed off. I was allowed to help with the model railways, though I was less interested than he in engines and points and tended to dribble off into laying out station gardens and approaches. Once I frightened them all gloriously by pretending to be suffocated when we were playing hide-and-seek in a hay loft. I helped to lay on the brown grease paint when Jack went to a fancy-dress party as a Sikh soldier, his turban expertly wound by one of my mother's many Indian army cousins. It was in many ways a happy household, with devoted parents—perhaps a too devoted and demanding mother—with the best of the period's standards of diet and health, and plenty of books.

299

Below it, of course, was the underworld of obsessive acts and witch-craft; at Cloan, our Haldane grandmother's house in Perthshire, Jack and the older cousins drove me and the other younger ones into panicky terror, which eased up somewhat after they had put a dummy head, used for making and trimming Granniema's bonnets, into my bed. I went into screaming hysterics, and it was realized that they were going too far; my twin cousin Graeme bore it silently, and it was thirty years later before I knew that they had made him suffer just as much as I. Was it a deep Haldane rationalism and anti-superstition in Jack which allowed him to tease me so painfully or was he experimenting on me, his, so to speak, other half? Or was it the normal love of power? Perhaps all mixed.

I cannot write of his childhood separately from my own since the overlap makes disentanglement virtually impossible. Yet, he would have asked for objectivity—although as aware as anyone that this is not a sensible demand in human relationships where the emotions are involved. Let me, then, set forth a few facts. We were brought up with our ears untrained for music; later Jack was to pride himself on being tone deaf, but I doubt if this is ever true of normal humans with normal childhood contact with music. We were both clumsy and accident-prone—bad accidents at that—but both of us felt we had to be brave and do the things which might hurt us. We were never good at organized games or sports, though fiercely competitive in the exam room.

Jack had the base of his skull fractured when he was still a small boy, and I fell right down the stairs and stopped myself yelling because I knew he must be kept utterly quiet. When he recovered consciousness he wanted to see me, and I came in wearing my red wooly dressing-gown and he murmured that I was a lobster. It seems likely that skull injuries (I had a concussion, just from falling in the street) do something curious to the personality; you are a slightly different person before and after. Some drugs do the same. This interested Jack later, and I am inclined to think that he pursued it intermittently and that it may have been one of the things which drew him toward India where rather subtler thinking about the human personality exists. When we were in our teens, we tried a few mild experiments, including sniffs at the chloroform bottle, but we had the good sense to do this standing. When we had to sit down, we stopped.

Just before going to Eton as top scholar of his year, Jack broke his arm and so went with it in a sling. The combination in a new boy of intellectual arrogance with a physical disability was too much for the young toughs in College who combined to hurt him to the limit of their doubtlessly minor power. He was to some extent protected by his fag masters, of whom one was Julian Huxley and the other was Geoff Wardley, who was in turn

my husband's best friend—this bringing them together. The then au-
thorities at Eton, however, no doubt thought this was all for the best and
part of the English way of life and probably had little control of Chamber.
He came home from his first half desperately miserable and longing not
to go back. He told me some of the tortures and I made up my mind (I was
approaching eight) that I must convince my parents that they should
take him away. I tried, but it was no use; this was good for him. . . .

Whether it was or not, it did something which had to come out sooner
or later. Perhaps it was the cause of a deep resentment against my mother
and against the established order. Later, he came to terms with Eton,
learned a lot, including a vast amount of Latin poetry, and enjoyed being
a member of Pop, and having the power of the pop cane, but he made few
friends, other than the Huxleys and Dick Mitchison.

When he came up to Oxford however, where he sailed triumphantly
through all his exams, he spread himself in friendships and light and the
golden air of the pre-war years for the upper classes. His friendships were
very wide, with young men of completely varied interests. Later, from
1914 onward, most of them were killed. After World War I, he came
back, expecting somehow that the world of post-war peace might be the
same as that of pre-war peace—as did I—but almost all our friends were
dead. He never made friends in the same spacious way again. His friends
were men and women in his own discipline, work friends. The play world
was gone for ever.

It had been glorious and romantic. Not fancying other games, he
rowed in Torpids though never made it for Eights; he had to have a
special oar built as he cracked an ordinary one. At the end of the training
period there were bonfires and much drink; when with liquor he could
and did speak entirely in blank verse—or sometimes in rhyme. He was
expert at climbing in and out of College, though he broke a few of the
heavy Stonesfield slates with which New College cloisters were roofed
and once got a spike into himself, which was expertly doctored by one
of the young science dons. When he became a don himself, after World
War I, he had some of the easier routes closed, as he felt they did not
create sufficient problems to be of educational value.

There were College tea parties with Fuller's cakes and heavily buttered
and anchovied toast, and here I could come unchaperoned. I dragged
them all into acting, for at that time I was forever writing plays, first
Saunes Bairos about an imaginary country in the Andes where eugenics
was highly organized by the priesthood. In this Jack, as a respectable
pater-familias strode on stage saying, "Twins, my God, twins!" Some of
the audience then left. Later, he was magnificent as a Sarmatian king, in a

great wolf-skin rug. In both these plays I cast myself as his daughter, whether or not this has any significance. Anyhow, I was always the heroine! It seems that it was possible in Oxford in those days to get Firsts in Greats, to dance and flirt and play games and speak at the Union; nowadays one apparently has to choose. Or did we have all that extra energy because we did not cook or wash up or even make our own beds? Jack and I, oddly enough, did a lot of dancing together, but almost always Viennese waltzes, in which we felt it was cheating to reverse; the big interest was which of us first would get too giddy to stand. In spite of no musical ear and all that, we did feel the beat of dancing, as we did of poetry, perhaps of drumming.

What led him to science? Mostly I suppose, our father. As children we were both in and out of the lab all the time, but probably nobody explained to me what was happening, or else I did not take it in. As my mother tells in her book, *Friends and Kindred*, my father took Jack, at twelve, to do secret work with him on a submarine for the Admiralty. A year or two later, he was allowed to go diving in the deep-diving experiments in the Kyles of Bute. I was madly envious, but would have fitted an adult diving dress even worse than did Jack, for whom it leaked at the wrists, though that was not going to stop him going on with it.

There were scientists constantly at the house; in the days when children were seen and not heard, we listened to a lot of grown-up conversations. There were Nils Bohr from Denmark, "the great wild boar," and Miss Christiansen. There were colleagues from Germany and Austria. Above all, there were mine managers and such. Whenever there was a serious mine accident, my father used to pack his mine clothes and go; this was reality.

My brother shared his father's scientific thought more and more, and when, about 1906, we moved to the house at the end of Linton Road, and my father had his own laboratory and his own colleagues and pupils, Jack was inevitably drawn in. I was perhaps more pulled into my mother's orbit of politics, though the politics into which I finally came were not hers. I used to do "lab-boy" quite a bit for my father, but never with complete interest or understanding.

How did he get into genetics? We must have known Bateson and Punnett; in fact, I named guinea pigs after both of them. Then there was Karl Pearson, of whom it was written:

> Karl Pearson is a biometrician
> And this, I think, is his position:
> Bateson and co,
> Hope they may go
> To monosyllabic perdition.

Certainly Jack was interested in genetics while he was still at Eton. Our first joint scientific experiments began when I was about twelve. I had by that time a number of guinea pigs and was making my own observations on their lives and loves. I could separate and mimic, so that they would answer back, at least a dozen calls and cries; I was on intimate terms with them; I knew them as individuals. Once I got one of them to nibble off a wart on my finger, which never returned. Then came Mendelism, which at that time was easily understood, even by someone such as myself with no scientific knowledge except, of course, what I had picked up and usually transmuted to my own ends, as in *Saunes Bairos* which had some fine scientific gossip of the period embedded in it.

Early genetics was relatively unmathematical; we talked in terms of dominants and recessives. Chromosomes had not come into their own; the cell mechanism was still obscure; but guinea pigs were a mine of information: we had to arrange marriages, which sometimes went against the apparent inclinations of the partners, though I rather enjoyed exercising power over them. My interests went as far as sucking a teat to get the particular flavor of guinea pig milk. But there were more and more guinea pigs, and then we began to detect something that didn't quite fit in: linkage. We were just beginning to puzzle about this when World War I came. By that time we were already thinking in terms of rats and mice. I took over in 1914, when, at sixteen, I began to attend lectures and so on as a home student. My fellow worker was my best girlfriend, Frances Petersen, granddaughter of the Warden of Wadham, who intended to be a doctor. We had the rats and mice in the animal house of the zoology department at Oxford; long after I had made my name as a writer, the older technicians lamented that I ever left science, but I doubt if I could ever have left facts alone to speak for themselves; I would have tampered.

I remember very well the excitement of reading Morgan's book when it first came out; it may have been the last scientific book that I could understand. After Morgan, the mathematics crept in. Early on, any of one's observations suddenly might fit in and have a point. Our first paper, on color inheritance in rats, was published in 1915, the first thing in public print that I had my name on. But I never liked the rats much; they were unsympathetic and bit me. And the mice unaccountably escaped—and mated.

Meanwhile my brother, joining the family regiment, the Black Watch, was getting the reputation, which Eric Linklater remembers as the way he first heard of him, as a first-class regimental officer—just, patient, careful of his men's welfare and feelings, above all, in the days of trench warfare, brave but no taker of undue risks. He trained at Nigg and we swam together in the cold North Sea and I kept taking omens and bargaining with whatever powers had our lives now in a choking hold.

We had, of course, been brought up without religious beliefs, although we went to New College chapel sometimes, and, indeed, both of us used to get prizes for scripture knowledge, so useful for games of Nebuchadnezzar and such. My mother used to read to us out of Montefiore's *Bible for Home Reading* with the dirty bits left out, so that they were an unexpected pleasure later. We had a set of strict ethical principles which were slightly harder to live up to because there was no supernatural sanction behind them. We had no religious conflicts with our parents, but in time we began to wriggle in our ethical bonds, but lying, for instance, was apt to make us both rather uncomfortable. I remember when, just after World War I, a love letter arrived for my brother but addressed J. Haldane, and so, naturally, was opened by my father, who was a distinct puritan in these matters, possibly never having slept with anyone except my mother. Knowing nothing of this affair, I had to decide on a course of action within seconds, and managed to produce a convincing lie about a highly suitable and marriagable friend which, I think, pacified my father.

The Third Battalion of the Black Watch went to France in early 1915, into the horrors of trench warfare, treading on the faces of one's own half-buried dead. My brother took to making his own bombs and going out with them along the mazes of old water-logged trenches, listening for German conversation, lobbing in his bomb and watching the resultant shower of enemy arms and legs. He became immersed in this savage life where in summer one wore only a kilt and boots; he must have killed a lot of people, though, of course, nothing compared with what the man who operates the bomb hatch in a modern plane has as his responsibility. Perhaps it is easier to come to terms with those one has killed in this nearly hand-to-hand way, though it may involve one in an almost Jainist attitude to life. Nearly half a century later, when I watched him letting a horsefly suck from his hand while he watched her beautiful eyes, I asked him whether *this* had anything to do with *that*. He disclaimed it so fiercely that it may have been true.

His other way out during World War I was in writing verse; he also wrote a short story which I admired very much at the time, a highly romantic story about the near loss of a young soldier's virginity. We still read poetry in those days. He and I used to play capping verses or dodging one another through the obscurer poets. We did this all through our teens. Then he stopped reading the moderns. After Yeats they began not to mean much to him, even Graves, whom I had expected him to like. Besides, he couldn't any longer beat me at the poetry game and as one of our chief pleasures was always one-upping one another, it ceased to have much point. But he went on reading the classics, at which I was never much good.

Most of the officers of the Third Battalion of the Black Watch were killed; the only reason he escaped was that my father asked for him to help in his work at Headquarters, countering the gas attacks at Ypres. Going back into battle after that, back to his men, he was hit by a shell; a car picked him up and took him back to the dressing station. That car was itself far too near the front line, the occupant, then Prince of Wales, having disobeyed orders again. He was sent back with a blighty and his kilt crawling with lice, some of them no doubt the darkish "Ghurkie lice" from the Ghurka battalion next to the Black Watch.

I wonder how many now know the Black Watch songs, the one about the behavior of the regiment during the Peninsular Wars and the one about the R.S.M. "Wha wisna there when the Prussian Guard brak through?" He knew them all.

A. LACASSAGNE
Fondation Curie,
Paris, France

APPENDIX B

RECOLLECTIONS OF HALDANE[1]

Almost from the time we were first acquainted, Professor Jack Haldane honored me with his friendship, and so it was with pleasure that I accepted an invitation from Dr. Dronamraju (whom I had met in 1960 at the Haldanes' home in Calcutta) to contribute to this memorial volume. As the paths along which my own work has led me have been so different from the chosen domains of Haldane, I shall content myself with relating three anecdotes that spring to mind as I recall the moments spent in his company.

I had had occasion to encounter Professor Haldane in the days before World War II, when, ever a willing visitor to Paris, he used at times to attend a session of the Société de Biologie; but it was not until toward the end of 1944 that I really came to know him, and the scene of our meeting was London.

Paris had been liberated only three months earlier, and the war was still on. My trip to England was in connection with a medical consultation I was called upon to give concerning the case of a highly placed personality; and so it was that November 25 found me at Le Bourget airport, boarding a Croydon-bound Royal Air Force plane, with, in my wallet, an Order of Mission from the Presidency of the Provisional Government of the French Republic. After spending three days in a small English town where my VIP patient was hospitalized, I proceeded to London. There my first concern was to meet the members of the Mission scientifique française, many of whom were good friends of mine. Most of them had spent several years in various laboratories in the United States, and now with the end of the war in sight, they had gathered together in London.

From the headquarters of the French Delegation, Rapkine, the biochemist who was then representing France on the executive committee of the Society for Visiting Scientists, introduced me to that admirable organization. I was given a warm welcome, a membership card, and a

[1] Translated by Miss Patricia F. Boshell, M.A. Oxon.

room; and that same evening I joined my fellow-countrymen in the Cantine française where they all dined. Here were to be found all manner of scientists, old and young, representatives of various disciplines who among them had held every variety of post, but the discussions that arose in the course of conversation were on the level of the purest *cama-raderie*. Little wonder that Haldane should feel at home in such a gathering, for he was on close terms with several of his *emigré* colleagues, especially René Wurmser, the biophysicist. He took a lively part in the discussions: he loved to speak French. I had the good fortune to find myself seated beside this brilliant *causeur*.

The main items of interest to us both at the time were scarcely of a scientific nature; mostly we were concerned with the ways and means of subsisting, in London and in Paris, under the drastic conditions of that tragic period. Haldane's pronouncements were frequently caustic, at times vehement, but always profoundly human. By the time the meal came to an end, we had experienced such a community of ideas that a very real friendship was born between us. He offered to accompany me to my lodgings, and our talk continued as we made our way through the blacked-out streets. Although Haldane appreciated better than anyone how extremely long-drawn-out were the processes of evolution, he proclaimed his disappointment at the lack of any signs of moral progress in present-day man, who seemed to be just as ferocious as in prehistoric times. He spoke ironically, with some bitterness and with compassion, of the decadence of the human condition, and of the people's attitude of resignation. He wanted to show me two examples. Firstly, a pub. In the semi-darkness of some narrow premises, the air thick with pipe smoke, men were standing around, most of them middle-aged or elderly, scarcely speaking a word, slowly imbibing their beer; watching them quench their thirst at this Lethe brought to my mind scenes from Zola's "L'Assommoir."

Next we descended to a tube station, temporarily converted into a public dormitory. This was V-2 time, when a motley crowd of Londoners of all ages and of every section of society sought shelter underground and slept there on their makeshift beds.

Wurmser, who was aware of the friendship that had sprung up between Haldane and myself, did his best to encourage it by inviting me to dine at his home whenever Haldane was passing through Paris. The last occasion was when Haldane was on his way to India, in which country he intended to live henceforth.

In 1960, on my journey back from Japan where I had been taking part in a symposium, I decided to make brief halts in several cities in India. I knew, of course, that Haldane was by then living in that country, but couldn't recall exactly where. I thought I could get the necessary information on my arrival in Calcutta.

The director of the Alliance Française had advised me to write to the various local secretaries of that organization in the different places I intended to visit. I had duly informed the secretary of the Calcutta branch that I would be arriving at 10.45 A.M. on Saturday, November 5, on the plane from Bangkok. My flight was so uneventful that we landed half an hour early.

Walking to the airport buildings, I noticed among the small group of people awaiting arriving passengers, a well-built gentleman whom I took at first for a Bonze; he was bareheaded, clothed in a saffron-yellow robe, and was waving wildly in my direction. To my astonishment I realized it was Haldane. He laughed at my surprise, refusing to tell me how he knew about my arrival. In the lounge was Mrs. Haldane, and both wanted to carry me off straightaway to their home. Whereupon the Cultural Attaché of the French Consulate appeared, with the firm intention of escorting me to the hotel where a room had been booked for me. Eventually we agreed that I would spend the first of my two days in Calcutta in town, where I had several people to see, and that the second day would be devoted entirely to Haldane, who lived in the suburbs, close to the Indian Statistical Institute where he had his laboratory.

So the next day—a Sunday—I turned up, bag and baggage, in a taxicab, at the Institute where we had made an appointment for 11 A.M. Professor and Mrs. Haldane were on the threshold, and with them three of their pupils, one of whom was Dr. Dronamraju.

It was to be a day of charm and of exceptional interest. Haldane had planned it with great care, so that within the short time at our disposal I could get some idea of the work he was presently engaged in, of the local mode of life, of the art and mythology of India, and could see typical specimens of the fauna and flora of the country. In such a diversity of domains, he was the perfect cicerone, dispensing with bounty and good nature the inexhaustible treasures of his prodigious memory.

Our visit to his laboratories was brief; they were simple, and there was no costly modern equipment. His real work bench was provided by nature itself, especially by the adjoining flower beds and cultivated plots, which formed a sort of experimental garden. His young disciples, trained in many different disciplines, were charged with the statistical study and mathematical interpretation of the genetic characteristics manifest in the plants under specific conditions of culture, in the butterflies with their predilection for a particular color of flower, and in a certain group of people among whom intermarriage had long been the custom. I could not fail to be struck by the admiration and devotion of these young Indian students for their Master, whose diligence was an example to them all, whose enthusiasm was contagious, and who waged constant battle for the advance of scientific research in India.

This impression was enhanced in the course of the patriarchal lunch to which we were all convened in the Haldanes' home a few hundred yards from the Institute. Not only did Haldane dress as an Indian, not only had he adopted their customs (he was by then a vegetarian), he had even taken Indian nationality. In the living room of his small villa, a variety of dishes, seven or eight of them, were brought in and placed on a side table (with, in addition, some meat and fish solely for me). Each of us helped himself at will, then carried his plate to a chair or sofa, or even squatted on the floor. The whole atmosphere of the house was unpretentious, homely, somewhat disorganized even; and one couldn't help feeling moved by the warmth and friendliness of the hospitality of our host and hostess.

Lunch over, we left to visit the wonderfully rich Indian Art Museum. There I had the revelation of Haldane's great humanism and encyclopedic knowledge. He guided me through halls of sculpture and bas-relief, with a running commentary as we stopped before more and more remarkable objects. Every halt produced a fresh lesson which covered art, history, folklore, and mythology. Greek influences launched him into comparisons between the Hellenic and Hindu Gods, into considerations on the filiation of the fables which constantly crop up in successive religions. I couldn't help thinking of that other erudite, Anatole France, whom I had been fortunate to meet fairly often some forty years earlier.

Our day ended at the Zoological Gardens, whose director, warned in advance by Haldane, greeted us at the entrance. He was kind enough to accompany us throughout our visit, which lasted until nightfall, showing us his most characteristic and rarest "inmates." Haldane missed not a single opportunity to add some pertinent remark.

The next morning he, his wife, and Dr. Dronamraju escorted me to the airport whence I was flying to Benares. I was never to see him again.

Three and a half years later, I had a letter from Professor Haldane dated March 11, 1964. In it was the well-known epigram which he himself used to quote often: "Cancer's a funny thing." He had learned that two years previously I had myself been operated for a lesion of the same nature. I reproduce here, just as he wrote it in French and in his own hand, the opening paragraph of his letter:

Mon cher collègue,

Wurmser m'a donné la bonne nouvelle que vous vivez et travaillez encore. On vient de m'enlever une carcinome rectale. Il parait donc que nous avons fait, tous deux, des tentatifs de reproduction asexuée. Moi je préfère la méthode normale. J'espère que nous sommes tous deux membres de la groupe qui exigent deux, ou encore plus, cancers pour nous tuer.

Je vous envoie des vers que j'ai fait pendant mon séjour à l'hôpital. J'ail dû être anasthésié quatre fois, mais l'anesthésie moderne n'est pas quelque chose à craindre. Je crois qu'il faut prendre l'offensif contre le cancer sur le plan psychologique, et mes vers ne sont pas donc tout à fait dépourvus d'utilité. . . . J'espère que l'on fera des vers semblables en français.

His poems and this letter depict well the stoic irony with which he faced his fate. He was serene as are all those for whom a return to nothingness appears as an inescapable and natural occurrence. He was conscious of having made good use of his life: the task he had set himself was to further, through the medium of scientific progress, the possibility of all mankind to acquire a minimum of wellbeing and happiness—which is what no religion, philosophy, or legislation has yet achieved.

RENÉ WURMSER
University of Paris,
Paris, France

APPENDIX C

Haldane as I Knew Him

I first met J. B. S. Haldane at the Congress of General Physiology in Stockholm in 1926. Haldane presented some experiments on tetany by overbreathing, making the demonstration on his own person. The scene was a bit painful and no doubt surprising for those unaware of Haldane's practice of running personal risks, a habit which his father had inculcated in him during his childhood.

I was not specially interested in this functional physiology, but Haldane had already an established reputation—he was known as a writer. He had published his first parascientific book, *Daedalus*, in which a constant trait of his preoccupations appeared: the sense of living in an epoch where science affects human life more than ever. Reader in biochemistry in the laboratory of Hopkins, he was known as an extremely stimulating teacher. As an investigator he had published papers in two quite different fields: the mathematical theory of natural selection and the kinetics of enzymes. I was attracted by the style of these works, and generally, by his approach, rare at that epoch, toward the problems of biology, his tendency to the use of mathematical formulation, his idea that giving a figure for a property is by itself improvement. At that time I was occupied by relations between cellular redox potentials and metabolism. My own inclination toward quantitative biology played a part in the start of a friendship which subsequently became so precious for me.

Haldane did indeed show the apparent rudeness and Etonian self-assurance about which so much has been said. It is also true that he did not take the trouble to make a conquest of people who did not interest him, but he could be intensely kind to those he loved. For them, he had the most delicate attentions. His generosity and fidelity toward friends knew no limits.

I have many recollections of Haldane, from his Cambridge days to Bhubaneswar, not forgetting those in war-time London. In Paris and elsewhere, we passed together many evenings that lasted late into the night. I cannot, however, add anything to what has already been said

313

about his personal life. Besides, this exceptional man has aroused such passionate and clairvoyant curiosities in all those near him that a true image of his personality is already on record. What I write here is just a tribute of admiration and affection.

Perhaps the kind of friendship I had with Haldane let me know better than many others the affective and poetic side of his nature. Under most circumstances he was a prey to the passion for knowledge which was the great affair of his life. Having refused to specialize in a particular branch of science, he could not keep from asking questions about everything. There was no *detente* for him. Relaxation came sometimes when he travelled; and it was then that he seemed to be in high spirits, his attention diverted to unhabitual subjects by the scenery and events along the road. Moreover, Haldane had a stock of stories ready at hand on any subject matter which were masterpieces of intelligence and humor. My wife and I preserve incomparable souvenirs of some travels we made together. Once he took us, with his wife, to the famous sites of British prehistory. Another time we travelled by car, visiting Roman churches and pleasant inns from London to Scotland where we enjoyed the splendid hospitality of the Mitchisons, the brother-in-law and sister of Haldane. Once again, in France, descending into the Loire Valley, we saw his pleasure in visiting this region marked by history. More lettered than many men of letters, he would recite entire passages of Rabelais or some regional poet. This culture, Haldane never ceased to widen. He had long been interested in Hindu philosophy. At the period when he was preparing for his departure to India, he was giving much thought to the pre-Christian religions of Europe, particularly their relation to certain forms of Hinduism. He wrote to me once, "though not a Christian myself, if only for my European culture, I think I ought to be able to tell a picture of St Peter from one of St Sebastian."

It would not be right to say that Haldane's scientific contribution has not received just recognition. He was generally considered the founder of biochemical and population genetics, the creator of many ideas on the origin of life; he was indeed considered, to cite Julian Huxley, as one of the great scientific figures of the century.

It seems to me, however, that his contribution has not been recognized sufficiently in one field, that of enzyme kinetics. One of the rare features that has been added to the Victor Henri theory (more commonly known as Michaelis theory) came from Haldane. This theory assumes that the combination of enzyme and substrate corresponds always to an equilibrium. Haldane considered this an improbable assumption. In a paper with Briggs, he derived the basic law of steady state kinetics still used for treating enzymatic catalysis. His book *Enzymes* (1930) has conserved, in my opinion, all its didactic value, although many years have passed since its publication. I cannot but cite a passage. It deals with the temperature dependence of the Michaelis constant for saccharase. The temperature coefficient is very small, "but this may not be universally the case. If it is not, we should expect to obtain the true energy of activation only in high substrate concentrations. Submaximal substrate concentrations should give a spuriously low or high temperature coefficient, the increase in the velocity of transformation of the enzyme-substrate compound being partly counteracted by the decreased formation of the compound or augmented by its increased formation." Here, in a few words, is an outline of much modern work on the activation process. Similarly, on Quastel's theory, "the theory will probably be capable of development so as to admit a consideration of the orientation of the substrate molecule and the finer structure of the activating field." Is this not the essence of some recent ideas on catalysis? Setting apart the concept of transconformation, which was derived by measurements of the entropy of activation (itself suggested by the absolute rate theory), it seems to me that all the essential notions of enzymology are still to be found in Haldane's book. In any case, this book has played a considerable role in the formation of two generations of biochemists.

This, again, is but a small part of Haldane's influence on his contemporaries. Science has now become a matter of collective effort, and not much is achieved in solitude. It is still true, however, that progress is due to the animating influence of a few individuals. Haldane was justly one of these few, a wonderful dispenser of ideas. His genius for expounding ideas counted for much in this role, and we in France very often benefitted from his lectures at the Sorbonne, at the Institute Henri Poincaré, and at Roscoff. He had the rare quality of getting enthusiastic about other people's work and of liking to direct attention to it, often adding much from his own imagination. He visited the Institut de Biologie Physico-chimique each time he was in Paris, listening attentively to everything our young workers had to tell him, and sometimes he would write back to me from England his reflections on the research problems of our workers.

He took particular interest in a study my wife and I undertook during the years immediately after World War II. There may have been several reasons for his interest. Firstly, the work led to some unexpected biological facts discovered by using the type of quantitative methods he liked. A second reason might be that we used no expensive or complicated equipment; all was obtained through simple hematometric counting. We were

315

engaged in the study of isohemagglutination with the hope of getting favorable conditions for applying thermodynamics to an antigen-antibody reaction. We were able to show through simple hematometric counting that the fixation of agglutinin on the red cells is reversible; we could also measure the heat of the reaction. It became evident from the results that all anti-B isohemagglutinins were not alike but that they differed according to the genotype of the persons who formed them. These differences on the heat of reaction and entropy change corresponded to different molecular dimensions. Thus, anti-B isohemagglutinins of types OO, A_1A and A_1O, while having molecular weights of 170,000, 250,000, and 500,000 gave heats of reaction, respectively, of 1.7, 8, and 16 kcals per mole.

We were thus faced with, for us, unfamiliar problems. Haldane closely followed this laborious and time-consuming work, and his interest was a source of encouragement for us. From a physico-chemical point of view, we did get a satisfactory explanation of the observed differences between the three anti-B agglutinins, the entropy variation corresponding to molecular transconformations occurring in course of the reaction. From the point of view of genetics, we had supposed that the genes A and O, or genes closely linked to them, co-operate in an individual of genotype A_1O in the formation of anti-B agglutinin, imprinting therein its characteristic structure. In his book *The Biochemistry of Genetics*, Haldane proposed another hypothesis, namely, that the formation of agglutinin may be determined by the nature of the antigens present, these latter being the primary gene products. I relate this story because Haldane's hypothesis has proved to be correct, as shown by Dr. Charles Salmon's experiments in a Paris hospital, when he alternated group A_1O cells with group O cells in transfusing an erythroblastopenic child.

We had the occasion, in the spring of 1963, to pass a few days with Haldane and his wife in their Bhubaneswar house, where they lived with several young scientists, in the Indian way. He appeared to us to be quite at home and offered us the warmest hospitality. While visiting with him the many beautiful temples of the region, we could appreciate again his universal culture which we had admired before on our travels together in Europe.

It was only a few months later that Haldane felt the first symptoms of the illness that was to overcome him. This was in Cleveland where he went to visit our common friends, Boris and Harriet Ephrussi, at their genetics laboratory.

Back in London, he sent from University College Hospital the text of the poem on cancer which, he said, had gained him some fame. He also wrote about a test he was working on, together with Jayakar, which was more precise than that of Student. He also mentioned some observations being carried out at Bhubaneswar in his absence and which he said "pose problems for future biochemistry."

I find the true dimensions of this man reflected in these last letters. Instead of just surviving, which happens to many scientists of his age, he preserved all his passion and scientific imagination, all his intellectual and physical courage. One can rightly say that he remained, up to his last days, an exceptional man from every point of view. The word "exceptional" comes repeatedly when one talks about him; he is, in fact, a striking example of that inequality of man on which he has written, as on so many other topics, pages full of reason and originality.

A. E. MOURANT
Serological Population Genetics Laboratory,
St. Bartholomew's Hospital,
London, England

APPENDIX D

SOME ASPECTS OF THE INTERNATIONAL BIOLOGICAL PROGRAMME

I do not know whether Professor Haldane ever expressed any views on the International Biological Programme (IBP). He must have known of its existence, for he was present at the Eleventh International Congress of Genetics, held at the Hague in September, 1963, during which a discussion was held on the proposed Programme. Certainly he would have approved of its aims. It is less certain how far he would have agreed with its methods—whatever they were, he would certainly have found in them many points of detail to criticize.

Since the International Biological Programme is a very powerful tool for furthering those aims to which Haldane devoted his life, however, I am dedicating this article on the Programme to his memory, and to the continuation of his work, which was almost entirely biological, outstandingly international and, which, like the proposals for the Programme, overlapped many formal boundaries between the sciences.

SOME REMINISCENCES OF PROFESSOR HALDANE

Though it has no direct connection with the main subject of my article, I feel it is appropriate that I should record here some of my memories of J. B. S. Haldane. I first became aware of his existence when, as an undergraduate at Oxford in 1923, I attended the lecture inaugurating R. A. Peters as professor of biochemistry, and the latter expressed approval of the interchange of young scientists between Oxford and Cambridge, he having just come from Cambridge and Haldane having just gone there.

From that time on, no scientist, and certainly no British scientist, could fail to be aware of Haldane's activities, but it was not until 1940 at Cambridge that I first saw him and heard him lecture. I forget the subject of the lecture—it probably had to do with co-operation with Russia—but Joseph Needham was in the chair, and he spoke of a meeting with Haldane—I think he said it was their first meeting. At the foot of the stairs of the biochemistry department he met Haldane, staggering and looking ill, and asked if he could help him, but Haldane declined his offer, saying that he was not ill but was about 75 per cent (or some other figure) sodium haldanate. He had, for the purposes of an experiment, swallowed what he had calculated to be the maximum "safe" dose of sodium bicarbonate! It was, therefore, no surprise to me to read of Haldane's daring experiments carried out on himself during World War II in connection with safety in submarines, to mention only one example of his courage in self-experimentation.

I did not, however, meet him personally until 1946 when we were both working in London, and I was introduced to him in the staff refectory at University College. Thereafter, I came across him frequently at scientific meetings, and I gained the impression that he was interested in my work on blood groups. This was, however, no special compliment to me, for he was interested in everything scientific. I attended the farewell meeting of the Genetical Society just before he left for India, and I think it was on that occasion that he invited me to stay with him and Mrs. Haldane if ever I visited India. Thus when, in 1960, I spent two days visiting the Indian Statistical Institute at Calcutta, I stayed in their charmingly unconventional household which was at that time shared by K. R. Dronamraju. It was then that I came to appreciate Haldane's unselfish consideration for other people, and that of Mrs. Haldane as well. This was shown in many little details but especially in their concern to show me anything which might interest me scientifically. I was shown the southern stars from the roof of the house and, on the outskirts of Calcutta, something of the natural vegetation of the region, as well as the rice paddies where he was carrying out his genetic experiments. I have a delightful photograph taken there of Haldane carrying a small grinning Indian boy on his back.

I again met him in 1962 at the Human Population Genetics Conference in Israel and at the International Congress of Human Genetics at Rome which followed. In Israel he strode around the countryside dressed in Indian costume: with his tall figure and impressive bald head, he lacked only the beard to make him the complete Hebrew prophet! Presiding at the meeting, he showed his extraordinary memory by declaiming long passages from the Psalms. In Rome at one of the formal sessions, a physicist castigated geneticists for not knowing enough mathematics—this was a meeting attended by Haldane, Fisher, and Penrose!

My last meeting with him was at the International Genetics Congress in 1963, as already mentioned. I well remember his masterly address on human genetics, and I think that the last time I ever saw him was when we dined together at a small restaurant in Scheveningen. In the course of a typical, widely ranging Haldane conversation he said, to my surprise, that he had a great admiration for St. Paul, not, he hastened to add, that he agreed with his opinions.

It is not for me to attempt to assess the scientific work of Haldane; I am far from competent to do so, but I do know that he was one of the most impressive personalities I ever came across, and a man who, despite his many peculiarities, inspired in me a great admiration and affection.

The Beginnings of IBP

International co-operation in the sciences, which Haldane did so much to foster, is no new thing. It is, indeed, as old as the sciences themselves, but in recent years the vast increases which have taken place in the speed of communication and of travel have made possible a new kind of co-operation, through the closely integrated organization of a series of expeditions to different places and observations carried out at central laboratories.

The first subject to benefit from these possibilities was geophysics, through the International Polar Years, then the International Geophysical Year (IGY), and now the International Years of the Quiet Sun. Biology, however, because it is something which affects all mankind, especially at the present time with the biological problems which face the whole human race, was clearly a strong candidate for similar treatment, which now is being realized in the International Biological Programme.

There are two main reasons why the IBP, or something along very similar lines, should be carried out in the near future. One is that, because of the control of disease without any substantial control of conception, man is rapidly reaching the point where starvation will be the limiting factor of his numbers. Before there can be any fundamental alleviation of this situation, it is necessary that a comprehensive survey be made of the biological resources of the earth as well as a full study of man's own biology. Also, as a result of the rapid advance of industrialization, habitats of plants and animals are being destroyed and organisms are becoming extinct at a vast and increasing rate. Moreover, the ways of life of many simple peoples, living in close equilibrium with their surroundings, are being destroyed. A great deal of information about the organic world, including man himself, will be lost forever if it is not retrieved in the near future. Thus, behind the Programme are the twin urges of humanitarianism and the desire for knowledge, each of relatively little effect without the other. The IBP has the important task of helping to ensure the continued existence of man.

The first tentative plans for an International Biological Programme were put forward by Professor G. Montalenti in 1959 when he was president of the International Union of Biological Sciences (IUBS).

The plans subsequently were taken up by the International Council of Scientific Unions (ICSU), which is the international body ultimately responsible for the IBP, as it was for the IGY. It has appointed and acts through the Special Committee for the International Biological Programme (SCIBP). In each country details of the national contribution to the IBP are the responsibility of the National Academy of Sciences, which in Britain is the Royal Society.

The Organization of the IBP

The IBP was officially launched at its First General Assembly held in Paris in July, 1964. The official title, which defines the scope of the whole Programme, is "The Biological Basis of Production and Human Welfare." It is intended to promote the worldwide study of (*a*) organic production on the land, in fresh waters, and in the seas, and the potentialities and use of new as well as existing resources, and (*b*) human adaptability to changing conditions.

The emphasis of the IBP is on productivity. This is a vital issue at the present moment in the history of humanity, and there can be no doubt that it is largely because of the stress laid upon it that governments are willing to supply the money needed to carry out the Programme. However, the Programme must be, and indeed is, something very much more than a mere cataloguing of the food resources. Most scientists appreciate that any long-term practical benefits can be realized only if fundamental investigation is made of the general biology, and especially the ecology, of natural communities, including their human components.

One of the subjects to be studied is the nitrogen cycle. It is, of course, most important to know how and in what quantities nitrogen is now being fixed in various environments and how it is passed around the biological community, some of it ultimately emerging as protein edible by man. It is likely, however, that some of the laboratory work done on this subject will be of a fundamental biochemical nature, and that the biochemistry of fixation by different kinds of organisms will be compared, thus clarifying our ideas about the way in which the process was evolved. Since nitrogen-fixing bacteria often contain hemoglobin; it could happen that such a study would lead us back in the chain of causation, and in time, through the study of hemoglobin to a clearer idea than we now have of the origin of free oxygen and its utilization. Thus, although fossil plants and animals can be regarded only in the most marginal sense as part of the earth's biological resources, yet a knowledge of paleontology, especially the growing subject of biochemical paleontology, has much to offer in helping us to understand the biology of modern organisms and the productivity of the organic communities of the present time. Already the IBP is associated with an international meeting on paleolimnology, for it is realized that an understanding of the conditions under which sediments have been laid down on the floor of lakes may be important in under-standing the present-day productivity of their waters.

There are in the world today still many organic communities that have changed little for thousands, or even millions, of years and, almost without exception, these are being threatened with early disruption by the advance of civilization and industrialization. Perhaps the most important of these is the tropical rain forest. It was in these communities, or similar ones, that most of the evolution of present-day animals and plants took place, and, if we do not study the ecology of these communities now, it is unlikely that we shall ever understand the forces which shaped the organisms which emerged from them. Many individual species of animals also are threatened with early extinction, including a number which show unique primitive features. A detailed study of these also is vital for our understanding of the organic world as a whole.

Then, too, nearly every simple human community throughout the world is threatened by the advance of industrialization. Many of those still untouched by that advance are exposed to extremes of environ-mental conditions, such as great heat or cold or low partial pressure of atmospheric oxygen, and they have not the means which we possess of largely isolating themselves from their natural environment. It was probably under similar conditions that much of human evolution took place through constant interaction between environmental stresses and the genetic constitution of the individual and the population as a whole. Thus, an early study of physiological adaptation and population genetics in such communities is essential to an understanding of the evolution of mankind.

It is unlikely that any fossils, except deep-frozen ones, retain sufficient intact DNA ever to permit even a partial reconstruction of their molecular genetics. Even where an organism has survived but its original environ-ment has been destroyed, it would appear at present impossible to reconstruct the process whereby that environment shaped its genome. Krooth (1965), however, has made a most ingenious suggestion, namely, that when it becomes possible to make a complete biochemical map of every chromosome, not only will it be possible to confirm what is now widely believed—that every minute detail of the genome has been determined by evolution in relation to some past environment—but it will become possible, presumably through the interpretation of the total genome by a computer, to reconstruct in great detail the whole of the process of evolution. (Here, perhaps, is a task for the IBP of 2567!)

There will, however, be no IBP even in 2067 if man does not survive or if he reverts to barbarism. The most important immediate need is an increased supply of food; therefore, while the IBP will be carrying out pure scientific research, it will mainly be oriented toward increasing food production. Much can, of course, be done to increase food production without any scientific research at all, or perhaps only with what may be called operational research—by taking the necessary financial, administrative, and psychological steps to introduce the best practices of one country to another. I remember that Haldane was greatly impressed with the intensive cultivation going on in the Jordan valley south of the Sea of Galilee, and that he remarked that this showed what could be done in large areas of India which had a similar climate. Perhaps indeed psychological research, in the form of social anthropology, may prove an important part of the IBP in relation to nutrition. Many populations could be much better nourished than they now are, if they would only agree to cultivate and eat foods which are perfectly well adapted biologically to their region, but the eating of which is contrary to their traditions. If, as appears likely, the IBP sponsors the development of totally new kinds of food, such as blue-green algae, giving a very high yield of protein per acre, the hindrance to their utilization is likely to be mainly psychological. Plans are, in fact, being developed for anthropological teams, as an adjunct to their investigations under the aegis of the human adaptability section, to introduce experimentally to the populations being studied novel foods developed by other sections of the Programme. There is, however, much that can be done to increase production of the standard and well-accepted foods. Haldane was engaged in India in research designed to increase rice production. Another way in which the IBP is likely to facilitate food production is through the study of arid-zone ecology. It is interested in the progress of work in this field at a number of places, including a new research station now being established at Azraq, in Jordan, which has already given hospitality to a multidisciplinary British expedition. Here, again, was a subject which interested Haldane and which inspired a long quotation from the Scriptures which I heard him make at the conference in Israel, already mentioned, about "the desert blossoming as the rose."

The planned five-year duration of the IBP began in July, 1967, and if, as all concerned hope, the Programme is a success, it will surely lead, as did the IGY, to follow-up programmes, and perhaps in the long run it may be found that its most important contribution to human welfare will have been the establishment of a tradition of international co-operative biological research for the benefit of mankind as a whole.

REFERENCE

KROOTH, R. S. 1965. The future of mammalian cell genetics. Birth defects. Original article in series of National Foundation, March of Dimes, New York, 1(2):21–56.

T. A. DAVIS
Indian Statistical Institute,
Calcutta, India

APPENDIX E

BIOLOGY IN THE TROPICS

The late Professor J. B. S. Haldane felt that studies concerning natural populations have a prominent role to play in the development of modern biology in developing countries in Asia and Africa (Haldane, 1965). He suggested many projects in biometry, animal behavior, and ecology that could be undertaken without using expensive and complicated apparatus. The rich tropical fauna and flora, he believed, offer excellent opportunities for quantitative studies of variation. Some examples of my work in this sphere are discussed below.

FOLIAR ASYMMETRY IN THE COCONUT

The leaves in the coconut palm (*Cocos nucifera L.*) are arranged along five distinct spirals which are either right-handed (counter-clockwise) or left-handed. In a palm bearing nuts, if the spiral is right-handed, the bunch hangs on the left side of the leaf, and conversely in a left-handed palm.

The coconut palm is usually cross-pollinated, but the pollen parent is generally unknown. In the years 1950–52, at the Central Coconut Research Station, Kayangulam, Kerala, in India, controlled hand-pollination was effected on 25 seed parents using four pollen parents of the tall variety. All the pollen parents were used as seed parents as well. Observations of the leaf spirals of all the surviving progeny were made in 1958. There is no suggestion that the direction of the spiral is inherited from the parents or genetically determined in any other way (Davis, 1962, 1963).

The two kinds of foliar spiral in palms are distributed almost at random in many centers in India. Data were collected from other regions of the world, too (Table E–1). The 45,443 palms represent 33 regions. The aggregate figure from different countries of the southern hemisphere gives 47.39 per cent lefts and from that of the northern hemisphere 51.35 per cent, the difference being statistically significant at the 1.0 per cent level.

327

T. A. DAVIS

TABLE E-1
Cocos nucifera: Distribution of Left- and Right-Spiralled Palms

Country/Region	Lefts	Rights	L + R	L − R
1. Tonga Is.	234	266	500	−32
2. American Samoa	516	484	1,000	32
3. Western Samoa	96	104	200	−8
4. Fiji	223	277	500	−54
5. New Hebrides	265	235	500	30
6. New Caledonia	216	334	550	−118
7. Br. Solomon Is. Protectorate	1,461	1,621	3,082	−160
8. Trust Territory of Pacific Is.	275	247	522	28
9. Papua and New Guinea	406	398	804	8
10. Netherlands New Guinea	414	586	1,000	−172
11. Philippines	726	774	1,500	−48
12. North Borneo	244	332	576	−88
13. Sarawak	275	325	600	−50
14. South Vietnam	1,833	1,478	3,311	355
15. Malaya	272	228	500	44
16. Andaman Is.	658	505	1,163	153
17. Assam	254	252	506	2
18. East Pakistan	499	586	1,085	−87
19. Ceylon	1,803	1,754	3,557	49
20. Bengal, Orissa, and Andhra	2,258	2,084	4,342	174
21. Madras	2,042	2,018	4,060	24
22. Kerala	2,875	2,722	5,597	153
23. Mysore, Gujarat and Maharashtra	997	875	1,872	122
24. Mauritius	15	19	34	−4
25. Zanzibar	244	216	460	28
26. Nigeria	222	278	500	−56
27. Dahomey	520	510	1,030	10
28. Ghana	568	557	1,125	11
29. Ivory Coast	505	554	1,059	−49
30. Sierra Leone	784	749	1,533	35
31. Surinam	475	335	810	140
32. Br. Guiana	416	239	655	177
33. Jamaica	467	443	910	24
Total	23,058	22,385	45,443	673

The exact cause for the above situation is not yet known. Grote Reber, an astrophysicist of Tasmania, who examined my data, suspected that the foliar asymmetry was influenced by the magnetic inclination of the earth.

In the course of these studies a surprising finding was made. The palms having left-handed foliar spiral yielded 20.9 per cent more nuts than the right-handers in a population in Central Kerala (Davis, 1963). Differences in the weight of copra and number of nuts were also found in the Trust Territory of the Pacific Island and in Tanzania as well.

328

FLORAL ASYMMETRY

The arrangement of the parts in flowers in most species of Malvaceae, Sterculiaceae, and other natural orders is a distinctly twisted one and is noticeable in the buds as well as in the open flowers. In about half the number of flowers of any plant, the petals are twisted clockwise and the rest counter-clockwise. Over 80,000 flowers from 34 species of Malvaceae were examined. The proportions of left- and right-spiralled flowers differed significantly only in two species (*Hibiscus rosa sinensis* and *Abutilon indicum*) in which the left-handers predominated. A similar significant excess of left-handers was found in the case of *Bombax ceiba*, the red silk cotton (Table E-2).

TABLE E-2
LEFT- AND RIGHT-SPIRALLED FLOWERS OF SOME BOMBACACEOUS SPECIES

| SPECIES | No. OF PLANTS | AESTIVATION OF COROLLA | | | | Chi-Square |
		Left	Right	L + R	L − R	
Adansonia digitata	5	213	204	417	9	0.019
Bombax anceps	2	93	94	87	−1	0.005
Bombax ceiba	27	19,664	18,826	38,490	838	18.245
Bombax insignis	2	46	28	74	18	0.438
Ceiba pentandra	8	804	771	1,575	33	0.691
Ceiba rosea	1	30	28	58	2	0.007
Chorisia insignis	1	49	48	97	1	0.010
Pachira acquatica	1	83	102	185	−19	1.951
Pachira cyathophora	2	87	78	165	9	0.491
Pachira insignis	1	11	14	25	−3	0.360
Pachira longifolia	1	36	32	68	4	0.236
Pseudobombax grandiflorum	1	27	39	66	−12	0.218
Salmalia insignis	2	39	24	63	15	0.357
Total	54	21,182	20,288	41,470	894	23.028

VARIATION IN VERNATION AND PTYXIS

The study of pre-foliation offers much scope for observing variation in plants. Phyllotaxy, vernation, and ptyxis of a number of species have been studied.

In *Pothos scandens* the lamina of a leaf rolls in bud in a left-handed (clockwise) or in a right-handed manner, or it involutes. Not all the leaves of a plant or even of a shoot have the same type of ptyxis (Davis, 1967). Data relating to 577 leaves from these plants are presented in Table E-3. The ptyxis of each leaf was noted. The conditions of the laminae of every two consecutive leaves were estimated and summarized. It is clear that a leaf with left convolution is followed more frequently by

329

one having right convolution, and vice versa. On the other hand, an involute leaf has a greater chance of being followed by another involute leaf. There is also some indication that a leaf with left convolution has a greater chance of succeeding an involute leaf.

TABLE E-3

Pothos scandens: PTYXIS OF LEAVES

FIRST LEAF	SECOND LEAF			
	Left	Right	Involute	Total
Left	20	155	44	219
Right	150	21	34	205
Involute	47	16	90	153
Total	217	192	168	577

OBSERVATIONS ON A SOCIAL WASP

Sixteen colonies of the social wasp *Ropalidia variegata* (Smith) were closely watched from November, 1963, to July, 1965, on the premises of the Indian Statistical Institute, Calcutta. This wasp is active throughout the year and colonizes both on *Diospyros discolor* and *Musa sapientum*. A nest normally has two rows of cells built downward, the uppermost cell having the single pedicel. It was found that the number of vertical rows of cells differed in the nests of the two species, which is thought to have been caused by the pronounced differences in the morphology of the leaves (Vecht, 1962). When the position of the smaller *Diospyros* leaf was slightly altered, the stability of the tilted nests was restored by adding new cells or rows of cells along the side nearer to the line of gravity. In nature the leaf may be subjected to further deflections in different directions, and the number of cell rows may increase. On the other hand, since the banana leaf is adapted to vertical movements, the nests on it do not differ greater from the two-row pattern. In changing the structure of the nest to suit different sites and trees, the wasp demonstrates adaptability to ensure survival under varying conditions (Davis, 1966).

Unlike most *Polistes* wasps, a founding female of *R. variegata* is helped substantially in the feeding of the developing larvae and to a lesser extent in the construction of cells by workers arriving from older nests of the same colony or from different colonies.

NESTING SITES OF THE BAYA WEAVERBIRD

The Baya weaverbird (*Ploceus philippinus*), a non-migratory bird of the family Ploceidae, is distributed in Burma, Ceylon, Malaysia, Pakistan, and India. The active nesting season of the Baya extends from May to September in India. The nests are very large and the colonies are not concealed from predators. Nests are made of thousands of leaf fibres. Nestlings are brought up as carnivores, although adults are usually granivorous. These factors demand certain requirements in the nesting season, nesting trees, and suitable siting locations on nesting trees. A detailed survey was made in several Indian States. About 10,000 nests from 1,241 colonies on 35 different species of plants were observed (Table E-4). Trees having prominent thorns, prickles, or similar natural protective mechanisms which act as deterrents to predators are most attractive to the Baya. Colonies on the unarmed (with no branches) coconut and areca palms account for an appreciable 16.7 per cent. The tall, unbranched, and slippery nature of the stems, the long and swaying leaves providing long nest-building fiber seem to have made these palms suitable for colonizing. Species of *Acacia* seem to be the most favored hosts (Ali, 1931). It is also interesting that the most favored host is characteristic of a certain geographic region. In Assam and North Bengal, over 84.0 per cent of the colonies observed were on the areca palm, while about 60.0 per cent in Andhra were on the wild date. In northeastern India, palmyra is preferred most often. In Southern India, 62.0 per cent of the colonies were on the coconut. Thus, the nest building behavior of the Baya reveals a great deal of variation.

Tongue Pigmentation in Man

A certain proportion of Indian men and women of all age groups have dark tongue pigmentation. These pigments may appear as isolated spots, small patches, broad or narrow streaks covering different areas, or be distributed throughout the upper surface and rim of the tongue. Data on the incidence of the trait were collected from several Indian states and Ceylon. In total, 12,080 men and 4,552 women were examined; 19.17 per cent of the women and 10.52 per cent of the men were affected. The permanent dark pigmentation is noticeable from birth in most affected cases and becomes clear by the age of five years. It does not disappear in later life. Thus, it differs from the types of transient discoloration of the tongue that occur under certain pathological conditions. The highest percentage was found in Ceylon, 27.8 per cent, and the lowest, 2.8 per cent, in Jammu and Kashmir. The frequency increases steadily as one proceeds from North to South with some departures in the states of Gujerat and Mysore. There may be some positive correlation with skin color, but the implications are not yet clear.

TABLE E-4
HOST PLANTS OF BAYA COLONIES IN DIFFERENT INDIAN STATES

SITING PLANTS	ASSAM AND N. BENGAL	ANDHRA PRADESH	BIHAR	GUJARAT	JAMMU AND KASHMIR	KERALA AND MYSORE	MADHYA PRADESH	MADRAS	MAHARASHTRA	ORISSA	PUNJAB	RAJASTHAN	UTTAR PRADESH	S. W. BENGAL	TOTAL
1. Acacia sp.	—	77	—	33	9	—	33	9	6	2	53	42	106	6	376
2. Phoenix sylvestris	—	190	7	—	1	—	20	—	5	9	5	—	10	—	247
3. Borassus flabellifer	—	27	16	—	—	17	—	7	4	15	—	—	12	64	162
4. Areca catechu	109	—	—	—	—	—	—	—	—	—	—	—	—	—	109
5. Cocos nucifera	4	2	—	—	—	64	—	23	—	3	—	—	—	2	98
6. Zizyphus jujuba	—	—	—	5	2	3	10	—	6	—	3	—	12	—	41
7. Dalbergia sissoo	2	—	—	—	—	—	—	—	—	—	10	5	13	—	30
8. Prosopis sp.	—	14	—	—	—	—	2	—	—	—	2	—	2	—	20
9. Butea frondosa	—	—	—	—	5	—	—	—	—	—	7	—	5	—	17
10. Tall grasses	—	—	—	—	1	—	—	4	—	—	—	—	9	—	14
11. Inside wells	—	—	—	1	—	—	1	—	5	—	4	3	—	—	14
12. Telegraph lines	8	—	—	—	—	—	—	—	—	—	—	—	3	—	11
13. Pithecollobium dulce	—	8	—	—	—	—	—	—	—	—	1	—	—	—	9
14. Others: thorny plants	3	—	4	—	1	3	—	2	3	—	—	2	14	4	37
15. Others: unbranched plants	3	3	6	2	—	7	—	—	—	2	—	2	22	—	47
16. Unidentified species	—	—	—	1	1	2	—	—	—	—	4	—	1	—	9
Total	129	321	33	42	20	96	66	45	29	31	89	54	210	76	1,241

Further studies are in progress on this and other polymorphisms including abnormalities of toes, among others. I hope I have given some indication of the scope of quantitative studies of biological variation in Indian populations in which Haldane was deeply interested.

References

ALI, S. 1931. Nesting behavior of the Baya (*Ploceus philippinus L.*). *J. Bombay Nat. Hist. Soc.*, 34:947–64.

DAVIS, T. A. 1962. The non-inheritance of asymmetry in *Cocos nucifera. J. Genet.*, 58:42–50.

———. 1963. The dependence of yield on asymmetry in coconut palms. *J. Genet.*, 58:186–215.

———. 1966. Nest structure of a social wasp varying with siting leaves. *Nature*, 210:966–67.

———. 1967. Prefoliation in *Pothos Scandens Linn. Bull. Jardin Botanique de l'Etat.*, Bruxelles (in press).

HALDANE, J. B. S. 1965. Biological research in developing countries, p. 222. *In*, G. E. Wolstenholme and M. O'Connor (eds.), *Man and Africa*. CIBA Foundation Symp., J. A. Churchill, London.

VECHT, J. VAN DER. 1962. The Indo-Australian species of the genus *Ropalidia* (Icaria) (Hymenoptera, Vespidae). *Zool. Verhandel.* Leiden, no. 57.

Designed by Arlene J. Sheer

Composed in Monotype Baskerville and Baskerville Display Types
by Baltimore Type and Composition Corporation

Printed offset by Universal Lithographers, Inc.
on 60 lb. P & S, R

Bound by L. H. Jenkins, Inc. in Columbia Milbank Vellum